Veterinary Pharmacy

Veterinary Pharmacy

Edited by

Steven B Kayne

BSc, PhD, MBA, LLM, MSc (Med Sci), DAgVetPharm, FRPharmS, FCPP,
FIPharmM, MPS (NZ), FNZCP, FFHom

Independent Consultant Pharmacist and Visiting Lecturer,
School of Pharmacy, University of Strathclyde, Glasgow, UK

Michael H Jepson

BPharm, MSc, PhD, FRPharmS, MCPP, MInstPkg, FIPharmM, DHMSA,
MBIRA(Hon)

Former Head of Pharmacy Practice, University of Aston, Birmingham,
UK
Course Director, Royal Pharmaceutical Society of Great Britain Diploma
in Agricultural and Veterinary Pharmacy
Member, Veterinary Products Committee 1994–2001

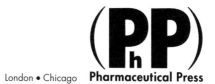

London • Chicago **Pharmaceutical Press**

Published by the Pharmaceutical Press
Publications division of the Royal Pharmaceutical Society of Great Britain

1 Lambeth High Street, London SE1 7JN, UK
100 South Atkinson Road, Suite 206, Grayslake, IL 60030-7820, USA

© Pharmaceutical Press 2004

(**PᴴP**) logo is a trade mark of Pharmaceutical Press

First published 2004

Text design by Barker/Hilsdon, Lyme Regis, Dorset
Typeset by Mathematical Composition Setters Ltd, Salisbury, Wiltshire
Printed in Great Britain by TJ International, Padstow, Cornwall

ISBN 0 85369 534 2

A catalogue record for this book is available from the British Library

Contents

Preface

There are many aspects of veterinary pharmacy, be it in relation to pets or companion animals, or in relation to commercial livestock, that are analogous to mainstream pharmacy. There are also some very major differences, and it is our aim to address as many of those aspects as possible that are particularly relevant to the pharmacist. This book is certainly not designed to encourage practices that might contravene the Veterinary Surgeons' Act (see chapter 6).

Many pharmaceutical formulations and presentations for human and animal use are similar in application. Of course dosage, normally for animals directly related to weight and route of administration, will vary according to species, to habitat, and as to whether the animal is food-producing or not. There can be the matter of scale, thus a modified release tablet formulation for a dog may not appear too different to one for a human, but an anthelmintic bolus for a cow with its internal 50 gallon fermentation tank, may weigh in at 150 g. Environmental factors may have to be considered whether in the context of treating cat flea problems or disposing of the contents of a dip bath used to control external parasites of sheep – maybe after dipping 2000 sheep – which of course, will have necessitated bath top-up calculations at regular intervals.

One important trend in veterinary medicinal product development relates to the ever wider use of immunological products, vital to maintaining and improving health status in modern farming methods. As very many of these are for disease prevention, which is seen as prophylactic use, many of those for commercial livestock are not restricted to prescription and are available through pharmacies and merchants. The importance of ensuring that any supply is backed by well-informed information should be self-evident. At first, the chapter on nutrition may seem rather specialised but as background knowledge, even very relevant to some recent human health related issues, it is essential reading in this context.

It is not always recognised that veterinary medicines, although they are subject to strict standards of quality, safety and efficacy, can still produce unwanted reactions in humans as well as animals, often as a consequence of incorrect use. The reporting of suspected adverse reactions and issues of zoonoses and the closer working of all health professionals, especially doctors, pharmacists and veterinarians, are all matters which deserve to be addressed more determinedly.

It is hoped that the book will assist with the maintenance of good health in the community, both human and animal, by covering extensively the potential zoonotic risks of associating with animals. To highlight this, potential risks for humans are flagged with a hazard symbol. A second aim is to provide a resource for pharmacists to answer enquiries from animal owners about veterinary matters in an informed way. It is hoped that this book. intended as a reference source as well as for study, will meet some of these challenges. Examples of products available in the UK are given, many with trade names, manufacturers and legal status; lists may not be exhaustive and the mention of a particular product does not indicate any recommendation on our part.

We also hope that the appearance of this book will be a factor in kick starting the Royal Pharmaceutical Society's Diploma in Veterinary Pharmacy back into life after two or three years of quiescence and will also stimulate Schools of Pharmacy to include some exposure to veterinary pharmacy in their undergraduate courses. In the latter we share the desire of the Veterinary Pharmacists' Group of the Royal Pharmaceutical Society, who have been supportive of this endeavour, to promote and encourage all those both at postgraduate level or undergraduate level to take more and renewed interest in this long-established area of pharmacy which stretches back over the centuries.

The book is designed to be a source of reference to be consulted whenever the occasion presents. To facilitate this aim and provide complete chapters for the convenience of busy community pharmacists, there is some repetition of material to obviate the necessity of flicking back and forth when searching for different aspects of a particular topic.

The ready willingness of the contributing authors to this first edition is enormously appreciated. Their response when asked to assist was greatly uplifting and encouraged the belief that a specialised title like this had a modest place alongside *The Veterinary Formulary*, first published by the Pharmaceutical Press in 1991 and now in its fifth edition and the product of an enlightened and courageous initiative. We have a lot to live up to!

Steven B Kayne
Michael H Jepson
December 2003

About the editors

Dr Steven B Kayne spent almost 30 years as a Community Pharmacist in Glasgow, with a special interest in pet care. He completed the Society's Diploma in Agricultural and Veterinary Pharmacy in 1991 and contributed to the course thereafter. He writes and lectures widely on veterinary subjects of interest to pharmacists and was Editor of *The Veterinary Pharmacist*, the newsletter of the Veterinary Pharmacists Group for several years. Dr Kayne is a visiting lecturer at the University of Strathclyde, Glasgow and holds a number of advisory positions as well as being a member of the Scottish Executive of the Royal Pharmaceutical Society of Great Britain (RPSGB) and Chairman of the College of Pharmacy Practice in Scotland.

Dr Michael H Jepson, a Visiting Fellow at Aston University, was formerly head of Pharmacy Practice in the School of Pharmacy. He has been Course Director for the RPSGB Diploma in Agricultural & Veterinary Pharmacy since its inception in 1981. He has held numerous appointments as External Examiner for UG and PG degrees and research degrees and he has also undertaken several consultancy assignments by invitation. Dr Jepson was a Nominated Member of the Veterinary Products Committee, 1994–2001.

In 1986 he was awarded the 26th RPSGB Silver Medal, in 1997, awarded by examination a Diploma in the History of Medicine of the Society of Apothecaries, and in 1999, nominated an honorary member of the British Institute of Regulatory Affairs. Since 2001, he has been Acting Course Director for the BIRA diploma and MSc in Regulatory Affairs. Dr Jepson serves on several councils and committees associated with various aspects of pharmacy, notably of the Veterinary Pharmacists' Group, the Institute of Pharmacy Management and the British Society for the History of Pharmacy. He is a recently appointed member of the Veterinary Formulary Advisory Committee.

Contributors

Gordon Appelbe LLB, PhD, MSc, BSc (Pharm), FRPharmS, Hon MPS (Australia), FCPP
Independent Pharmaceutical and Legal Consultant, London, UK

Tom Alexander BSc, PhD, MVSc, DPM
Formerly Deputy Head, University of Cambridge Veterinary School, UK

Andrew Cairns BSc, MRPharmS
Chairman of the Veterinary Pharmacists' Group of the Royal Pharmaceutical Society of Great Britain, London, UK

Graham Cawley MSc, MS, BVMS, MRCVS
Consultant Veterinary Surgeon on Drug Trials and Technical Enquiries for Companies, Cumbria, UK

Colin Chapman BPharm, BVSc(Hons), PhD, FPS (Australia)
Dean and Professor of Pharmacy, Victorian College of Pharmacy, Monash University, Australia

Sarah Cockbill BPharm, PhD, LLM, BPharm, MPharm, DAgVetPharm, MIPharmM, FCPP, FRPharmS
Senior Research Associate, Welsh School of Pharmacy, Cardiff University, UK

Francis Hunter MRCVS, VetFFHom
Arun Veterinary Group, Pulborough, West Sussex, UK

Michael H Jepson BPharm, MSc, PhD, FRPharmS, MCPP, MInstPkg, FIPharmM, DHMSA, MBIRA(Hon)
Former Head of Pharmacy Practice, University of Aston, Birmingham, UK; Course Director, Royal Pharmaceutical Society of Great Britain Diploma in Agricultural and Veterinary Pharmacy; Member, Veterinary Products Committee 1994–2001

Steven B Kayne BSc, PhD, MBA, LLM, MSc (Med Sci), DAgVetPharm, FRPharmS, FCPP, FIPharmM, MPS (NZ), FNZCP, FFHom
Independent Consultant Pharmacist and Visiting Lecturer, University of Strathclyde, Glasgow, UK

Martin Shakespeare BPharm, MRPharmS, DAgVetPharm, DipCP(DES), RNR
Ministry of Defence, Whitehall, London, UK

Lucy Whitfield MA, VetMB, CertLAS, MRCVS
Named Veterinary Surgeon, for Huntingdon Life Sciences Ltd, Suffolk, UK

Barrie Wilton
Consultant on the management and healthcare of pigeons; former Director of Petlife International Ltd; pigeon fancier for 50 years, Wiltshire, UK

Abbreviations

ACP	Advisory Committee on Pesticides
ABPI	Association of British Pharmaceutical Industry
ADI	Acceptable Daily Intake
AMELIA	Animal Medicines European Licensing Information and Advice (VMD Guidance Notes series)
ATC	Animal Test Certificate
BIBRA	British Industrial Biological Research Association
BKA	Bee Keepers' Association
BP(Vet)	British Pharmacopoeia (Veterinary)
BSAVA	British Small Animals Veterinary Association
BVA	British Veterinary Association
BVetC	British Veterinary Codex
CFS	Chronic Fatigue Syndrome
COT	Committee on Toxicity of Chemicals in Food, Consumer Products and the Environment
CP	Centralised Procedure
CPMP	Committee for Proprietary Medicinal Products
CSL	Central Science Laboratory
CSM	Committee on Safety of Medicines
CVL	Central Veterinary Laboratory
CVMP	Committee of Veterinary Medicinal Products
DEFRA	Department for Environment, Food, and Rural Affairs
EMEA	European Agency for the Evaluation of Medicinal Products
FAO	Food and Agricultural Organization of the United Nations
FEDESA	European Federation of Animal Health
FMDV	Foot-and-Mouth Disease Virus
FPS	Finished Product Specification
GMP	Good Manufacturing Practice
JECFA	Joint FAO/WHO Expert Committee on Food Additives
LOD	Limit of Detection
MA	Marketing Authorisation
MAFF	Ministry of Agriculture, Fisheries and Food (see DEFRA)
MAVIS	Medicines Act Veterinary Information Service

MCA	Medicines Control Agency
MFS	Medicated Feedingstuff (prescription)
MIC	Minimum Inhibitory Concentration
MRL	Maximum Residue Limit (for vet drug residues)
MRL	Maximum Residue Level (for pesticide residues)
NBU	National Bee Unit
NOAH	National Office of Animal Health
NOEL	No Observable Effect Level
NPIS	National Poisons Information Service
OP	Organophosphorus Compound
PhEur	European Pharmacopoeia
PL	Product Licence
PPE	Personal Protective Equipment
PSD	Pesticides Safety Directorate
PSU	Periodic Safety Update
PSUR	Periodic Safety Update Report
QP	Qualified Person
RAPS	Retail Animal Products Surveillance
RCVS	Royal College of Veterinary Surgeons
RMS	Raw Materials Specification
RPSGB	Royal Pharmaceutical Society of Great Britain
SAR	Suspected Adverse Reaction
SPC	Summary of Product Characteristics
STA	Special Treatment Authorisation
TAS	Target Animal Safety
TDI	Tolerable Daily Intake
TGE	Transmissible Gastroenteritis
TSE	Transmissible Spongiform Encephalopathy
VMD	Veterinary Medicines Directorate
VPC	Veterinary Products Committee
VPG	Veterinary Pharmacists' Group (of RPSGB)

Part 1

Animals and human health

1

Keeping animals – implications for human healthcare

Steven B Kayne

The centuries'-old bond between people and animals has contributed to a variety of human needs. Animals first provided basic resources for living: food, clothing, transport and material for shelter. Folklore has highlighted the value of many animals as models of probity to which humans may wish to aspire (Gunter, 1999).

> ... 'honesty from the ant which does not steal from the stores of other ants, decency from the cat which covers up its excrement, chastity from the dove and piety from the stork which guards the purity of its family and is kind to its fellows' (Levinson, 1972).

Later, the relationship developed to meet psychological needs of humans for companionship and security. This activity differs from most other forms of ownership in that its primary aim is the development of a complex relationship.

Farmers run a business and keep animals to provide saleable commodities. They keep working dogs, horses, beef cattle and dairy cattle (Figure 1.1), sheep, pigs, poultry, and sometimes goats. With the possible exception of the sheepdog, decisions on whether to treat or slaughter animals are usually taken on economic grounds. Animal welfare and good husbandry are both overwhelmingly important to farmers and repaid by optimised productivity.

The situation with small animals is quite different. The rewards derived from keeping animals as companions arise from the relationship itself. This is not to say that larger animals cannot also be part of a special relationship. Occasionally, a favourite cow, such as the Highland cow pictured in Figure 1.2, or a horse becomes a family pet or tourist attraction, and therefore a return on investment may not be a factor in its welfare.

There is evidence that humans have treated pets more as friends and enjoyed their companionship since prehistoric times, spending

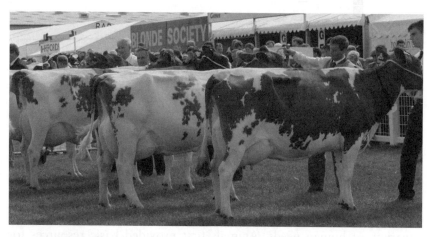

Figure 1.1 Ayrshire dairy cattle (Royal Highland Show, Edinburgh 2003).

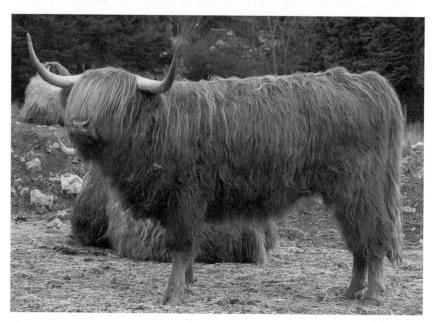

Figure 1.2 Highland cow (Fort William, 2003).

considerable resources on maintaining their health and general well-being. Many generations of Chinese emperors kept dogs that as puppies were suckled by human wet nurses and tended by their own servants. In mediaeval Europe keeping pets was frowned upon, the feeling being that extra food available, whatever its quality, should be given to the poor.

Modern attitudes to keeping animals vary across the world. Cows are considered sacred in India and wander at will; cats and dogs in some Far Eastern countries may be consumed as food. Most research has centred on Western attitudes to animal ownership and it is within this context that this chapter has been written. There is a view amongst non-pet-owners that pets fulfil some need for human social interaction or child substitution and that pet owners are therefore emotionally inadequate. In fact, research shows that pet owners are generally perfectly normal people whose pets enhance their existing relationships.

What is a pet?

A pet is a domestic or tamed animal usually kept in the owner's house for pleasure or companionship and treated with affection. This definition does not cover some of the more exotic pets (e.g. snakes and spiders) which many people would find less attractive. It also does not recognise that some animals (mainly dogs and sometimes horses) start out as working animals and subsequently become a family pet.

Keeping pets

Before obtaining a pet, the prospective owner should think carefully about why he or she wants an animal. Pet ownership is great fun but a huge responsibility.

Some things for potential pet owners to consider:

- Are you overly house-proud? Cat and dog hairs can get everywhere and some pets never stop chewing furniture (even if they have toys) and scratching paintwork on doors.
- Are you squeamish? Pet owners need to worm their animal, treat it for fleas or other conditions and generally clear up after it.
- Have all members of a household been consulted before committing to pet ownership?
- Are you acquiring this animal out of pity?

Keeping a pet may help to fulfil some of the owner's basic psychological needs. The names people give to their pets are likely to be associated with the nature of the human–pet relationship. Most owners consider pets to be part of the family, responding to their behavioural profile at any given time. Dogs seem to sense when their owners are unwell or unhappy, and often offer comfort. Pets are taken on holiday or away for the weekend, for which some hotels cater (see below). From early in the year 2000, pets from specified countries (including the UK) have been able to travel to and from other specified countries without having to undergo substantial quarantine requirements, much to the delight of many British pet owners who are now able to avail themselves of the facilities at a hotel conveniently located near the Channel Tunnel terminal in Calais. The hotel provides a canine guest service, including doggy welcome bags, a dog-walking service, pet grooming, lots of toys and dog-friendly staff.

Reasons other than companionship for which pets are acquired include:

- To perform certain tasks (guide dogs or hearing dogs).
- For protection.
- For education of children.
- Receipt as a present.
- To conform to popular local trends.
- For ornamental purposes (exotic birds or tropical fish).
- For the sounds they make (song birds or parrots, macaws).

When a decision to buy a pet is made, potential owners usually spend time finding out the scope of their new responsibilities, e.g. the amount of exercise required, special health requirements, the costs of feeding, and the costs of healthcare (see Box 1.1). When a pet is received as a present these considerations are absent and a pharmacist's proactive intervention may be appropriate, especially when the client is known by the pharmacist.

Choosing a pet

People publicly identified with a companion animal are making a symbolic statement of their personality and self-image. Similarly, the presence of a pet and the way it is treated can influence the image others form about individuals. The kind of pet that one chooses is a way of expressing one's personality. Thus the Great Dane may be a symbol of masculinity, power, strength and virility; conversely, a Chihuahua serves as a symbol of femininity. The German Shepherd Dog and the Rottweiler may be considered ideal for protection (Hartley and Shames, 1959). Pets can also reflect status, as some pets are expensive or 'fashionable', e.g. the Vietnamese pot-bellied pig or African pygmy goat (see Figure 1.3).

Miniature pot-bellied pigs originated in the jungles of China and Vietnam and were first introduced as pets in the USA around 1985, arriving in the UK shortly after. Since that time, the animal has achieved a limited popularity among pet owners looking for something different through its general cleanliness, intelligence and unique appearance.

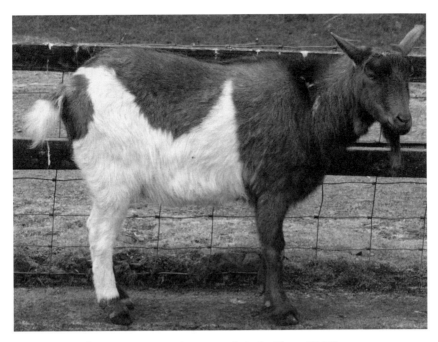

Figure 1.3   African pygmy goat (Rare Breeds Park, Oban, 2003).

Unfortunately for many owners, pot-bellied pigs grow to be adults the size of which precludes their presence in the average family home. The problem of disposal can be significant – a local zoo might assist. A report in the London *Times* in August 2002 highlighted the problem of large unwanted exotic pets that had been turned loose by German owners and that had adapted to the local environment. Near relatives of the piranha were found swimming in a river, and a 25 kg turtle that had lived for 10 years in a lake was recovered by divers after complaints from local residents. King pythons have been found eating cows near Hamburg and mammoth ox frogs munching on fish and amphibians in lakes and streams near Karlsrühe.

Ideally, prospective owners should review all the characteristics of intended pets and ensure that the animal fits in with their environmental and family circumstances and its needs (space, exercise, quantity of food, etc) can be accommodated. They should also remember that small animals soon grow into much larger animals – and choose the species accordingly. If one knows the age and weight of a puppy it is possible to predict the eventual adult size by consulting special growth-curve tables that may be found in small-animal veterinary text books. Breed is also important. Amongst dogs, greyhounds, whippets, basset hounds and English pointers are said to be the most placid breeds with low levels of aggression. At the other end of the scale is a group of belligerent snappers that show high levels of aggression. This group includes such breeds as Jack Russells, corgis, cocker spaniels and border collies that might be inappropriate in a house with young children. However, it is possible for owners to modify a dog's natural character most easily during the first 14 weeks of life. This should be borne in mind when choosing 'rescue' dogs from cat and dog homes. The very best homes (for example Battersea Cat and Dog Home in London) carefully screen stray animals for health and temperament before making attempts at rehousing them.

Box 1.1   Choosing my perfect pet

I married recently and with the prospect of settling down and buying our first home on the horizon, I thought I would make yet one more life altering decision – I would buy a pet. We always had dogs in my house while I was growing up and I always knew that I would have to have one of my own as soon as I could afford to live somewhere bigger than a shoebox. Now, despite the fact that said house had yet to be purchased I was eager to begin the process of choosing my perfect pet.

This should be easy, I thought – all I wanted was something small, cute and cuddly. A dog – yes it must be a dog. Cocker spaniels are awfully cute; maybe I should get one of them. But then I remembered a cocker spaniel who used to live down the road from us. He barked constantly! And he hated strangers ... and children ... and the neighbours. So I considered a beagle. They're supposed to be quite friendly. I also discovered they need huge amounts of exercise. Then I made the mistake of asking my husband what kind of dog he would like. I was trying to be polite, but I should have known he would have some very definite opinions on the subject! He wanted a cairn terrier. Not that this was a bad suggestion. Cairns are small, loveable and extremely playful. They're also scruffy, they love to dig and they bark a lot. I agreed we could have one eventually, but it wasn't my 'perfect pet'. Clearly I needed to do some proper research.

There were numerous resources at my disposal, but before I looked at any of them I decided to make a mental list of all the qualities I did, or did not, want in my dog. I highly recommend this as it facilitated my research considerably. I did not want a dog that was likely to bark constantly, slobber, be overly wary of strangers or other pets, weigh more than 10 kilos or need high levels of exercise. I did want a dog that was likely to be friendly and affectionate (I love a dog that likes to cuddle!), playful (to keep my husband occupied in the evenings), good with children (must think ahead a couple of years) and last but not least, I desperately wanted one with a sweet face.

Armed with this new material, I decided that I would confine my research to various breeds of terriers and spaniels. Even having narrowed it down this far, however, there was still a flood of information at my disposal. There were books,

(continued)

Box 1.1 (continued)

CD-ROMs, TV specials and literally thousands of web sites. I admit it was somewhat overwhelming, but I was determined to be organised and methodical. So I immediately logged on to my computer and started searching for everything I could find on terriers. After getting some 10 000 'hits', I went back and tried to be a bit *more* organised and methodical.

I found a book with large colour photos and brief descriptions of about 150 different breeds of dogs. It was just what I needed to help me narrow my search further. Based on these summaries of the most likely physical and emotional characteristics of different breeds, I was able to select just a couple of likely candidates.

It was at this point that the Internet really came in handy. Searching for just one breed at a time, I was able to find detailed information on personalities, physical traits, potential health problems, history of the breed, locations of breeders and of course, lots and lots of pictures. There were sites run by professional kennel clubs and breeders, sites developed by vets and dog lovers and others created by folks who simply wanted to share the wonders of their particular family pet with the whole world. There were some sites devoted to a single breed, with everything you might ever want to know about that type of dog, and other sites that let you enter characteristics and search for your ideal pet. Each of these different types of web sites provided a unique perspective and was extremely useful in helping me come to my final decision.

I've chosen my perfect pet, a cavalier King Charles spaniel – it seems to satisfy my requirements. All I need now is a house!

Rebecca Kayne

The Royal Society for the Prevention of Cruelty to Animals (RSPCA) has called for a drastic tightening of pet trade controls after a surge in the number of exotic animals found abandoned. Neglect and cruelty convictions involving exotic pets more than doubled from 58 to 126 in the year 2000. Among unwanted animals found abandoned were Burmese pythons, a snapping turtle, iguanas and bearded dragons. In Somerset, England, a young squirrel monkey that had been fed on a diet of Cornish pasties and chips was handed in to the local RSPCA office by its owner who was unable to cope. In another case a 2-metre Burmese python was fed on chicken and slept in the owner's bed before it was rescued from a one-bedroomed flat. A Burmese python can reach 5 metres in length and needs a room-sized enclosure.

Responsibilities of pet owners

It is an offence under the Protection of Animals Acts 1911 to 1988 to cause an animal 'unnecessary suffering'. Failure to take appropriate action in the event of illness or injury, or to provide adequate footcare and worming, could all be construed as 'unnecessary suffering', although it is accepted that the courts would need to define the words 'appropriate action' and 'adequate' in any given set of circumstances.

Owners also have a responsibility within the law to ensure that their animals are not dangerous (Box 1.2). Britain, like the USA, seems to be in the grip of a fad for designer pet wolves and although it is illegal to keep any wolf or wolf hybrid in the UK without a special licence or outside a specified enclosure, people will still keep trying. The decision by a Newcastle judge to keep a suspected wolf hybrid confiscated from its Durham owner under the Dangerous Wild Animals Act is reported to have been influenced by a chilling tape recording of wolfish night-time howling. The owner's case was not helped by the fact that he had claimed his pet to be 78% Canadian timber wolf. There have been at least four other similar prosecutions recently. The main danger with hybrids is that they can be extremely unpredictable, exhibiting the strong predatory instincts of a wolf without its normal inhibiting fear of humans.

Box 1.2   When is a dog dangerous? – A case of canine aggression (1998)

An action was brought under Section 2 of the Dogs Act 1871, as amended by the Dangerous Dogs Act 1989, which provides for a court to direct that a dog must be kept by the owner under proper control or destroyed if it is considered to be dangerous. The judgment hinged on what exactly was meant by the word 'dangerous' when applied to a dog.

The facts of the case were as follows. The defendant was the owner of two large Japanese Akita dogs named Hank and Hannah with a combined weight of 102 kg. While walking the dogs one evening in May he met a neighbour's children who were exercising Toby, their family's Jack Russell terrier. As Hank approached Toby, despite restraining action by the appellant, the powerful dog slipped his collar and broke free. A vicious dogfight ensued. The Jack Russell sustained severe multiple bites and shock and subsequently died, despite prompt emergency treatment.

It was argued on behalf of the defendant that Section 2 of the Dogs Act was never intended to apply to dogfights. A dog owner was liable in damages for injuries caused to cattle and sheep by his dog but nowhere does it specify a similar liability for damage to another dog. However, this argument was unacceptable to the court and it was concluded that Hank and Hannah were indeed dangerous and had not been kept under proper control when poor Toby was attacked. In the absence of any statutory definition of the word 'dangerous' in the 1871 Act, the 'ordinary everyday meaning' was applied. This decision was upheld on appeal.

Dangerous obviously *does* mean dangerous!

Owners also have a responsibility to look after their animals properly by attending to their needs in terms of appropriate diet, exercise and treatment. Modern hectic lifestyles mean that stress in humans is a well-documented factor and one that is recognised as a significant cause of health problems. But, while pets are known to relieve this stress, pet owners rarely stop to consider how their pet is feeling. Unlike humans, pets are unable to tell us when they are stressed! Pet owners therefore need to be able to understand the causes of stress in their pet and recognise the warning signs. In a new leaflet entitled *Stressed Pets* the Pet Health Council encourages pet owners to prevent stress by learning to modify those factors that make an animal feel nervous.

Pet behaviourists have emphasised that prevention of stress should start from the moment a new puppy or kitten is brought into the family home. Pets need to learn how to interact with people and with other animals, a process called socialisation. Without this interaction the animal may grow to feel threatened by simple challenges such as the noise of a vacuum cleaner or the arrival of guests. In most pets, stress is a minor problem and by following responsible pet-ownership practice it can be avoided. Pets can suffer stress through the loss of another animal within the same household with whom it has learnt to co-exist while other pets, e.g. Syrian (or Golden) hamsters, become stressed if kept other than singly.

In some cases medication may be necessary. Clomipramine (Clomicalm, Novartis) can be used to treat separation anxiety in cats and dogs. Canine sufferers display behaviours like barking, chewing and what is euphemistically called 'inappropriate elimination' when their owners leave them alone in the house. Feline urine spraying may also be treated with clomipramine.

Selegiline tablets (Selgian, Ceva) can be used to treat cognitive dysfunction syndrome, an age-related mental deterioration. Both drugs are prescription-only medicines (POM) and also used in human medicine; clomipramine is an antidepressant and selegiline is a treatment for Parkinson's disease.

Advantages of keeping pets

Therapeutic benefits

There may be significant therapeutic benefits derived from companion animals. In a 10-month prospective study to examine the behaviour and health status in 71 adults following the acquisition of a dog or cat, there was a significant reduction in minor health problems during the first month compared to a non-pet-owning group. This effect was sustained in dog owners to the end of the study. Walking a dog is a compelling stimulus to patients requiring exercise, particularly in cardiac rehabilitation or diabetes.

Physiological benefits that have been demonstrated include reduced blood pressure in a person patting and talking to a dog compared with that experienced with only human conversation. The patient and animal must be carefully matched. With the chronically mentally ill patient, pet therapy is based on the personality and animal experiences of the patient concerned. The inclusion of animals as a positive therapeutic approach for the development, treatment and rehabilitation of people is still a relatively new innovation; however, orthopaedic benefits of horse riding are well known.

As a group, pet owners may have lower blood pressure and lower cholesterol levels than non-pet-owners. One study has shown that people who suffer heart attacks are likely to make a swifter recovery if they have a pet. As a result, a variety of pet-therapy schemes have been introduced in the USA (e.g. 'Pet-a-Pet' and 'Caring Canines' in children's hospitals and nursing homes); a number are also being introduced in the UK. The Children in Hospital and Animal Therapy Association (CHATA) was founded in 1994 and works principally with terminally ill children in London hospitals. Volunteers must have qualifications associated with medicine or be qualified to work with children in some capacity. Some patients have claimed that contact with animals has reduced pain.

Emotional and social benefits

Pets, especially dogs, can enhance human emotional and social well-being and have a relaxational effect upon their owners, although tendencies towards humanisation of the animal are inappropriate. Even at preschool age, children derive psychological benefits from rodents, fish and birds.

Pets can influence human development, but whether the effect is due to the presence of a pet or to the person's relationship with the pet is uncertain. Female dog owners may exhibit less physiological reactivity during stressful tasks than comparative control women who do not own pets. Similarly, fish tanks in dental surgeries are common and are intended to soothe the nerves of waiting patients.

A pet may enhance social contact with other people, stimulating conversation. Owners as 'animal lovers' are often perceived as 'nice' people. There are also social benefits for people confined to wheelchairs, particularly as eye contact, meaningful conversation, and social interaction may be enhanced in the presence of a companion dog. Acknowledgements from passers-by when people in wheelchairs have a dog may help reduce feelings of social ostracism. There is considerable evidence that a residential or nursing home pet increases social interaction and alertness among patients and staff.

Assistance benefits

The enormous assistance given to the blind by more than 4000 guide dogs is widely recognised. Fundraising to cover the cost of training guide dogs is well organised, and many pharmacies act as collecting depots (e.g. for stamps and newspapers) and have collecting boxes on the premises. Such 'seeing-eye' dogs are exempt from many public health regulations that govern dogs in general. Such animals are allowed into restaurants and public buildings, as well as establishments operated by and for blind people. These exemptions recognise not only that these dogs are vital to their owners' mobility, but also that they are usually in excellent health, highly trained, and stay close to their owners. Blind people have a very close relationship with their guide dogs. As well as providing a valuable working function for its owner, a dog can help to decrease anxiety and boost confidence. The support is psychological as well as practical, and enhances a blind person's mobility. Separating the dog from its owner is often confusing and disorienting for both, and should be avoided whenever possible. To promote their special status, organisations for the blind emphasise that guide dogs are safe, hardworking, healthy animals, not merely pets. Owners are encouraged to ensure that the dog is kept in good condition (Hardy, 1981).

However, it is recommended that visiting a hospital with a guide dog should be restricted when:

- Patients are in isolation for an infectious disease or are immunocompromised.
- Patients are in intensive care, coronary care, undergoing renal dialysis, or are being treated in other restricted areas.
- The patient suffers from a dog allergy or phobia.
- Patients are in a severe psychotic state.

'Dogs for the Deaf' is a related scheme that provides specially trained dogs to people who are hard of hearing. The animals can warn of a phone or doorbell, or a baby crying, by touching the owner gently with its paw and then leading them to the source of the sound. Similarly, dogs and cats may be able to warn epilepsy sufferers and their families of an impending seizure. They are thought to be able to detect electrical disturbances or minor body odour and behavioural changes.

The following guidelines to ensure the quality of life of the animals involved in providing practical assistance or therapy were adopted by the International Association of Human–Animal Interaction Organizations at a meeting in Prague in 1998:

- Only animals that have been trained using techniques of positive reinforcement and that have been, and will continue to be, properly housed and cared for may be involved.
- Safeguards must be present to prevent adverse effects on the animals involved.
- The involvement of assistance and or therapy animals must be potentially beneficial in each case.

Basic standards ensure safety, risk management, physical and emotional security, health, basic trust and freedom of choice, personal space, appropriate allocation of programme resources, appropriate workload, clearly defined roles, confidentiality, communication systems, and training provision for all persons involved.

The process of incorporating animals as a therapeutic approach for the development, treatment, and rehabilitation of people is still in its infancy. Subject to precautions relating to hygiene, there may be significant health advantages from owning pets. Pharmacists should become an even more important source of pet-care information and advice in the future, given this apparently important link with healthcare.

Disadvantages of keeping pets

Disease and injury to owners

Zoonoses

Definition   Pets can create special health problems for humans. The word zoonosis is derived from the Greek word *zoon* for animals; *zoo* is the combined form, which together with *nosos* (diseases) gives the word for animal diseases. Zoonosis is singular and zoonoses the plural form. The term, used to describe animal diseases that are transferable to man, first appeared in the literature in the 1950s.

> 'Zoonoses are infectious diseases, the agents of which are transmitted naturally between vertebrate animals and humans.'

This definition fits in with the concept of zoonoses and was accepted by the World Health Organization (WHO, 1959). However, early definitions omitted the word 'infectious' and were criticised as being too wide ranging, as they included not only diseases that man acquired from animals but also diseases produced by non-infective agents such as toxins and poisons (Steele, 1985). Neither definition includes reference to ectoparasites. A more comprehensive definition is:

> 'Zoonoses are infectious animal-associated diseases that may be transmitted to man from vertebrate animals by bites, scratches, injection of saliva from ectoparasites, and inhalation of airborne agents.'

This definition includes human diseases acquired from animals and those produced by non-infective agents (e.g. toxins and poisons). Strictly speaking, this definition also excludes ectoparasites, which act as intermediate hosts and can both transmit zoonotic diseases and cause them from allergic reactions or bites. More than 200 zoonotic diseases may be transmitted from animals to humans, but comparatively few involve pets and farm animals; the risk is greater from contact with wildlife (Simpson, 1999). Chapter 2 details the potential risks from food-borne zoonoses.

The most spectacular implication of zoonoses in modern times has been associated with the spread of acquired immunodeficiency syndrome (AIDS). Researchers have shown that human immunodeficiency virus (HIV)1 and HIV 2 were introduced into the human population by zoonotic cross-species transmission of the Simian immunodeficiency virus (SIV) from chimpanzees and sooty mangabeys, respectively. These zoonotic transmissions probably occurred in the course of butchering apes for food. However, it is unclear exactly what set off the life threatening AIDS epidemic in the late 1970s after an extended period of time during which apparently 'peaceful' co-existence between humans and HIV had occurred in many isolated communities in Central Africa.

Another zoonosis that has assumed renewed importance in recent times is plague. Plague is an infectious disease caused by the *Yersinia pestis* micro-organism, which is transmitted to the human host from a natural reservoir (different rodent species) by a fleabite (Grygorczuk *et al.*, 2002). Plague is still encountered in humans in the areas of its enzootic prevalence in local rodent populations. Infection by fleabite results in a bubonic or septicaemic plague, possibly complicated by secondary pneumonia. The person with pneumonic symptoms may be a source of a droplet-borne inhalatory infection for other people who consequently develop primary pneumonic plague. Plague is a severe infection characterised by a short incubation period, rapid onset and quick progress, with mortality if not treated properly. As *Y. pestis* can be easily obtained and cultured and is highly pathogenic for humans, a serious threat exists of its being used for bioterrorism purposes.

Since Severe Acute Respiratory Syndrome (SARS) emerged in November 2002, scientists speculated that the disease may have originated when a previously unknown virus mutated in a way that allowed it to jump from an animal to humans. The long-sought discovery came when a team of researchers from the University of Hong Kong and the Chinese government tested 25 animals from eight species being sold at a live-animal market in the province of Guangdong, where the disease first emerged (WHO, 2003). The tests found a virus that appeared virtually identical to the SARS virus in saliva and feces of six catlike animals, known as masked palm civets. The researchers directly isolated the virus from four of the animals and found pieces of genetic material from the microbe in two others. Tests also showed genetic evidence of the virus in feces of another animal, known as a racoon dog, and an eighth animal, a Chinese ferret badger, had antibodies to the virus in its blood. None of the animals showed any symptoms of being unwell. At the time of writing, 8500 cases of SARS have been diagnosed worldwide with 804 deaths. Four cases were reported in the UK; all recovered.

It is fully acknowledged that we do not have such direct and serious sources of animal infection in this country. Nevertheless there are still some zoonotic risks associated with pet ownership.

Classification of zoonoses

By complexity of life cycle The agents may be transmitted either directly (a simple life cycle) or indirectly by intermediate vectors or environmental contamination (a complex life cycle). The surrounding environment may be the reservoir of some diseases that may be shared by several animals and humans (e.g. soil is the reservoir for mycoses and mycobacterioses; water supports free-living pathogenic amoebae). One of the most complicated life cycles is associated with the tick-borne Lyme disease (see chapter 13).

By type of life cycle Within this simple/complex life cycle description, there is a classification based on the type of life cycle of the infecting organism. It divides the zoonoses into four categories, each with important shared epidemiological features of clinical importance:

- Direct zoonoses, which are transmitted from an infected to a susceptible vertebrate host by direct contact, and undergo little or no propagative changes.
- Cyclozoonoses require more than one vertebrate host species in order to complete the development cycle of the infective agent.
- Metazoonoses are transmitted biologically by invertebrate vectors in which they develop or multiply.
- Saprozoonoses have both vertebrate hosts and a non-animal development site or reservoir (including soil and water).

By type of causative organism   Another system of classification refers to the causative organism (bacterium, fungus, mites, protozoa or virus).

Bacteria   Infections from *Salmonella* are chiefly acquired through food-borne sources, but can also be transmitted directly by animals (see chapter 2). Many birds, mammals and reptiles harbour *Salmonella* spp. in the gastrointestinal tract, either as pathogens or as part of the normal flora. Common pets that can serve as reservoirs for the microorganism include tortoises, turtles, chickens, cats and dogs. The infection is usually characterised by a self-limiting gastroenteritis, with watery stools that may contain mucus and blood. The acute illness subsides within 24 hours and treatment involves electrolytes and possibly antibiotics.

An unusual pet, the African pygmy hedgehog, has recently made an appearance in Canada. Not only is stroking the animal's spikes unlikely to calm the owner's frazzled nerves, but the hedgehog may also be a source of *Salmonella*. Confirmed laboratory reports have indicated a link between the animal and infection with the bacterium.

Reptiles can harbour *Salmonella* in their intestinal tract without showing ill effects. It is possible to test for the presence of these bacteria by means of a fecal sample. Even if they are affected careful hygiene precautions should minimise the zoonotic risk. Contaminated litter should be disposed of with care and feeding bowls should not be washed close to utensils for human use. Observing strict hygiene standards would probably prevent such transmission. It is possible for reptiles to acquire *Salmonella* from infected food – raw chicken carcasses for example. *Salmonella* infection associated with keeping terrapins and tortoises has been widely reported.

Tyzzer's disease is a clostridial infection found in many species of pet and wild rodents (see chapter 14). Although there are no records of humans having any symptoms of a Tyzzer's infection, almost all species of mammals tested can become infected and serological tests of humans frequently show antibody counts that suggest that there has been an active infection that has gone unnoticed. It is important to remember that whilst Tyzzer's disease is a common cause of illness in rodents there are other conditions in which *Listeria*, *Salmonella* and *Escherichia coli* can be implicated. The latter are all potentially dangerous for humans and can even be fatal to young, ill or elderly people. For this reason rodent diseases should be treated promptly and carefully.

Fungi The most common fungal infections transmitted from pets to humans are the dermatophytes, *Trichophyton mentagrophytes*, *T. verrucosum* and *Microsporum canis*. They cause ringworm, which is a skin disease acquired by contact with infectious humans or animals. The disease occurs worldwide. There are other species involving human or soil reservoirs of infection. *Trichophyton* infection in humans is acquired from horses and cattle; *Microsporum* is acquired from dogs. Zoonotic transfer of ringworm is also possible from gerbils (as well as from farm animals).

Although *Histoplasma capsulatum* can be isolated from many different animals, including cats and dogs, zoonotic transmission to humans usually occurs in persons involved in breeding birds. The most commonly implicated pet is the pigeon. The fungal spore is usually spread by inhalation of dust from soil rich in animal feces. Outbreaks have occurred following soil and dust disturbance during building works. Symptoms in humans include influenza-like symptoms with cough, headache and muscle pain. With heavy infection, breathing difficulties can develop. Clinical disease is treated with amphotericin B. Exposure to dust contaminated by bird droppings should be avoided in endemic areas; masks should be worn and infected soil sprayed with formalin.

Mites Mites cause various skin conditions in pets including allergic responses and mange. The zoonotic transfer of *Notoedres cati*, responsible for military dermatitis of the pinnae, head and neck of cats, has been reported and care should be taken by owners when treating affected animals.

Protozoa Toxoplasmosis is caused by the intracellular protozoan parasite *Toxoplasma gondii*. *Toxoplasma* infection is common in cats, but rarely causes clinical symptoms. The condition is discussed in greater detail in chapter 13.

Encephalitozoon cuniculi is a protozoal organism in the microsporidia family that can infect a number of species of animals, including humans. In humans infections are rare except in immunocompromised individuals such as AIDS patients or those suffering from tropical diseases. Some species, such as dogs and cats, either die from the disease or survive the infection and completely clear it from their bodies. In rabbits and mice, however, the infection is persistent throughout their lives and may or may not cause obvious signs of disease. Even within species it appears that some genetic strains are more resistant to infection than others.

Viruses   Influenza may be spread by zoonotic transfer (Kaplan, 1982). Aquatic birds throughout the world are reservoirs for all influenza A viruses (Webster, 1997). The virus spreads by fecal–oral transmission in untreated water. There is evidence that transmission of avian influenza viruses or virus genes to humans may occur through pigs acting as an intermediate host. It is believed that this may then be transmitted to other mammals, including humans and domestic pets, by the airborne route. It is more likely to be a problem in farm environments; such transfers have been reported only rarely.

Rabies is probably the best known animal-borne viral disease as it has well-known symptoms (Cockrum, 1997). Untreated, the disease is fatal to humans, cats, dogs (see chapter 13), gerbils, guinea pigs, hamsters, rabbits and wild mammals. People going to countries where the disease is endemic should avoid stroking seemingly docile pets (especially dogs) and any wild animals. In Western Canadian parks, racoons appear very tempting to feed and pet, particularly if they are in family groups; but racoons can carry rabies. Travellers should be advised to seek assistance as quickly as possible from local health authorities if bitten, to allow tests on the animal to determine the presence of rabies.Widespread testing of bats for rabies began in Scotland in March 2003 following the death of a bat conservationist from the disease (English, 2003). Comprehensive sampling of the bat population was carried out to see how widespread rabies was among Scotland's eight bat species, which include 550 000 pipistrelles and 40 000 thumb-sized Daubenton's bats. The work focused on colonies in the east of the country. Daubenton's are the only species of bat in Britain that have been found carrying this form of rabies, which has been identified three times in recent years.

Most canine viruses are usually specific to dogs and therefore do not pose a zoonotic risk. As dogs seem to be susceptible to subclinical infections with certain human enteroviruses and coxsackie viruses, they may play a part in the epidemiology of these infective agents.

Other causative agents   The rickettsial infections, cat scratch fever and the *Spirochaete* infection Lyme disease are discussed in chapter 13.

Exposure to zoonoses   In examining the causal factors of potential zoonotic disease, the following risk factors have been identified (Kranz, 1983):

- Residence in a pet-owning household theoretically represents the most intimate and prolonged contact many people have with animals. However, some zoonoses can be transmitted without either prolonged contact (e.g. rabies), or even without direct contact with the animal (e.g. toxicariasis). People may also interact with pets belonging to relatives or neighbours, and with strays, thus demonstrating that residence in a pet-owning household is not the only factor. Furthermore, residence in a pet-owning household does not necessarily imply intimate or prolonged contact for every family member.

- Exposure to diseased animals.
- Exposure to a specific animal pathogen.
- Exposure resulting from a bite wound.
- Exposure as the result of a membership of a high-risk group (e.g. veterinarians, farmers, and farm workers).
- Residence in a country with large numbers of animals. In some ecological studies, rates of human disease have been correlated with the population densities of particular species in each country.

Mode of transmission of zoonoses   Problems may result from intended or unintended contact with animals as follows:

- Contact through petting a companion animal.
- Contact through involvement with an animal casualty.
- Unintended contact with 'friendly' neighbours' animals.
- Physical damage (mainly bites) resulting from attack.

Dogs and cats live in close proximity to their owners and can transmit diseases (e.g. echinococcosis and toxoplasmosis). Even greater danger is associated with exotic pets (e.g. parrots and monkeys) that may harbour potentially fatal infections (e.g. ornithosis and herpes infections). New lifestyles sometimes create special hazards. Both agricultural and urban developments may encroach into previously fallow ground, where new contacts may be made with wildlife that can be a reservoir of infection; plague and various types of viral encephalitis are examples of this.

Direct transmission   This involves spread of the infective agent by direct contact with the infected animal. This may occur by:

- A bite or scratch.
- A spray of infected urine.
- Inhalation of discharged respiratory droplets from coughing or sneezing.
- Contact with infectious reproductive discharges.
- Contact with infected fur or hide (Weber and Butala, 1999).

Indirect transmission   This involves an intermediate vector:

- Transmission by a flea, mite, mosquito, sand fly, or tick (e.g. Lyme disease).
- Transmission through environmental contamination (e.g. toxocariasis, see chapter 13). Airborne spread (e.g. droplets or dust). Cryptococcosis is a

dust-borne disease associated with pigeons which is caused by species of the fungus *Cryptococcus*. It can invade skin, lungs, joints and subcutaneous tissue. Humans are relatively resistant to the organism unless they are taking corticosteroids or have diabetes mellitus. Treatment and control are as for histoplasmosis (see above). Food-borne disease, especially foods of animal origin (see chapter 2).

In some cases there may be more than one route of infection. Psittacosis (parrot fever) is a potentially serious febrile bacterial disease caused by the Gram-negative bacterium *Chlamydia psittaci*, found in birds of the parrot family, and in pigeons, budgerigars, ducks and turkeys. In birds, it is mainly a latent infection. There are two direct mechanisms of transfer of the organism to man: (1) by inhalation of air contaminated with feces or plumage, or (2) by direct contact with dead birds, usually during postmortem examination. However, a history of close contact with birds cannot be found in up to 20% of cases, and in other cases may have been very brief. The infective agent may survive in dust for many years, and indirect infection may occur in these instances by inhaling dust-borne organisms. Outbreaks of the disease are usually confined to aviary and quarantine workers, poultry processing workers and veterinarians, although pet owners may also be infected. Control is exercised through import licences, where appropriate, and quarantine. Well ventilated poultry-processing plants and safe disposal of infected carcasses are also advised.

Chlamydial infection in pregnant women can be life threatening, causing abortion or neonatal death (Vivian, 1986). As a precaution, contact with birds during pregnancy should be minimised. Symptoms range from a mild influenza-like condition, with joint and muscle pain, atypical pneumonia, diarrhoea, and vomiting, to endocarditis, myocarditis and renal problems with immunocompromised patients at risk of encephalitis and meningitis. In animals, most infections are asymptomatic, except for respiratory disease in parrots. The condition is treated with antibiotics; tetracycline and erythromycin are effective within 7–10 days. If thought appropriate by a veterinarian, pet birds may be given oxytetracycline in their feed. Transmission of infective agents directly or indirectly to another susceptible individual of the same generation is said to be horizontal transmission. When transmission occurs from one generation to the next, either prenatally *in utero* or neonatally via colostrum, it is called vertical transmission. Prenatal toxoplasmosis is a serious disease of human infants.

Factors affecting the emergence of zoonoses Many elements can contribute to the emergence of a new zoonotic disease (Hugh-Jones *et al.*, 1995):

- Microbial/viral determinants (e.g. mutation, natural selection and evolutionary progression).
- Individual host determinants (e.g. acquired immunity and physiological factors).
- Host population determinants (e.g. host behavioural characteristics and societal, transport, commercial and iatrogenic factors).
- Environmental determinants (e.g. ecological and climatic influences).

Emergence of new zoonotic pathogens seems to be accelerating for several reasons, including the following:

- Global populations of humans and animals have continued to grow, bringing increasingly larger numbers of people and animals into close contact.
- Transportation has advanced, making it possible to circumnavigate the globe in less than the incubation period of most infectious agents.
- Ecological and environmental changes brought about by human activity are massive.

Principles of prevention and control of zoonoses Prevention and control are sometimes referred to as 'primary prevention' (preventing the occurrence of disease) and 'secondary prevention' (damage limitation after a disease has already occurred). Rehabilitation after the failure of primary and secondary prevention has been called 'tertiary prevention'. The methods for prevention and control of zoonoses include the following:

- Neutralising the reservoir of infection by isolating infected individuals from the healthy population, treating infected individuals to reduce the risk of transmission (this could involve slaughter of animals if treatment is ineffective, impracticable or too costly), or 'cleaning up' the environment in which the animal lives.
- Reducing the potential for contact with the reservoir (e.g. by isolation) through strict quarantine regulations (e.g. for rabies), or by more drastic population control methods (e.g. reducing the number of stray dogs and cats on the streets).
- Increasing host resistance. In veterinary medicine, genetic selection favouring resistance, and reducing stress by improved nutrition or better shelter are routine procedures that ensure increased resistance to disease. Chemoprophylaxis and immunisation are other important measures.
- Public health protection. Prophylactic immunisation (when available) and education are two major weapons against zoonotic disease. Simple measures (e.g. maintaining personal hygiene, washing hands, or wearing protective clothing) can reduce the possibility of disease transmission.

- Health reporting procedures. These involve passive reporting of disease clusters and active surveillance to identify areas of potential danger.

This chapter has considered those zoonoses derived from companion animals and pets that pharmacists might encounter in community practice. In rural areas, however, clients can present with a variety of other conditions resulting from contact with farm animals (see chapter 10) and wildlife. Fortunately, there are few wildlife zoonoses in the UK compared with many other countries, but some of these are of considerable importance. For example, badgers are considered to be a major reservoir of *Mycobacterium bovis* infection for cattle; magpies are responsible for infecting bottles of milk with *Campylobacter jejuni*. *C. jejuni* has been known to cause severe disease in animals for more than 70 years, but it is only comparatively recently that modern culture methods have facilitated more intense study (Hone, 1986). Wild birds (e.g. collared doves) are also often heavily infected with *Chlamydia*. Wild pigeons have also been thought to carry disease. Chance encounters with injured or dead wild animals may lead to unfortunate consequences if simple rules of hygiene are not observed.

Injury

When either humans or pets are injured it is important that prompt first aid is administered. An English court case has established that owners are legally responsible for their pets' actions with respect to other pets. Proper control must therefore be maintained at all times, particularly with large, powerful dogs. Appropriate immunisation should be considered if the skin is broken.

Tarantulas are becoming increasingly popular as pets, and ocular injury resulting from them has been reported. Tarantulas are widely available, easily maintained, and considered harmless as many are non-venomous. Unfortunately, the popular American varieties have evolved highly urticarious hairs to leave on their webs and flick at predators. There is evidence to support the theory that the transfer from spider to human hands and then eyes may result in serious ocular inflammation (Blaikie *et al.*, 1997). People who handle Chilean rose tarantulas regularly should wear gloves, avoid rubbing the eyes during handling, and thoroughly wash their hands to minimise the transfer of hairs.

Dozens of families were pestered by an escaped tame badger in south-west England in May 2003 (Studd, 2003). This followed earlier attacks by another animal that resulted in five people being taken to hospital with injuries.

The mite *Cheyletiella parasitovorax* responsible for the 'creeping dandruff' that infects rabbits may cause bites on the arms or abdomen of owners following close contact with the animal during grooming.

Toxins

People who purchase reptiles, spiders, and other exotic pets may be at risk from toxic secretions or venoms. In such cases, owners should ascertain where treatment would be available should an accident occur. In practice, most venomous attacks are no worse than a bee sting, and a pair of sturdy gloves would offer adequate protection.

Cancer

There have been suggestions that keeping pet birds increases the risk of lung cancer. A number of studies in the Netherlands, Germany, Sweden and Scotland have attempted to demonstrate a correlation between lung cancer and keeping pet birds, but more work is required to confirm the findings. There is some circumstantial evidence that pigeons may be implicated, but the keeping of budgerigars, canaries, and parrots does not seem to constitute an appreciable risk (Britton and Lewis, 1997).

Allergies

Allergic symptoms resulting from contact with animal hair and dander are well known and include acute rhinitis, lacrimation and urticarial skin eruptions. Significant respiratory symptoms together with atopy have been reported in children after exposure to furry pets (Yarnell *et al.*, 2003).

Some people consider pet ownership to be sufficiently important to warrant ignoring chronic allergy symptoms and medical advice to remove a pet from the household. In a study on the consequences of lifestyle on health, 341 adults (mean age 38.4 years) were recruited who had been diagnosed as being allergic to dogs or cats (Coren, 1997). Each recruit had been specifically advised by their doctor to stop sharing their living quarters with their pets, but only 21% had complied. Such low compliance might be expected because of the large human emotional investment in a pet. It was even more interesting for a subset of 122 of these people, the allergy had been diagnosed sufficiently long ago that the animal they were living with at the time had died. In this group, 70%

had replaced the deceased animal with a new dog or cat despite the presence of allergies.

Treatment of allergic conditions is normally with oral and/or topical antihistamine or steroid preparations. Isopathy, in which a sample of the animal's hair is made into a homeopathic dilution, has also been used orally with some success (Beattie and Kayne, 1997).

Extrinsic allergic alveolitis (bird breeder's lung or pigeon fancier's lung) is a disease caused by the inhalation of antigens found in avian droppings. It is characterised by systemic and pulmonary symptoms of cough, dyspnoea, and restrictive lung disease. A similar condition (farmer's lung), the symptoms of which usually appear 4–6 hours after exposure, has also been described (Schatz et al., 1979). Diagnosis is with the aid of immunological tests.

Behavioural problems

Some people may inadvertently acquire pets that cannot be easily accommodated at home. Forming a bond with a puppy and then having to find it a new home can be extremely traumatic, affecting an owner's health and quality of life. The death (or loss) of a companion animal can also greatly affect the owner, causing a profound sense of bereavement. Assistance from the pharmacist could include advice to obtain a new pet or (in severe cases) medical referral. Communicating with an owner whose animal is ill with a chronic illness or where the animal is lost may be even more difficult.

Several pet tracking devices are now available to facilitate lost pets' retrieval. One example is a two-part system incorporating a passive 5 mm microchip which is injected under the skin of the pet and activated when swiped by a hand-held scanner. The resultant short-wave radio signal provides a unique number that can then be cross-referenced with a confidential database of owners. Both the Kennel Club and the RSPCA, who are currently managing this database in Britain, see the device as a means of making a significant impact on the rising figures of lost and stolen animals. Although the technology for this system has been available for some time, there have been delays in its release due to attempts to finalise a technological standard that can be used internationally. Pressure for this has come about as a result of changing quarantine regulations throughout Europe. Another important reason is the spate of 'dognapping' that is proving difficult to contain in southern Europe. Italian criminals have turned to kidnapping dogs in the hope of extorting cash from their distraught owners. According to the police, gangs are using the same ruthless tactics as the worst Sardinian and Calabrian kidnappers. Indeed dognapping seems to have caught on in England, with newspapers reporting the removal of a Jack Russell puppy and several much larger dogs from owners' back gardens.

Euthanasia

For owners and veterinarians, 'putting a pet down' is one of the most difficult things they will ever do. Euthanasia continues to be an option for many pet owners who do not want a terminally ill pet to suffer, or who may find the veterinary costs for continued treatment of their pet to be prohibitive. An owner's emotions at this time often make it hard for them to think, communicate and make decisions. Therefore, it is often helpful for owners to discuss the process of euthanasia with the veterinarian well in advance of its occurrence. Knowing when euthanasia should be considered depends on the pet's health; it is appropriate to look at the quality of life that the pet is experiencing.

Three questions to be considered in making the decision to put a pet down are:

1. Does the pet still enjoy eating and other simple pleasures?
2. Is the pet able to respond to contact in a normal way?
3. Is the pet experiencing more pain than pleasure?

In an emergency, under the Protection of Animals Act 1911, a police officer may authorise the humane destruction of certain animals to terminate unreasonable suffering. There are procedures for cats and dogs recommended by the Royal College of Veterinary Surgeons. Under normal circumstances veterinary surgeons will seek the signed consent of the owner to put an animal down, but if the owner is not present or refuses and the animal is suffering, the vet may take appropriate action.

Methods of euthanasia These are commonly categorised into three main groups:

- Inhalants
  - The inhalant agents include anaesthetic gases, ether, cyclopropane, nitrous oxide, halothane, methoxyflurane, enflurane, isoflurane, nitrogen gas, and hydrogen cyanide gas. They are administered to the animal via a closed chamber, container, or facemask.

- Non-inhalants
  - The non-inhalant agents are controlled drugs and include various brands of pentobarbital sodium (200 mg/mL) administered to cats and dogs in doses of 120–200 mg/kg by intravenous, intraperitoneal or intrathecal injection. A compound preparation containing secobarbital sodium

(400 mg/mL) and cinchocaine (25 mg) is also available in 25 mL vials given slowly to horses and cattle (0.1 mL/kg) and cats and dogs (0.25 mL/kg). This formulation is claimed to stop the incidence of gasping that occurs with pentobarbital. Ornamental fish may be euthanised by using an overdose of anaesthetic followed by a lethal dose of pentobarbital into the heart.

- Physical methods
  - Physical methods of euthanasia include the use of the captive-bolt pistol, gunshot (used for horses), cervical dislocation, decapitation, electrocution, microwave irradiation, and rapid freezing (most of which are not used for pets). Ornamental fish may be anaesthetised as above and the fish put down by severing the spinal chord just behind the gills or by delivering a sharp blow to the head with a blunt instrument.

Personnel administering an agent for euthanasia must know:

- Whether the agent is appropriate for the species.
- What route, dose or concentration of the agent should be administered.
- If the agent may result in fear, struggling or other signs of distress.
- If the animal shows signs of experiencing pain.
- How rapidly the agent results in unconsciousness.
- If the agent causes tissue changes.
- The technical skills for appropriate administration.
- If the agent is economical.

The emotional needs of the pet owner should be addressed throughout the process of euthanasia. Has the pet owner been informed of any alternatives? Has the owner received a complete explanation of the euthanasia procedures? Should the owner be present during euthanasia and should family members be allowed to view the body afterwards? Arrangements for disposal of the carcass should be as dignified as possible. Various wooden and cardboard pet coffins are available for those owners who wish to take their pet away with them for personal burial. Return of ashes after cremation is also possible and miniature urns in wood, marble or granite are marketed for the purpose.

When the animal is finally 'put to sleep' the act may cause considerable despair, and owners do sometimes require support from family members and friends. Pharmacists may well be consulted in which case homeopathic or flower remedies may be of assistance. In severe cases prescription medicines may be necessary.

The pharmacist's involvement with pet care

It has been suggested that well over half a million pet owners visit a pharmacy daily, giving plenty of scope for new professional and business opportunities (Kayne, 1995). Much of pet healthcare is of a prophylactic nature and it is possible to satisfy requests for assistance without contravening the Veterinary Surgeons' Act 1966. This restricts diagnosis and treatment of animal diseases to veterinary surgeons or owners. Pharmacists are able to advise on availability of medicines when approached with questions such as 'My dog has XYZ, what is available to treat it?', providing the owner makes the final choice, but not to suggest cures in response to 'Can you tell me what's wrong with my dog and give me something to help?'. The community pharmacist could again become an important source of information and supply to pet owners. If a pet arrives unexpectedly, for example as a present, pharmacists can suggest proactively the need for regular routine worming or flea treatments as part of their extended role as healthcare providers. This is a particularly effective role in suburban or rural communities. General hygiene advice, for example, washing hands after contact with animal feces or cleaning fish tanks (Kayne, 1993), and explaining how pet owners can guard against risks from ecto- or endo-parasites), can be extremely important. The majority of zoonotic diseases result from contact with animal excreta, but risks can be minimised by good hygiene procedures. Health advice can be particularly important for pregnant women.

The companionship that a pet can provide is often seen as something that has special value for the elderly. Under the Royal Pharmaceutical Society of Great Britain (RPSGB) Code of Ethics, animals, other than guide dogs, are banned from pharmacies. However, such action may be difficult to enforce with elderly owners who cannot bear to be parted from their pet for even short periods. As with all aspects of pharmacy practice, some degree of flexibility is appropriate. The fixing of hooks on outside walls to which dogs (or even ponies!) can be tethered has proven effective in some pharmacies.

In the early days of pet involvement all that is required is sufficient knowledge and a small dedicated section with a discrete notice. In order for us to develop this often neglected but potentially rewarding, extension of pharmacists' activities the inclusion of appropriate training in the undergraduate pharmacy course would be invaluable. The business aspects of pet care are explained in chapter 7.

References

Beattie N, Kayne S B (1997). The use of subjective outcome measures to assess the effectiveness of isopathy in the treatment of allergies. *Pharm J* 259: (PPR Suppl 8 Nov), R13.

Blaikie A, Ellis J, Sandfers R, MacEwan C (1997). Eye disease associated with handling pet tarantulas: three case reports. *Br Med J* 314: 1524.
Britton J, Lewis S (1997). Pet birds and lung cancer. *Br Med J* 313: 1218–1219.
Cockrum E L (1997). *Rabies, Lyme Disease, Hanta Virus.* Tucson: Fisher Books.
Coren S (1997). Allergic patients do not comply with doctors' advice to stop owning pets [letters]. *Br Med J* 314: 517.
English S (2003). Rabies testing for Scots bats. *The Times* 8th February.
Grygorczuk S, Hermanowska-Szpakowicz T (2002). *Yersinia pestis* as a dangerous biological weapon. *Med Pr* 53: 343–348.
Gunter B (1999). *Pets and People: The Psychology of Pet Ownership.* London: Whurr Publishers.
Hardy G (1981). The seeing-eye dog: an infection risk in hospital? *Can Med Assoc J* 124: 698–700.
Hartley E L, Shames C (1959). Man and dog: a psychological analysis. *Gaines Veterinary Symposium* 9: 4–7 (quoted in Gunter B (1999). *Pets and People: The Psychology of Pet Ownership.* London: Whurr Publishers).
Hone R (1986). Pet associated illness in Ireland: a review. *Irish Med J* 79: 176–179.
Hugh-Jones M E, Hubbert W T, Hagstad H V (1995). *Zoonoses: Recognition, Control and Prevention.* Iowa: Iowa State University Press, 4–7, 79–120.
Kaplan M M (1982). The epidemiology of influenza as a zoonose. *Vet Rec* 110: 395–399.
Kayne S B (1993). Fish and the pharmacist. *Pharm J* 250: 542–544.
Kayne S B (1995). The pharmacist's role in pet care. *Pharm J* 254: 515–517.
Kranz J M S (1983). Defining and measuring exposure to epidemiologic studies of potential zoonoses. *J Am Vet Med Assoc* 183(12): 1454–1458.
Levinson B M (1972). *Pets and Human Development.* Springfield: C C Thomas (in Gunter B (1999). *Pets and People.* London: Whurr Publishers, 1).
Schatz M, Patterson R, Fink J (1979). Immunologic lung disease. *N Engl J Med* 300: 1310–1320.
Simpson V R (1999). *Potential Wild-life Zoonoses in Britain.* Symposium on zoonotic diseases of UK wildlife, BVA Congress, Bath 23 September 1999.
Steele J H (1985). The zoonoses. *Int J Zoo* 12: 87–97.
Studd H (2003). Another rogue badger upsets families. May 27.
   http://www.sarsnewswire.com/newspage.asp
   http://www.cdc.gov/ncidod/dvbid/lyme/
Vivian M (1986). Pregnant women and chlamydia infection [letter]. *Vet Rec* 135: 619.
Webster R G (1997). Influenza virus: transmission between species and relevance to emergence of the next human pandemic. *Arch Virol Suppl* 13: 105–113.
World Health Organization (1959). Animal borne disease. *WHO Tech Rep Serv* 169: 6.
World Health Organization (2003). SARS update. 23 May.
   http://www.who.int/csr/don/2003_05_23b/en/
Yarnell J W, Stevenson M R, MacMahon J, *et al.* (2003). Smoking, atopy and certain furry pets are major determinants of respiratory symptoms in children: the International Study of Asthma and Allergies in Childhood Study (Ireland). *Clin Exp Allergy* 33: 96–100.

Further reading

Bell J C, Palmer S R, Payne J M (1988). *The Zoonoses*. London: Edward Arnold.

Gunter B (1999). *Pets and People: The Psychology of Pet Ownership*. London: Whurr Publishers.

Pearce J M (2000). *Animal Learning and Cognition: An Introduction*, 2nd edn. Hove: Psychology Press.

Robinson I, ed. (1995). *The Waltham Book of Human–Animal Interaction: Benefits and Responsibilities of Pet Ownership*. Oxford: Pergamon Press.

Wilson C C, Turner D C, eds. (1998). *Companion Animals in Human Health*. Thousand Oaks: Sage Publications.

2

Food-borne zoonoses

Martin Shakespeare

Farm animals are distinct from animals kept as companions, or employed in other social roles, such as guide or hearing dogs. By their very nature they are kept to provide revenue for the farmer from the sale of products, the majority of which are consumed as food.

Because of this role, the diseases that are transferred to humans following the consumption of this produce are significant. These diseases are described as 'food-borne zoonoses'.

Definition of food-borne zoonoses

Food-borne zoonoses are defined as 'those diseases contracted from eating foods of animal origin'. This definition is sufficiently wide as to cover the broad spectrum of pathogens, including prions. The most important however are still the traditional culprits, responsible for the majority of food poisoning cases, the bacteria. Of particular significance are *Escherichia coli, Listeria* and *Salmonella* spp.

Food-borne zoonoses and society

The systems used in the agricultural industry are important in reducing the societal impact of these diseases. When the systems work efficiently they prevent the transmission of disease into the food chain. The prevention measures necessary are not solely applicable to producers, as opportunities for the spread of disease occur at every stage of the food products' transit from farm to table. Hence, safety measures have to be applied rigorously at every stage of production and transit. The system carries with it considerable monetary costs and an inspection and enforcement burden for both local and national enforcement bodies.

When the system fails, for whatever reason, the effects on health can be profound, with illness or death as dramatic outcomes. The producer, transporter and retailer are not the only fallible links in the chain, people often fall ill because they abuse the food they eat through incorrect storage, handling or cooking.

The infective pathway

An animal contaminated with a pathogen, which may or may not produce clinical signs of disease in the animal, produces a food item such as milk or meat. The pathogen is transferred to the product that, if consumed without adequate cooking or other forms of processing, results in the consumer becoming ill.

Food-borne zoonoses associated with meat

Most people in the UK still eat meat or meat products. There are several pathogens associated specifically with meat. These now include the prion protein associated with variant Creutzfeldt–Jakob disease (vCJD). The following sections describe the most significant pathogens.

E. coli

E. coli is a normal part of most mammals' gut flora. It has several distinct serotypes of which *E. coli* 0157 is the most infamous and dangerous. This serotype is variously known as enterohaemorrhagic *E. coli* (EHEC) or vero cytotoxin-producing *E. coli* (VTEC) 0157. The organism carried in animal fecal material contaminates foodstuffs which are then consumed, or transferred by direct contact with infected animal feces. The organism is particularly associated with ruminant animals, especially cattle, sheep and goats (Tarr, 1995).

Most cases of clinical disease occur in children, the elderly, or the immunocompromised. The most notable recent outbreak of *E. coli* poisoning was that stemming from J Barr, butcher and baker of Wishaw, Scotland. The outbreak is believed to have followed cross contamination between cooked and raw meat. The outbreak was serious and extensive. There were 272 confirmed cases, of which 60 were classified as probably linked and 164 as possibly linked. A total of 127 people were admitted to hospital, 13 of whom required dialysis, and 18 of whom died. Three further patients died later from complications associated with infection, giving a final figure of 21 fatalities for the outbreak. Of the dead, eight people had attended the Wishaw Church luncheon, and six were residents of Bankview Nursing Home to which cooked meats from J Barr had been supplied. The 18 people who died during the outbreak were all over 69 years of age.

Prevention centres on reducing fecal contamination of carcasses as the inoculum necessary to initiate progression to clinical disease has been estimated at less then 100 viable organisms. Once in the gastro-intestinal tract, the organism adheres to the gut wall where it proliferates and produces a toxin capable of damaging the gut lining to varying degrees. Although the toxin may cause solely fluid loss and diarrhoea, in more severe cases haemorrhage into the gut lumen, known as haemorrhagic colitis (HC), may also occur. The condition can progress to haemolytic–uraemic syndrome (HUS), especially in children, with kidney damage that may progress to full renal failure with associated haemolytic anaemia and occasionally death. It may be that the development of HUS may be linked to the use of antibiotics, with the drugs rapidly killing the bacteria and producing massive toxin release. In adults, especially the elderly, but also occasionally in infants, the course may be slightly different with the development of neurological disturbances in addition to the HUS symptoms. This complex is known as thrombocytopenic purpura (TTP), and fatalities follow its development (Wong *et al.*, 2000).

Rehydration is essential and dialysis may be necessary. If kidney failure occurs, short-term dialysis, followed by later kidney transplantation, is the only treatment option. The use of antibiotics is considered to be inappropriate.

The Pennington report

Following the outbreak at Wishaw, Professor Sir Hugh Pennington was commissioned to investigate and make recommendations for future control of the disease. The group chaired by Professor Pennington produced a report that was published by the UK government on 8 April 1997 and made 32 recommendations. The main points were that there should be enforced separation of cooked and raw meat at catering premises, a programme of lessons on food handling for children and an *E. coli* awareness programme for farm workers. Additionally it was recommended that all butchers should be licensed, with one of the conditions of gaining and maintaining accreditation being mandatory staff training.

Listeria monocytogenes

Listeria monocytogenes is found in soil and water. Milk or milk products made from unpasteurised milk may contain the bacterium. The disease may also be contracted by direct contact with infected fecal matter. Refrigerated products can pose a risk, as *L. monocytogenes* is capable of slow growth at low temperatures. The main significant risk group is pregnant women, with the disease affecting both mother and baby. Fetal or neonatal death can follow consumption of contaminated products. Immunocompromised patients and elderly patients can also suffer serious illness with fatalities (Lorber, 1997).

In most cases, infection occurs following ingestion of contaminated foodstuffs. There is a prepatent period of up to 10 weeks following infection. Clinical onset usually follows fever, headache, nausea and vomiting and symptoms similar to a severe chill. Abdominal cramps, stiffness of the neck and photophobia may also be present. The condition may progress with organ involvement including endocarditis, internal lesions, metritis, septicaemia and meningitis. As central nervous system (CNS) involvement becomes more widespread, there may be convulsions, confusion and vertigo.

Focal necrosis in the placenta may occur with spontaneous abortion, premature birth or infective transfer to the baby at birth. Babies may display a septicaemic infection within the first week after birth, with associated pneumonia within the first month of life. Penicillin or macrolide antibiotics, delivered either orally or intravenously, are the only effective treatment.

Prevention of infection involves thorough cooking of consumable products, especially beef, pork and poultry. Raw vegetables must be washed thoroughly in clean water before eating. Recommendations for persons at high risk, such as pregnant women and persons with weakened immune systems, are in addition to the recommendations listed above. In 1988 the following advice was issued by the Chief Medical Officer (CMO):

> 'The CMO has established that the incidence of listeriosis in pregnancy stands at 1 in 30 000 live and stillbirths. Pregnant women should avoid certain ripened soft cheese, feta, Brie, Camembert, blue-veined cheeses, such as Danish Blue, Stilton, and Gorgonzola, and Mexican-style cheeses. Additionally they should not consume meat-based pâté. Cheddar and Cheshire-type cheeses, soft fresh cheeses, such as cottage and cream cheese, fromage frais and processed cheeses in sealed packages do not pose a threat ... Pregnant women should reheat chilled meals and ready-to-eat poultry thoroughly until piping hot. They should not assist with lambing, milk recently lambed ewes, touch the afterbirth or come into contact with newborn lambs. These recommendations also apply to immunodeficient individuals. Healthy children more than 4 weeks old are not at risk.'

This advice is still current and valid.

Salmonella

In a major study on infectious intestinal disease (IID) carried out in England between 1994 and 1995, there were approximately 9400 cases of *Salmonella* food poisoning. On the basis of the outbreak data available from the Public Health Laboratory Service (PHLS) it is believed that 90% of all *Salmonella* infections affecting humans are derived from food.

Salmonella enteritidis is the main culprit in fish and poultry. Other *Salmonella* including *typhimurium, agora, montevideo* and *enteretia (paratyphi* spp.) are also clinically significant. *S. typhimurium* is primarily associated with cattle but has also spread to pigs, sheep and poultry. Certain of the 2300 serotypes appear to be particularly invasive, including *S. virchow* and *S. java*. Reported cases of *Salmonella* show a distinct consistent seasonal pattern, with a peak of infection observed in August (MMWR Report, 1996).

Comminuted meat products and eggs have been identified as the main source of infection, especially sausages and burgers, although the microbes have also been found in beef, pork, chicken and, surprisingly, cereals. Animals may be asymptomatic carriers of *Salmonella*. They may also suffer clinical disease with intestinal disturbance, septicaemia and death. Spread within herds or flocks can be rapid with disastrous results. *Salmonella* spp. are also an issue in companion animals, as dogs, cats and particularly reptiles can also act as carriers.

Transmission usually follows ingestion of infected food, or direct or indirect contact with animal fecal material. Symptoms include sickness, diarrhoea, abdominal pain and fever. The infection can also be inapparent and present as unexpected overwhelming septicaemia. Susceptible groups include the usual individuals, with the elderly, very young, infirm and immunocompromised being at the most risk. In the USA, recurrent *Salmonella* septicaemia is used as a marker for progress from human immunodeficiency virus (HIV)-positive status to acquired immunodeficiency syndrome (AIDS).

The most significant serotype in terms of mortality is *S. typhimurium* DT104, showing 3% mortality. It is especially dangerous in the elderly. Infection with DT104 appears to be on the increase, with 500 confirmed cases in 1991 rising to 4000 in 1996 (approximately 13% of total cases reported). There is also a threat from resistant serotypes, with 58% of *Salmonella* DT104 isolates being resistant to ampicillin, chloramphenicol, streptomycin, sulfonamides and tetracyclines. The R-serotype of this pathogen is additionally resistant to trimethoprim and quinolones (Wall *et al.*, 1995).

Treatment is usually symptomatic, using rehydration or antimotility agents such as loperamide. In severe or invasive cases ciprofloxacin or trimethoprim are used at doses related to the age and weight of the patient and the severity of disease.

There is now statutory surveillance in place for all breeding flocks of poultry, and voluntary monitoring for all other flocks. A slaughter programme is in place, and any breeding flock found to be infected is isolated and culled. This ensures chickens used for egg production commence their working lives free of *Salmonella* spp. Industry codes of practice complementing the statutory salmonella control programme are also in place. There is a vaccine available that can be used in laying flocks; this is used by many suppliers to the supermarket trade to ensure clean egg supply. These measures have resulted in a reduction in the number of human cases of infection associated with poultry and eggs.

The British Egg Information Service has issued the following guidelines for consumers relating to the consumption of eggs:

> 'consumers should avoid eating raw eggs; refrigerate unused or left-over egg-containing foods; discard cracked or dirty eggs; avoid cross contamination of food by washing hands, cutting surfaces and plates after contact with uncooked eggs; and look for the lion logo and best-before date stamped on eggs.'

Clostridium spp. (see also chapter 10)

Clostridium perfringens

Clostridium perfringens, the causative anaerobic bacterium of many cases of gas gangrene, may also cause food-borne disease. Widespread in the environment, and an inhabitant of the gastrointestinal tracts of man and animals, it is often found in foodstuffs as a result of fecal contamination.

As with other forms of clostridial disease, it is the production of exotoxins by the pathogen that causes the main damage, especially where the food ingested carries a large inoculum, or heavy toxin load. The usual pattern of disease is linked to the ingestion of a number of viable *C. perfringens* that may produce clinical symptoms of abdominal cramps, diarrhoea and fever. The symptoms begin within 24 hours of ingestion and the clinical course is usually of short duration. Elderly patients and young children are most affected by this pathogen.

A more serious form of disease, known as enteritis necroticans or Pigbel, is linked to ingestion of a massive inoculum of *C. perfringens* type C. This form can be fatal and is usually a result of inadequate cooking or slow cooling of cooked meats or meat products, with inadequate reheating, allowing the bacteria to multiply and produce exotoxin.

The clinical signs are linked to the effect of the exotoxin on the gut wall. Cell death and invasive necrosis lead to overwhelming septicaemia and damage to major organs, including the heart, liver and kidneys. Treatment is usually solely supportive.

Large outbreaks of food-borne disease are usually associated with communal events and mass catering, either from professional or domestic sources, especially where food prepared in advance is not correctly stored. One of the largest thoroughly documented outbreaks occurred at a factory in Connecticut, USA. An employee banquet, prepared for over 1300 people, resulted in 600 cases of food poisoning linked to previously prepared gravy which had been incorrectly stored and inadequately reheated (MMWR Report, 1994).

Botulism

Clostridium botulinum

Botulism as a complex of disease states arises from contact with *Clostridium botulinum* or its associated neurotoxin. As with other species of *Clostridium* it forms spores which can survive desiccation and high temperatures. It is often associated with ducks, geese and some other types of poultry. Cattle and horses have also been found to act as hosts for some strains of clostridia. The organism is found in the environment, and also in the gastrointestinal tract of infected mammals that may be asymptomatic carriers and amplifiers, although certain strains of the organism can affect them also.

Food-borne botulism is not infective, it is related solely to the ingestion of botulinum toxin and is normally associated with products such as duck pâté, sausages, and seafood, including smoked fish which have been inadequately heat treated, as the neurotoxin is destroyed at high temperatures. The amount of toxin necessary to cause clinical signs is measured in nanograms, thus although foods ingested may contain no active bacteria the residual toxin content can be sufficient to produce symptoms.

The disease usually begins 18–36 hours after the ingestion of the toxin, early signs include gait difficulties, dysphagia and impaired vision. Respiratory distress, muscle weakness, abdominal distension and constipation may appear progressively. In severe cases assistance to maintain breathing by mechanical ventilation is required to prevent death. Botulinum antitoxin is used to treat the condition and, provided respiratory support is maintained, the majority of cases will make a full recovery. The antitoxin may be obtained from locally designated centres throughout the UK, and in emergencies through the Department of Health Duty Officer. There are cautions related to its use, however, as hypersensitivity reactions are not uncommon (Lindsay, 1997).

Many cases of food-borne botulism are believed to go undiagnosed, as the symptoms may be transient, with confusion of clinical signs with Guillain–Barré syndrome (see below).

Yersinia enterocolitica

Of the same bacterial genus as plague, *Y. enterocolitica* is transmitted to humans by ingestion of foods as diverse as meat (pork, beef and lamb), oysters, fish and raw milk. It causes an acute onset of gastroenteritis, with diarrhoea and vomiting, marked fever and abdominal pain. The pain can be so severe that it mimics appendicitis and has also led to misdiagnosis of Crohn's disease. It is capable of producing clinical complications that include septic arthritis, colonisation of existing wounds, bacteraemia and urinary tract infections. Luckily it is rarely fatal.

Cryptosporidiosis

The *Cryptosporidia*, a family of spore-forming parasitic protozoans, occur widely in the environment and can be found in a variety of foodstuffs, with contamination arising from animal fecal matter. *Cryptosporidium parvum* is considered to be a particularly significant pathogen. Calves, lambs and deer have been identified as asymptomatic animal reservoirs, capable of shedding viable organisms in their feces (Current and Garcia, 1991).

Human infection follows either direct contact with animal feces, or consumption of inadequately cleaned or cooked products. There have also been incidents of individuals contracting the disease after swimming in contaminated water. Person-to-person spread has also been recorded, and is a particular risk in patient-care settings.

An inoculum of less than 100 encysted organisms can cause clinical disease. Following a prepatent period of between 2 and 14 days, and in individuals with no underlying risk factors, there is profuse self-limiting watery diarrhoea, with abdominal pain and cramps, and a low fever that may last up to 7 days. Loss of appetite and anorexia can follow with severe weight loss, especially in immunocompromised patients. There is also a high probability of relapse, with many patients having another bout of diarrhoea within 14 days of apparent cure.

In patients with HIV/AIDS, the disease may progress chronically, spreading to the bile duct, CNS and lungs. Unless treated swiftly, death will follow.

In low-risk patients treatment is purely supportive. Severe cases may need intensive care; however, treatment is difficult and as yet there is no specific therapy for patients infected with this pathogen. The strategy employed in HIV/AIDS patients centres around boosting the already damaged immune system with optimal retroviral therapy.

The pathogen can be destroyed by freezing, drying or heating materials to temperatures greater than 65°C, and irradiation. It is resistant to many disinfectants in common use (see chapter 10).

Campylobacter spp.

Campylobacter is a much under-rated cause of food poisoning. The pattern of infection for this pathogen in the UK is very different to that in the USA. In the UK, 80% of clinical cases relating to *Campylobacter* spp. are linked to contaminated food, whereas in the USA most cases are linked to waterborne sources of the pathogen.

This particular pathogen is widespread and present in many farm animals, with poultry in particular being very susceptible to a heavy bacterial load. Under normal circumstances the infected animals show no sign of disease, although there have been cases of abortion in sheep being linked to *C. jejuni*. The bacterium has been isolated from pigs, birds, cattle, dogs, cats, unpasteurised milk and water supplies. The two species considered significant in human disease are *C. jejuni*, and *C. coli*, with the infective dose considered to be less than 100 viable organisms (Peterson, 1994).

The organism is capable of surviving freezing and has been shown to survive for several months in frozen minced meat and poultry as well as in certain chilled foods. Thus cross-contamination could be a factor in infectious spread.

The most immediate symptom of *Campylobacter* infection is a self-limiting diarrhoea of 2–10 days' duration sometimes with bloody stools. *Campylobacter* mainly affects babies and young children, the immunocompromised, and the debilitated. Other symptoms include fever, nausea and abdominal cramps that may vary from mild to severe with occasional misdiagnosis as appendicitis, as with *Y. enterocolitica*. Symptoms may regress and reappear over a period of weeks. A septicaemic form has been seen in HIV/AIDS patients. Clinical cases of *Campylobacter* infection are associated with 20–40% of cases of Guillain–Barré syndrome. The triggering of reactive arthritis has also been associated with the disease. Following infection it is estimated that less than 1% of the population may become asymptomatic carriers (Molina *et al.*, 1995).

On average about 60 000 cases of *Campylobacter* infection are reported in the UK to the PHLS. In most cases the disease is controlled without resort to antibiotics; however, as it may be life-threatening in immunocompromised patients, antibiotics may have to be used.

Campylobacter spp. display high levels of resistance to fluoroquinolones, hence treatment with macrolide antibiotics is preferable; however, there are now some isolates dually resistant to both antimicrobial groups. In acute cases where resistance is suspected, tetracyclines, chloramphenicol and gentamicin have all been used. However, these treatment options are usually only initiated in secondary-care settings after sensitivity testing has been undertaken.

The main control measure is the reduction of fecal contamination of carcasses at and after slaughter. Hazard Analysis and Critical Control Point (HACCP) measures, including keeping raw and cooked meats separate and ensuring that temperature-controlled processing of products is correctly undertaken are effective in controlling spread through the food industry. They are summarised in Table 2.1 and considered in more detail below.

In the home, consumption of pasteurised milk and the thorough cooking of meat and poultry are recommended for everybody and

Table 2.1 Hazard Analysis and Critical Control Point (HACCP) principles

HACCP is a systematic approach to the identification, evaluation and control of food safety hazards based on the following seven principles:

Principle 1:	Conduct a hazard analysis
Principle 2:	Determine the critical control points (CCPs)
Principle 3:	Establish critical limits
Principle 4:	Establish monitoring procedures
Principle 5:	Establish corrective actions
Principle 6:	Establish verification procedures
Principle 7:	Establish record-keeping and documentation procedures

especially for members of high-risk groups. Pets can carry and spread the organism and should be excluded from kitchens. The organism is sensitive to heat and drying, therefore thorough cooking acts as an effective control measure.

Guillain–Barré syndrome

Guillain–Barré syndrome can affect any individual, and is often associated with diarrhoea. It is an acute inflammatory episode in which demyelination of multiple neurones occurs. Muscle weakness and paralysis can affect motor function, including breathing. Patients often require intensive care, especially if lung function is significantly impaired. Most patients recover, although convalescence may be prolonged. Fortunately, less than 5% of cases are fatal. Some theories suggest that this may be an autoimmune disease triggered by bacterial or viral pathogens, of which *Campylobacter* spp. form only one group of several possible culprits. However, there is as yet no clear scientific evidence to support this, although research is currently being undertaken (Bolton, 1995).

Variant Creutzfeldt–Jakob disease (vCJD) and BSE

In 1997 Professor Stanley Prusiner won the Nobel Prize for Medicine for his discovery of prions (proteinaceous infectious particles), which contain no DNA or RNA. Prions are defined as 'small proteinaceous infectious particles which resist inactivation by procedures that modify nucleic acids'. Prusiner postulates that prions may play a part in Alzheimer's disease, Parkinson's disease and other degenerative neural diseases.

Prions are unconventional as an infectious agent – consisting of protein alone, with no nucleic acid. The diseases they cause are also different to any other infection or disease, as the evidence in all species shows that both infective material and hereditary factors have to be present for disease to occur.

The physical symptoms of the disease spectrum caused by prion agents arise from the alteration of cell-wall proteins into insoluble forms following exposure to and incorporation of prion proteins. The process then becomes a self-sustaining chain reaction, which produces sheets of insoluble protein in neural tissue and particularly in the CNS, with inevitably fatal results.

It is now believed that following infection by a sufficient inoculum of aggressive prions, genetically susceptible individuals can develop the clinical signs of transmissible spongiform encephalopathies (TSEs). Their name reflects the finding on autopsy of brain and central nervous tissue riddled with holes like a sponge. The two most significant TSEs in the UK at present are bovine spongiform encephalopathy (BSE) and scrapie, which have an associated link to vCJD in humans.

BSE is a fatal neurological disease of cattle that was first identified in Great Britain in November 1986. The feeding of meat and bone-meal (MBM) to cattle is blamed for its appearance in the national herd and this hypothesis had achieved wide acceptance by the end of 1988. Changes in the way that animal carcasses were rendered before inclusion in the MBM appear to have enabled the prion agent to survive. The particular batches of MBM believed to be responsible for the outbreak is thought to have contained material from sheep carcasses infected with scrapie, and particularly brain and spinal tissue. After clinical onset is observed the disease is rapidly fatal causing death within a few weeks or months.

A ban was put in place in July 1988 by the UK, preventing the inclusion of ruminant-derived protein in cattle feed. In November 1989 a voluntary ban supported by animal feed manufacturers stopped the inclusion of MBM in ruminant feeds. In 1990 this became law.

By October 1996 BSE had been reported in ten countries outside the UK. Some countries in Western Europe reported cases in their native herds, probably arising from the importation of contaminated feed. Others where cases occurred were unrelated to imported feed; however, these countries had imported livestock from the UK for breed improvement, or other purposes. One case was reported in the USA in December 2003. Once into the cattle herd, BSE can spread by maternal transfer. The only solution has been to undertake a slaughter policy to eradicate the disease.

Variant Creutzfeldt–Jakob disease

Dr Robert Will first described variant CJD in a 1996 paper in *The Lancet*. He stated:

> 'In the past few weeks we believe we may have identified a new clinico–pathological phenotype of CJD which may be unique to the UK. This raises the possibility of a causative link between BSE and CJD. The identification of a form of CJD that might be causally linked to BSE will result in widespread anxiety and concern.'

This was an amazingly studied understatement. Initially known as New Variant CJD, the 'new' designation for the disease was dropped by the Spongiform Encephalopathy Advisory Committee (SEAC) in March 1999, leaving the disease to be designated variant CJD (vCJD) (Will *et al.*, 1996).

The identification of this variant arose from a series of deaths and postmortem findings which, although having many of the characteristics of classic CJD, did not fit the accepted case profiles. When compared with classic CJD cases, they were found to have an earlier age of onset of disease, with a much longer period from clinical manifestations to death. Classic (or sporadic) CJD affected patients aged 50–75 whereas vCJD affects a much younger group, with victims so far aged between 18 and 41 years. Additionally, the patients did not have the characteristic electroencephalogram (EEG) findings of sporadic CJD. At the time of the article in *The Lancet* no similar cases had been seen in any other European country, thus triggering the hypothesis of a possible link with BSE.

The two diseases of similar aetiology and clinical progress also occupied the same geographical location and time frame. It is now widely accepted that the diseases are linked, and that consumption of infected meat or other bovine material provides the inoculum. The evidence from studies in mice and monkeys support this hypothesis. The most likely scenario for the emergence of vCJD is shown in Figure 2.1.

It is still unclear how the prion invades the body after ingestion of infected material; however, a theory relating to Peyer's patches in the gastrointestinal tract of children and young adults is currently under development. Peyer's patches allow pathogens to be presented to the immune system in a controlled manner so that immunity can be developed. They recede in size and number as the child matures into adulthood. The theory proposes that the prion is absorbed from the gut via the Peyer's patch and is then ingested by mobile lymphoid cells which transport it to other parts of the lymph node system, where it is subsequently able to develop in susceptible individuals.

The cumulative number of definite and probable cases to the 6th of May, 2002 totalled 121. This included 18 fatalities for which no diagnostic confirmation will ever be possible, as the bodies were cremated, or the relatives refused permission for exhumation and autopsy.

Victims initially present with non-specific psychiatric symptoms. These include signs of progression from anxiety/depression to gradually worsening changes in behaviour. Altered perception and painful sensory distortion have also been seen in approximately 50% of patients. After

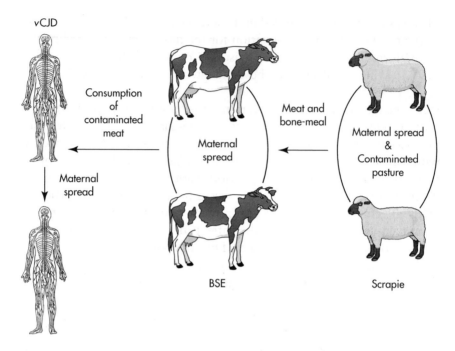

vCJD

Consumption
of
contaminated
meat

Maternal
spread

Maternal
spread

Meat and
bone-meal

Maternal spread
&
Contaminated
pasture

BSE

Scrapie

Figure 2.1 Diagrammatic representation of the most likely scenario for the emergence of vCJD.

weeks, or months, the disease affects coordination and patients may have difficulty walking and picking things up; involuntary movements and convulsions occur. Memory problems develop, and patients have reality perception difficulties, loss of motor control, dementia, paralysis and wasting. The patients deteriorate rapidly, and require intensive nursing. In the final phase of the disease total immobility occurs with the patient becoming mute. Death following overwhelming pneumonia is not uncommon (Will *et al.*, 1999).

Diagnosis in the initial stages of clinical onset is made difficult by the resemblance between this and other neurological and psychiatric disorders. Differential diagnosis relies on the use of magnetic resonance imaging (MRI), computed tomography (CT) scans, and an EEG.

Confirmation of diagnosis is usually obtained only on autopsy, where the characteristic spongiform changes are seen. There are some indications that testing tissue from the tonsils may allow definitive diagnosis to be made without invasive techniques.

In the interests of scientific research and public health, all patients suspected of suffering from a TSE are reported to the National

Creutzfeldt–Jakob Disease Surveillance Unit (CJDSU), based in Edinburgh. Doctors from the unit visit all people with the disease to take a detailed history from the patient and their relatives. Case notes are only closed after the death of the patient, when no further data are likely to be forthcoming.

The task of the CJDSU is to identify and investigate all cases of CJD and other TSEs in humans occurring in the UK. This work is aimed at determining the magnitude of the public health problem, and to produce informed prevention strategies and valid diagnostic tests.

Treatment

Drug therapies have been tried in an effort to slow the progression of the disease. Amantidine and amphotericin, although seen as effective at slowing or arresting the condition *in vitro*, have little or no effect on the disease in sufferers. Aciclovir, interferon, antibiotics, steroids and other antiviral agents have also been tried and have failed to alter the outcome significantly.

As patients deteriorate, rehydration and liquid feeds need to be used. Pain control may also be necessary. Clonazepam, or sodium valproate are used at normal doses initially to control spasm and spasticity after which dose is titrated to response. Sulfated glycosaminoglycans, and Congo red are also proposed as possible starting points for therapies, as they are both believed to affect prion protein metabolism. Vidarabine is also under evaluation.

Future hopes for therapies centre around protein stabilisers to prevent conversion of normal protein into prion protein. Antigene therapies are also proposed. Such agents would destroy the gene responsible for producing the prion protein; however, it is unclear if this modification would carry with it a risk if the gene responsible has other associated metabolic functions, currently unknown, within the normal healthy body systems. Even these therapies may only slow progression, and are not seen as a cure.

The BSE Inquiry

The UK government set up the BSE Inquiry in December 1997. The inquiry found that standards of care and support for families varied widely and suggested that improvements were needed, including speedy diagnosis with informed, sympathetic advice to relatives about the future course of the disease and the needs of the patient. It is now recognised that there is a requirement for rapid assistance for families to allow victims to be cared for in their own homes, and given access to hospice or similar care settings in the final phases of the disease's progress (BSE Inquiry, 2000).

Much of the health professional input in the care of victims of vCJD is palliative and relies heavily on good nursing practice. It has been found that many staff have become distressed and shocked whilst carrying out their duties in support of patients and their relatives, due to the nature and rapidity of the disease's progress.

Epidemiological clusters

Through the work of the CJDSU, two clusters of cases have been identified. A cluster of cases of vCJD was first identified in the Leicestershire village of Queniborough in November 1998. Between August 1996 and January 1999, five people developed the disease and subsequently died. All the victims lived in the area between 1980 and 1991. Therefore the investigation concentrated on this period, as this was the only time period when a common exposure could have occurred.

The investigation encompassed the farming practice prevalent in the late 1980s when BSE was first identified in cattle. At that time local beef cattle were raised alongside dairy cattle and were therefore fed MBM from the age of 6 days, rather than 6 months which was the norm for beef cattle, and therefore had a greater lifetime exposure to the BSE agent in MBM.

The investigation also covered slaughtering practice of large and small abattoirs in the area from the early 1980s. Cattle were slaughtered using a captive bolt; however, in some local abattoirs and butchers a pithing rod was also used to prevent the beast kicking after slaughter. The use of a pithing rod ruptures the brain structure and is more likely to release infective material into the work area or on to the carcass. Some local butchers also removed the brain from the head of the beast for further processing, increasing the chance of contaminating the rest of the carcass. Large slaughterhouses and meat wholesalers did not use meat from the heads of beasts, nor did they split the skulls to extract the brains.

As a result of the investigation, it was shown that the victims were 15 times more likely to have purchased and consumed beef from a butcher who removed the brain from a beast, compared with the control groups who purchased meat from outlets where cross-contamination with brain material was not a risk.

This careful and exhaustive investigation has identified the likely moment of infection, and for the first time has allowed the incubation period of vCJD in humans to be estimated. This is now believed to be within the range of 10–16 years.

Doncaster cluster   Currently there is also an investigation into three deaths in Armthorpe, near Doncaster. Two of the victims came from the same street, and the third visited the area frequently. Members of the CJD surveillance team have visited the town, and inquiries into possible common factors linking the cases are being undertaken. The likely parameters for this and any other investigation have probably been set by the Queniborough cluster.

Prevention of vCJD and BSE

The prevention of the passage of vCJD from sufferers to other humans is addressed in several ways. Regulations have been introduced covering the use of bovine materials in medicines and vaccines. The law came into effect on 1 March 2001 for human medicines, and from 1 June 2001 for veterinary medicines. All manufacturers of licensed medicinal products are affected and the MCA and VMD will ensure compliance.

Classic CJD has occurred by the transplantation of brain tissue or the use of brain-derived extracts. As a result, surgeons, especially neurosurgeons who treat CJD patients, are advised to destroy all surgical instruments after use.

Blood and blood products have been identified as carrying particular risk of transmitting vCJD. Therefore measures have been taken to treat blood used in the UK by leucodepletion to reduce any transmission risk. Canada and the USA have banned blood donations from people who have spent long periods in the UK, and other countries are considering introducing similar measures (Turner, 2000).

Prevention strategies   Guidelines have been put in place to prevent BSE reoccurring, and the prohibition upon feeding MBM to ruminants is rigidly enforced. Measures at slaughter to remove specified bovine material (SBM) from all cattle carcasses, and the strict inspection of meat at abattoirs, are aimed at preventing contaminated material from entering the food chain. SBM includes the head, spinal cord, tonsils, spleen, intestines and thymus gland. SBM must be rendered (temperature treated by boiling or steam heating) and then destroyed. The material must not under any circumstances be included in material for human consumption.

Any cattle suspected of having BSE are compulsorily slaughtered and their bodies destroyed. Milk produced by cows which are suspected of having BSE may not be used for any purpose other than feeding the cow's own calf. In addition to this very obvious measure there are several other measures in place to protect animal and, by implication, human health. All cattle reared for beef destined for human consumption have to be slaughtered at an age of less than 30 months.

It is uncertain what the future will hold. Estimates vary, with some predicting the condition reaching epidemic proportions with mass fatalities, and others suggesting that there will continue to be only a trickle of confirmed cases annually.

Milk-borne diseases (see also chapter 10)

Brucellosis

Brucellosis was named after Bruce, who in 1887 identified the bacterium that caused 'Malta dog', a disease familiar to many generations of seafarers. He named this pathogen, which he isolated from goats' milk, *Brucella melitensis*. This is only one of several species responsible for human infection which include *B. abortus* from cattle, *B. melitensis* from sheep and goats, *B. canis* from dogs, and *B. suis* from pigs. The diseases are distributed worldwide and are particularly prevalent in South America, Africa, the Mediterranean, Asia, and Eastern Europe where large flocks of animals are tended, and where eradication programmes are impracticable or unenforceable. The World Health Organization (WHO) has an ongoing programme of eradication by slaughter and vaccination aimed at controlling the disease in countries around the Mediterranean basin (Amada Gauci, 1995).

The UK declared eradication of *B. abortus* in 1993, and the use of pasteurisation, vaccination, and slaughter inspection has been successful so far in preventing recurrence. *B. melitensis* has never been isolated from animals in the UK and is therefore not considered to pose a threat.

The main symptoms of brucellosis in animals are focal necrosis of the placenta, abortion and infertility. The birth fluids and afterbirth are highly infective and cattle grazing on contaminated pasture are infected by consuming contaminated material. The disease is inapparent before the heifer aborts. Bulls may also be infected and can sexually transmit the pathogen, until ultimately becoming sterile. Cattle may be infected with any of the zoonotic strains, although horses appear to be resistant to all of the known zoonotic strains.

Disease in humans usually follows the ingestion of infected unpasteurised milk. An alternative route for infection is by contact with contaminated body fluids, membranes or the aborted young. There is some evidence for aerosol spread by infected droplets or dust. Human disease presents with lymph-node swelling, enlargement of the spleen, fever, testicular swelling, influenza-like symptoms, and lethargy, nausea and weight loss. Endocarditis or meningitis may follow, sometimes with fatal results (Corbel, 1997).

There is also a chronic undulant form of the disease which was often seen in cowmen and veterinary surgeons. Periodic bouts of high fever and other clinical symptoms are interspersed with periods of remission. This can persist for years or decades.

Treatment relies on the use of antimicrobials, usually in combination, to prevent resistance. The *British National Formulary* (*BNF*) and the WHO recommend the use of doxycycline plus rifampicin, or streptomycin. Therapy needs to be prolonged with the WHO recommending 6 weeks as a minimum duration. Longer-term therapy may be required in the undulant form of the disease. Recently, the quinolones in combination with rifampicin have been subject to trials and demonstrated to be effective. There is currently no vaccine available for human brucellosis.

Suitable protective clothing will reduce the risk from occupational exposure. The use of disinfectants, especially chlorinated disinfectants, iodine- or ammonia-based products can prevent environmental hazards. The mainstay of prevention, however, is eradication by animal vaccination or slaughter programmes. On a personal basis, travellers to areas where the disease is endemic should be encouraged to avoid unpasteurised dairy products and undercooked meat.

Q fever

Q fever, first described in Australia in the 1950s, is a disease that stems from cattle, although it usually causes no symptoms in the host animal. It is caused by a rickettsia, *Coxiella burnetii*, an obligate intracellular bacterium. The main significant zoonotic reservoir is considered to be cattle and sheep. Once infected the organism colonises and produces infective foci in the mammary glands and the placenta of pregnant animals. During birth, large quantities of the organism can be found in the amniotic fluid or on the placenta. The organism is capable of forming an environmentally resistant spore form (Maurin and Raoult, 1999).

The presence of the organism in milk results from the colonisation of the mammary system, and host animals can carry the disease for prolonged periods, with shedding occurring sporadically or constantly during lactation. The organism is resistant to heat and ideal pasteurisation conditions will remove it from milk; however, there is a risk from unpasteurised or incompletely pasteurised milk or milk products. It has been postulated that urine and feces from infected animals may also be a carrier medium for the organism.

There were 64 cases of Q fever reported in England during 1998, and 44 reported in Northern Ireland. Interestingly, the majority of the cases in Northern Ireland were in male agricultural workers who were probably exposed to the pathogen in the course of their work.

Transmission to humans usually follows exposure to infected material, and the Ministry of Agriculture (now the Department for Environment, Food, and Rural Affairs (DEFRA)) considers it to be an occupational zoonosis of agricultural and other workers involved closely with cattle and sheep. Further down the food-processing chain, transport drivers and abattoir workers may also be at risk.

A case of Q fever was reported by Aw and Ratti in 1997. It concerned an offal porter who developed Q fever while processing livers from sheep. The diagnosis was confirmed by an increase in specific serial antibody titre. The main clinical features were anorexia, nausea, headache, pyrexia and elevated gamma-glutamyl transferase. Twenty-four cases of occupationally-acquired Q fever were noted by the Communicable Diseases Surveillance Centre (CDSC) between 1984 and 1994.

The majority of individuals exposed to the organism display no signs of clinical disease. Infection rates and recording of clinical cases corresponds to lambing and calving cycles, allowing for the lag time of the organism's incubation period. After infection there is an incubation period of between 2–4 weeks, followed by an acute onset with high fever, associated chills, profuse sweating and severe headache. Unlike other rickettsial diseases in humans there is no skin rash. The patient may also present with anorexia, sickness and lethargy. The fever may last anything from 9–14 days and can recur at intervals with a total duration of up to 3 months. A dry cough may also be present with pain in the chest cavity similar to pleuritic pain. 'Cracking' in the chest may also be heard during respiration (Raoult et al., 2000).

Untreated cases can resolve within 5–14 days; however, symptoms may not regress for more than 7–8 weeks and relapses may occur. The untreated fatality rate is estimated at 1% of cases. Following a severe infection there may be a need for a prolonged convalescence. Elderly patients are particularly badly affected by this disease and may require prolonged supportive measures.

A chronic form of the disease also exists which causes a prolonged endocarditis leading to valvular damage, especially of the aortic valve. Recent figures show that this is more common in patients with pre-existing valve damage. The fatality associated with this form is estimated to be as high as 60% of cases unless corrective surgery is undertaken. Chronic hepatitis also occurs in a small number of cases.

C. *burnetii* can be difficult to treat as it can show a lack of response, rather than true resistance to antibiotics. The *BNF* recommends the use of tetracyclines at the usual clinical dose. The length of the course used may require adjustment with therapy extending for a period of days after the fever regresses to prevent relapse. Patients with endocarditis and valvular damage will need prolonged prophylaxis up to and beyond surgical replacement or repair.

As with many other zoonoses, prevention strategies revolve around good personal and environmental hygiene. Bedding contaminated by postpartum material, and the material itself, should be carefully handled, with collection and subsequent burying or incineration. Disinfection of housing and other areas should be carried out with DEFRA-approved products. Protective clothing including respirators, overalls, and gloves must be worn wherever feasible. All milk and milk products should be pasteurised, and monitoring of the process should be maintained to ensure that optimal standards are met.

Bovine tuberculosis

Although the prime cause of tuberculosis in humans is *Mycobacterium tuberculosis (var. hominis)*, there are still some cases recorded annually of the condition being caused by the closely related organism M. *bovis*.

The primary reservoir of M. *bovis* is cattle. Early control measures were focused on improving herd hygiene, culling out infected beasts and preventing spread within herds. The most effective control measure was the development of reliable pasteurisation of milk – the primary source of transfer of infection from cattle to man.

Within cattle herds the disease is transferred by aerosol inhalation with subsequent pulmonary infection, although infection from cow to calf has been well documented, as has re-infection of tuberculosis-free herds by infected humans. Badgers suffering from the disease have long been suspected of infecting cattle; however, the hard scientific evidence is sketchy and the mechanism of transmission is as yet unproven.

Cattle have been compulsorily and routinely tested using the tuberculin skin test since the 1950s. It is mandatory under the Tuberculosis

Orders (1984), made under the Animal Health Act 1981, that beasts with a positive test are slaughtered. The provision within the legislation for agreed valuation and compensation payments to farmers has been a major factor in achieving farmers' agreement to these measures. This has led to the UK achieving disease-free status. In 1998, of approximately 69 000 herds of cattle tested across the whole of the UK, there were just over 1800 individual confirmed cases within the national herd.

Clinical signs in cattle are variable, with some animals rapidly loosing condition, coughing and displaying udder lesions while others remain sleek and healthy. Ulcers are seen in a cutaneous form of the disease that can affect animals with advanced disease. Generalised symptoms include diarrhoea and enlargement of the liver and spleen. Pulmonary disease normally develops from a soft cough into haemoptysis, with physical examination of the walls of stalls for blood stained mucus being a very primitive method of determining infection in animals. Any of the major organs can become affected, and persistent, extensive lymph node swelling may be present. Skeletal involvement can also occur, with paralysis of the hindquarters occurring in some cases.

Transmission normally follows the ingestion of inadequately pasteurised or unpasteurised infected milk or dairy produce. Transmission may also follow inhalation of infected aerosols, or skin contact with cutaneous lesions on infected animals. In the UK only 25 cases of confirmed human infection were reported in 1998; however, in two of these cases multiple drug resistant *M. bovis* was responsible. There was nothing to link any of the cases with diseased cattle, hence these may represent reactivated disease contracted at an earlier date.

In humans, clinical symptoms vary depending on the source of contamination or route of infection. General symptoms include weight loss, pronounced fatigue and fever. Symptoms gradually worsen in active disease. The classic pulmonary pattern of the disease may be seen, with cough and haemoptysis. Ulcers or other lesions may be present in cutaneous disease. As with cattle, the organism can colonise any or all of the major organs or the skeleton and produce symptoms related to the site and severity of infected foci.

Patients may be asymptomatic for long periods after infection, with activation and progression of disease occurring when disease or age affects the immune symptom. Many of the current cases are among elderly people infected in their youth. The disease poses a considerable risk, along with other mycobacterial infection, to patients suffering from HIV/AIDS. Other people at an enhanced risk of contracting the disease are veterinary and animal workers. Migrant workers and members of other immigrant groups may also have the disease. As the treatment options for patients infected with M. *bovis* and M. *tuberculosis* are the same, drug therapy will normally eradicate both organisms if they are present together (Daborn and Grange, 1993).

Diagnosis follows a positive skin reaction to tuberculin purified protein derivative (tuberculin PPD). However, bacillus Calmette–Guérin (BCG) inoculation produces a positive test, so this must be excluded. Radiographical imaging, sputum testing, or enzyme-linked immunosorbent assay (ELISA) of samples supports the findings from skin testing. Differentiation of the causative *Mycobacterium* usually follows growth of the organism; however, this can be difficult. The polymerase chain reaction (PCR) assay has been used to this end with considerable success.

The regimens suggested by the Joint Tuberculosis Committee of the British Thoracic Society are normally used in the UK and are regularly updated to reflect the prevalence of resistant serotypes. For the latest recommendations the most recent *BNF* should be consulted.

Prevention in humans centres on immunisation. BCG vaccine is made from a live attenuated strain of M. *bovis*, and is routinely used to immunise people against contracting tuberculosis from both animal and human sources. The vaccine has been reported as causing cases of clinical disease in HIV-positive patients, and therefore these patients should not receive this immunisation. HIV-positive patients who travel to countries where M. *bovis* is endemic should be advised to boil all milk and abstain from any dairy produce that has not been pasteurised or cooked.

Another mycobacterium, M. *avium* subsp. *paratuberculosis (Map)* is found in raw milk and milk products. This organism is responsible for Johne's disease, a serious affliction of cattle worldwide, and can survive in unpasteurised hard and soft cheeses. In south-west England 1% of farms have cattle carrying the organism and an average of 2% of the herd is infected. It may be shed in the feces of infected animals (Hermon-Taylor *et al.*, 1998).

More heat resistant than Q fever or tuberculosis, due to the clumping of its cells, it can survive pasteurisation. M. *paratuberculosis* has been suggested as one of several factors in causing Crohn's disease, although the evidence is conflicting.

Tapeworm

The beef tapeworm (*Taenia saginata*, also known as *Cysticercus bovis*) and the pork tapeworm *(T. solium)* are very similar, both in overall appearance and life cycle. The definitive host for both worms is humans. The tapeworm only reaches maturity in the lumen of the human gut. The associated animal is an intermediate host which is necessary for the larvae to infect humans following the ingestion of infected inadequately cooked meat from a suspect carcass.

The adult worm is flat in cross-section and tapers wider from the head or scolex, through the proglottids or body segments. The scolex attaches to the gut wall of the host by means of suckers or hooks, depending upon the species involved.

If eggs hatch in the gut of the host, either primary or intermediate, larvae penetrate the wall of the gut and then migrate to a preferred site, usually in muscle tissue or other organs. In either pigs or cattle these normally migrate and encyst again in muscle tissue where the cyst may develop daughter cysts with multiple internal scolices. They may also migrate to other organs and cause a condition known as cysticercosis. The larvae encyst in sites as diverse as the brain or other areas of the CNS, eyelid and conjunctiva. The condition is also seen in humans when either eggs or larvae are ingested.

In cysticercosis, the cysts may be quiescent or active. Where active cysts are present they undergo a budding and proliferation process, leading to a series of connected cysts with multiple scolices in the vacuole. When the cysts are sited in the brain, complications including neurological disturbances, with epilepsy or paraesthesia, can occur.

Adult beef tapeworms can reach a size of between 12.5 and 25 metres in length; the pork tapeworm is much smaller reaching only a size of between 2 and 7 metres. Both species can live for up to 25 years. There are few symptoms associated with the adult worm, except slight irritation of site of attachment or vague abdominal symptoms with hunger pangs, loss of weight and general condition, indigestion, diarrhoea and/or constipation.

The beef tapeworm rarely causes cysticercosis; however, the pork tapeworm is capable of causing the condition in humans. Definite diagnosis of infestation follows either isolation of eggs or sections of the worm from the stool. Serological testing using ELISA confirms diagnosis, and in cases of cysticercosis imaging by CT, radiology or MRI is usually necessary.

For adult tapeworms treatment is undertaken using either niclosamide or praziquantel. The *BNF* states that niclosamide is available from IDIS Ltd on a named-patient basis. It is solely active against adult worms and does not kill larval stages. Side-effects are usually limited to gastrointestinal disturbances and itching with occasional rash.

To prevent any risk of cysticercosis by autoinfection following emesis, an antiemetic should be given at the same time as the niclosamide, on wakening.

Praziquantel is available from Merck on a named-patient basis. It is deemed to be as effective as niclosamide, and should be given as a single dose of 10–20 mg/kg of body weight after a light breakfast.

There is some controversy surrounding the treatment of cysticercosis. Usually surgical removal of the cysts is advocated in humans before damage ensues, with concomitant administration of anthelmintics. This is very important in infection associated with the eyes (Evans *et al.*, 1997).

The *BNF* makes no recommendations on the use of anthelmintics in neurocysticercosis; however, elsewhere in the world praziquantel or albendazole has been routinely used. Albendazole is approved for treatment of only hydatid disease and neurocysticercosis in the USA. It is teratogenic in animals, therefore a careful risk/benefit analysis must be carried out before its use in women who are pregnant or of childbearing years. It is hepatotoxic, and can also destroy bone marrow, therefore complete blood chemistry analyses and liver function tests should be routinely carried out before and during therapy.

Tapeworm infection is uncommon in the UK due to a strict system of meat inspection; however, this is not true of the rest of western Europe. Germany and France report significant numbers of cases annually associated with the consumption of infected meat in national delicacies. In non-Muslim developing countries there is a high incidence of the disease, causing more than a third of all cases of adult-onset epilepsy. Due to the longevity of the parasite, immigrants from these countries could present with symptoms of the disease long after their arrival in the UK. In the USA there have been sufficient cases among migrant workers for the condition of cysticercosis to be routinely tested for in cases of epilepsy amongst this sociological group. The number of tourists travelling from Great Britain to areas of risk, such as south-east Asia, the Indian subcontinent and Africa have increased dramatically in the past decade, therefore tapeworm infestation should be excluded in any diagnostic path relating to persistent abdominal symptoms or seizures following such trips.

Suspect meat or meat products should be thoroughly cooked and consumption of raw or undercooked meat from dubious sources avoided. Suspect carcasses or meat should be frozen for at least 3 weeks to kill any larvae. Viable eggs or embryos may also be present in water contaminated by fecal matter; therefore the usual precautions when drinking water of unknown quality should be applied.

UK Food Standards Agency (FSA) – scope and mission

In response to food scares, public concern over BSE, the Pennington report and a Department of Health study of the incidence of food poisoning in 1997, it was decided by the UK government to set up a Food Standards Agency.

The FSA is responsible for monitoring safety and standards of all food for human consumption, advising on diet and nutrition, and enforcing the law pertaining to food. It is also tasked with commissioning research into food safety. The Food Standards Act received royal assent in November 1999, and Sir John Krebs was appointed Chairman in February 2000. The Food Standards Agency is directed by an executive board, appointed to act in the public interest, and is established so as not to represent particular sectors of industry or government. Its members come from a wide and varied background, and bring to their work a wide range of relevant skills and experience.

The stated aim of the agency is to 'protect public health from risks which may arise in connection with the consumption of food, and otherwise to protect the interests of consumers in relation to food'.

The FSA has initiated a campaign called 'from farm to fork', aimed at making food less contaminated and safer for the ultimate consumer. Initiatives have also been launched to educate the public on food safety, nutrition, diet and clearer labelling.

The Agency is accountable to Parliament through the Minister of Health. As a safeguard for its independence it has the unique distinction of being given by statute the legal power to publish the advice it gives to the government. The Meat Hygiene Service is now accountable to the FSA.

Reducing zoonotic risks in food

Reducing the risks of zoonotic disease from foodstuffs is not just a process that begins and ends with the final consumer. Legislation and other physical measures to reduce or exclude pathogens from food are applicable to every step of the food chain, from field to table. Strategies for reducing food-borne zoonoses are illustrated in Figure 2.2.

Hazard Analysis and Critical Control Point (HACCP)

One of the major food industry schemes for recognising and identifying risk and its remedies is the HACCP process. This is now internationally

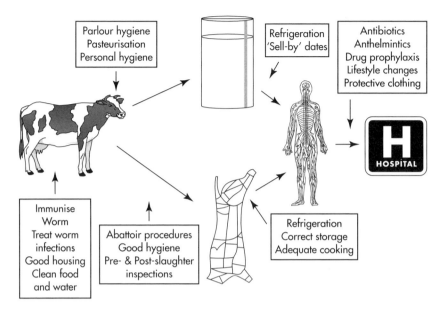

Figure 2.2   Prevention points and strategies for food-borne zoonoses.

accepted as the preferred system for the management of food safety in food businesses. It has seven principles that provide a structured format for food safety by controlling hazards inherent in the food-handling and production process.

HACCP applies to food producers and also to retailing and catering premises through current legal measures. The FSA has suggested that the principles should be extended to the agricultural process of food production, albeit in modified form. Until this is adopted widely, the current system of recommendation of a stepwise approach to infection control will continue (Notermans *et al.*, 1995).

General stepwise prevention strategies

Knowledge of zoonotic infections is the key to producing an effective stepwise programme. The application of our understanding of the likely routes of infection and the life cycle of the pathogen allows selective measures to be applied in a focused way, so breaking the transmission route at its weakest point.

Some of these measures may not be familiar or fully comprehensible to health professionals; however, they do form a non-medical system for prevention of disease, and are no less valid than more therapeutically orientated methods.

Step 1: control the disease in the animal

The incidence of zoonotic disease in animals may be reduced by the use of vaccination, clean foodstuffs and water, good housing and husbandry. Overcrowded or insanitary conditions can often lead to overt disease or unthrifty animals, requiring more therapeutic support to maintain sufficient health for them to attain slaughter weight or to continue to be productive. A reduction in infection rates has a dramatic effect on incidence of infection further down the food or product chain. The difficulties in implementing strategies at this point in the system are often economic, as although the measures may be available there may be little or no economic benefit to using them. In some cases those costs can become offset by higher prices for produce; however, that is not always the case. The lobby for animal welfare and organic produce has improved the willingness of producers and consumers to pay more for their food if it is of better quality. The converse is that there is also a need for food at the lowest price, and a bulk producer for a large supply contract may need to cut corners to stay in business, so increasing perceived, if not actual risks.

Step 2: reduce contamination at harvesting

When eggs are picked out, or cows milked, the application of sensible hygiene precautions is essential. Eggs should be free of droppings, cleaned and date-marked. In dairies, the udder of the cow, and the milking machinery should be as clean and hygienic as possible, with subsequent disinfection after each milking. Pipework and items such as clusters should be maintained and replaced as necessary to maintain adequate operating parameters. Milk should pass to the bulk tank and be subsequently chilled rapidly for later transport and pasteurisation.

At abattoirs, tight veterinary inspection both pre- and post-slaughter must be practised, with animals which display heavy fecal contamination being cleaned or rejected. Slaughterhouse controls should prevent or reduce onward transmission into the food chain, with rejection of suspect carcasses. Prompt refrigeration of meat and careful cleaning of the carcass can reduce bacterial contamination drastically.

Step 3: retailing controls

Disinfection of working tools and areas, along with personal and premises hygiene procedures, protects consumers and workers from zoonotic infection. Sourcing products from assured suppliers, temperature and environmental monitoring, and the separation of cooked and raw products reduces the possibility of amplification and transmission of infection. The tight control of 'use-by' and 'sell-by' dates is mandatory. Periodic inspection by public health officials, and the implementation of monitoring of refrigeration and freezer plants is also essential.

Step 4: domestic precautions

In the home, consumers should use common-sense measures, including disinfection of surfaces and equipment, personal hygiene procedures, and thorough appropriate cooking techniques. Using a refrigerator correctly and observing sell-by dates would prevent many cases of food poisoning.

General food hygiene recommendations

The FSA, the Food and Drinks Association and other public bodies have made various recommendations regarding food handling. These measures are designed to prevent cross-contamination of raw and cooked foods, and also reduce the risk of consumers eating products that are raw or undercooked (Box 2.1).

Box 2.1 Awareness of food hygiene

In surveys, respondents stated that:

- 23% never been taught to cook or prepare food
- 50% do not follow cooking instructions
- 15% admit not cooking meat fully or properly
- 25% do not always wash hands before cooking
- 10% do not separate raw meat from other foods
- 8% do not keep perishable items in refrigerator

People should clean surfaces, equipment and containers that have come into contact with raw meat. They must wash their hands after handling raw meat and before handling other utensils. The same plate should not be used for cooked and raw meat without washing the plate in between. Meat should be cooked until the juices run clear; this is especially the case with beef burgers. Barbecues are considered to be particularly risky, as meat may be not be fully cooked, and, if previously chilled or frozen, raw or undercooked in the middle.

These recommendations were made in the light of a number of surveys showing that public awareness of food hygiene was lamentable.

References

Amada Gauci A J (1995). The return of brucellosis. *Maltese Med J* 7: 7–8.

Aw T C, Ratti N (1997). Occupational infection in an offal porter: a case of Q fever. *Occup Med* 47: 432–434.

Bolton C F (1995). The changing concepts of Guillain–Barré Syndrome. *N Engl J Med* 333: 1415–1417.

BSE Inquiry Report (2000). London: Stationery Office.

Corbel M J (1997). Brucellosis: an overview. *Emerg Infect Dis* 3(2): 213–221.

Current W L, Garcia L S (1991). Cryptosporidiosis. *Clin Microbiol Rev* 4: 325–358.

Daborn C J, Grange J M (1993). HIV/AIDS and its implication for the control of animal tuberculosis. *Br Vet J* 149: 405–417.

Evans C, Garcia H H, Gilman R H, *et al.* (1997). Controversies in the management of cysticercosis. *Emerg Infect Dis* 3(3): 403–405.

Hermon-Taylor J, Barnes N, Clarke C, *et al.* (1998). Mycobacterium paratuberculosis cervical lymphadenitis followed five years later by terminal ileitis similar to Crohn's disease. *Br Med J* 316: 449–453.

Lindsay J (1997). Chronic sequelae of foodborne disease. *Emerg Infect Dis* 3(4): 443–452.

Lorber B (1997). Listeriosis. *Clin Infect Dis* 24: 1–11.

Maurin M, Raoult D (1999). Q Fever. *Clin Microbiol Rev* 12: 518–553.

MMWR Report (1994). Morbidity and Mortality Weekly Report (MMWR) on *Clostridium perfringens* gastroenteritis associated with corned beef served at St. Patrick's day meals – Ohio and Virginia 1993. *MMWR* 43 : 137–138, 143–144.

MMWR Report (1996). Morbidity and Mortality Weekly Report (MMWR) on multidrug-resistant *Salmonella* serotype *enteritidis* infection associated with consumption or raw shell eggs. United States, 1994–1995. Atlanta Centers for Disease Control and Prevention. *MMWR* 45: 737–742.

Molina J M, Casin I, Hausfater P, *et al.* (1995). *Campylobacter* infections in HIV-infected patients: Clinical and bacteriological features. *AIDS* 9: 881–885.

Notermans S, Gallhoff G, Zwietering M H, *et al.* (1995). The HACCP concept: specification of criteria using quantitative risk assessment. *Food Microbiol* 12: 81–90.

Peterson M C (1994). Clinical aspects of *Campylobacter jejuni* infections in adults. *West J Med* 161: 148–152.

Raoult D, Tissot-Dupont H, Foucault C, *et al.* (2000). Q Fever 1985–1998: clinical and epidemiologic features of 1,383 infections. *Medicine* 79: 109–123.

Tarr PI (1995). *Escherichia coli* 0157:H7: clinical, diagnostic, and epidemiological aspects of human infection. *Clin Infect Dis* 20: 1–10.

Turner M (2000). Universal leucodepletion to reduce potential risk of transmission of new-variant Creutzfeldt–Jakob disease. *Br J Haematol* 110(3): 745–747.

Wall P G, Morgan D, Lamden K, *et al.* (1995) Transmission of multiresistant strains of *Salmonella typhimurium* from cattle to man. *Vet Rec* 136: 591–592.

Will R G, Ironside J W, Zeidler M, *et al.* (1996) A new variant of Creutzfeldt–Jakob disease in the UK. *Lancet* 347(9006): 921–925.

Will R G, Stewart G, Zeidler M, *et al.* (1999) Psychiatric features of new variant Creutzfeldt–Jakob disease. *Psych Bull* 23: 264–267.

Wong C S, Jelacic S, Habeeb R L, *et al.* (2000). The risk of the hemolytic–uremic syndrome after antibiotic treatment of *Escherichia coli* 0157:H7 Infections. *N Engl J Med* 342: 1930–1936.

Further reading

Shakespeare M (2002). *Zoonoses*. London: Pharmaceutical Press.

Part 2

Introduction to veterinary pharmacy

3

Veterinary medicines

Steven B Kayne

The veterinary prescription originates with a veterinarian or it may be a farmer or owner who decides on a particular treatment; the administration of the prescription is again shared by the veterinary surgeon and the farmer or owner. Pharmacists cannot legally be part of this process (unless they own the animal in question). They are involved in the formulation and dispensing of veterinary prescriptions (albeit to a limited extent in the current situation in the UK). Pharmacists can, however, take a proactive role in the prophylaxis and treatment of a number of parasitic diseases and in advising clients as to what is available to treat their animals.

In this chapter the characteristics and control of veterinary medicines are discussed.

History

Development of veterinary medicine

Throughout many of the great epochs of human history there has been human interaction with animals. Even in ancient civilisations, such as those of Egypt, Greece and Rome, animals played major roles in religion, mythology, the military and agriculture. Gradually animals came to be used for travel, food sources and advancements in scientific study. Increasing dependence on animals made it imperative that doctors be trained to care for their health and welfare. Evidence discovered in the primitive societies of Mesopotamia and Egypt dates the beginning of the development of veterinary medicine to around 5000 years ago. The first evidence we have of the veterinary medical profession arises from ancient documents such as the Kahun Veterinary Papyrus, discovered in Egypt and dating around 1900 BC, the Hammurabis Code, arising from Babylonian society and containing codified prescriptions dealing with animals, and writings by famous philosophers such as Hippocrates and Aristotle. Generation after generation, there has continued to be development not only in the scientific and technological aspects of the field but also in the shaping of highly educated veterinarians interested in working to improve animal welfare. In ancient Mesopotamia the responsibility for protecting animals often fell under the jurisdiction of the priests, otherwise known as magi. Disease was seen as a sign of deities's displeasure, and the priests therefore intervened to appease the gods when faced with disease. There was encouragement for the development of specialists to be mediators between the gods and their human servants. Owners sought communion with the gods by asking priests to intervene in the hope of preserving the health of their ailing beasts. Due to their devout faith in animal gods, Egyptians developed prescriptions for animal protection. Ancient Greek and Roman societies began developments in veterinary medicine in similar, yet slightly different, directions to the Egyptians. The oldest relics of Greek veterinary medicine are seen in mythology. Varro, an early Greek philosopher, studied the numerous diseases of horses and gave evidence of primitive prognosis and treatment. He linked the causes of animal diseases to heat, cold, overworking, insufficient rest and food taken immediately after work. Treatments were remedial, often involving rubbing with cool water, dressing the animal in oil, feeding it or covering it. If the treatment did not work, the animal was often killed by piercing it in the head and allowing it to bleed to death. In Roman times *medica veterinaria* was practised in a *veterinaria*.

Claude Bourgelat opened the first school of veterinary medicine in Lyons, on February 13 in 1762. The school was founded by Louis XV and was designed mainly for the study of the diseases and treatments of livestock. The main focus of study was devoted to equine medicine due to the heavy dependence on horses by the military at that time. Studies were offered in anatomy, botany, zoology, pharmacy, therapy, surgery, legal veterinary studies, animal husbandry and animal care. The term 'veterinary surgeon' was so coined in 1796 by the British Army's Board of General Officers to distinguish them from human surgeons. Before this, animal doctors were known as 'farriers'. The literature records the story of an ox, labouring under 'hopeless constipation', to which was summoned an old farrier. A lively trout was taken from a stream and committed to the patient's gullet with a confident assurance that 'it would soon work its way through the impediment affording speedy relief'. Needless to say both trout and ox died.

The adjective 'veterinary' was popularised by the Frenchman Benôit Vial de St Bel whose plan for 'an institute to cultivate and teach veterinary medicine' developed into Britain's first veterinary school in

London that began issuing diplomas to practise the veterinary art in 1794.

Veterinary practice

Veterinary practice during the latter years of the 19th century and first three decades of the 20th century developed slowly; veterinarians rolled pills and folded powders from ingredients bought in bulk. Their armamentaria included turpentine, that acted as a universal stand-by, together with liquid paraffin and castor oil, common salt, soapy water enemas, iodine for wounds and carbolic acid for disinfection. A turning point was the arrival of prontocil, a sulphonamide used to treat blood poisoning, which was brought to the market by the German company IG Farber in 1935. Vaccines against several important diseases of farm livestock were available and by the end of the 1930s the sheep diseases braxy, lamb dysentery and louping ill were under control. Calcium borogluconate was also introduced at this time for the treatment of milk fever, a condition that had troubled farmers for decades.

The sulphonamides were first produced in 1932 and became available in veterinary medicine sometime later. Their effectiveness against bacterial disease led to significant improvements in animal welfare. Because of their efficacy and relative cheapness sulphonamides are still widely used today. The sulphonamides were followed by the introduction of penicillins.

A revolution in parasitic therapy occurred with the discovery of the benzimadazoles in the early 1960s the first being tiabendazole. Since then, structural changes in the core structure have improved efficacy and safety. This in turn has improved output for farmers and animal health.

Pharmacy involvement in distribution of veterinary drugs

According to veterinary pharmacist Douglas Davidson of Blairgowrie, Scotland, the bulk of animal medicines were distributed in the 1920s and 1930s through local rural pharmacies or sold nationally by pharmacy-connected companies, e.g. Hilstons, Day Son & Hewitt. Farmers diagnosed their animals' ailments and then bought the products over the counter (OTC) as necessary – of course there were no antibiotics to worry about at that time. Dips tended to be distributed by garages and hardware stores. Pharmacists had an important role in formulating dips, including arsenical sheep dips, compounding boluses and, certainly up to 1948, played a significant part in the practice of euthanasia where cats and kittens were unwanted or in cases where animals were seriously ill or suffering.

In the 1940s and '50s, when the expensive anthelmintics – phenothiazine and tiabendazole – came to the UK market, merchants became established by, in many cases, ex-staff from veterinary pharmacists' businesses. Following the implementation of the National Health Service Act in 1948, pharmacists (even in rural areas) saw great opportunities from the new dispensing arrangements and neglected the veterinary scene. However, a few pharmacy specialist-oriented businesses, such as Jearys, Cox & Robinson, and R D Jones survived. With the introduction of the Veterinary Surgeons Act, diagnosis and supply became the province of veterinarians. In recent years there has been a resurgence of interest in veterinary pharmacy helped by the fact that there has been a swing towards companion-animal medicine due in part to the depressed state of UK livestock production, with farmers having less money to invest in their livestock, and there being fewer livestock for them to invest in. In 1986 around 70% of animal medicines were used in farm livestock. The National Office of Animal Health (NOAH) represents companies who make around 95% of sales in the £357 million animal medicine market (2000 figure at ex-manufacturers price). The market is around one-twentieth the size of the UK market for prescription-only medicines (POMs) for humans, which for 1999 was worth £7246 million. Figure 3.1 details trends in the UK market in recent years.

As Figure 3.2 shows, by the year 2000, companion-animal medicine sales exceeded food-producing animal medicine sales by value and this sector continues to grow.

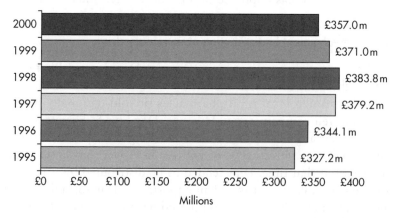

Figure 3.1   UK market values. (Courtesy of National Office of Animal Health (NOAH).)

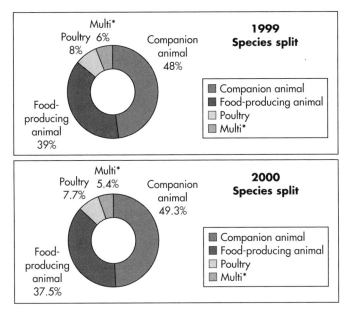

Figure 3.2 Species split of medicines (courtesy of NOAH). *Medicines used for both food-producing and companion animals.

Definition of veterinary medicines

Veterinary medicines are products that have been authorised by agricultural and health ministers under the Marketing Authorisations for Veterinary Medicines Regulations 1994 (which implements European Union (EU) single-market legislation) and the Medicines Act 1968 (see chapter 6).

Control of veterinary medicines and their use

The Veterinary Medicines Directorate (VMD) has primary responsibility for the authorisation scheme for veterinary medicines and their supply in the UK.

Responsibility for the use of these medicines at work falls to the Health and Safety Executive and local authorities through the Control of Substances Hazardous to Health (COSHH) Regulations and the Health and Safety at Work Act.

VMD

The VMD is an executive agency of the Department for Environment, Food, and Rural Affairs (DEFRA), responsible for:

- Authorising and controlling the manufacture and availability of veterinary medicines.
- Carrying out postauthorisation surveillance of suspected adverse reactions and for residues of veterinary products in meat and other animal products.
- Providing policy advice on these matters to the Agriculture and Health Ministers and implementing their decisions.

Each year the VMD publishes details on their work, as well as on general developments on the controls on veterinary medicines. These publications include:

- A series of guidance notes (Animal Medicines European Licensing Information and Advice (AMELIA) on various issues to assist in the interpretation and application of European Community (EC) legislation on veterinary medicines. Copies of these can be found online at www.vmd.gov.uk/amelia
- A quarterly newsletter, *Medicines Act Veterinary Information Service* (MAVIS), which can also be found online at www.vmd.gov.uk/mavis

The Veterinary Products Committee (VPC)

The VPC was set up in 1970 under section 4 of the Medicines Act with the following terms of reference:

- To advise ministers on the safety, quality and efficacy of veterinary medicines.
- To promote the collection and investigation of information relating to suspected adverse reactions to veterinary medicines.

There are two pharmacists on the Committee, at present appointed by relevant government ministers.

Supply of licensed and unlicensed veterinary medicines
(see also chapter 6)

A product authorised for veterinary use in the UK is one that is clearly labelled in English according to the requirements of the marketing authorisation and bears the UK authorisation number. Drugs imported from overseas are subject to authorisation by the VMD. There are exemptions for owners retuning to the UK with veterinary medicines prescribed for their animal while overseas (see PET scheme, chapter 13) providing the products concerned are not markedly different to those available on the UK market and that they are not considered dangerous to humans.

Categories of licensed veterinary medicines

At the present time veterinary medicines with market authorisations for veterinary use can be legally supplied according to regulations associated with four categories as detailed in chapter 6. These are:

1. POM: includes antibiotics and many parasiticides in pour-on formulations.
2. Pharmacy only medicine (P): very few veterinary medicines fall into this category. One example is Colombovac, a paramyxovirus vaccine for pigeons (see chapter 7).
3. Pharmacy and Merchants List medicines (PML): includes many parasiticides for prophylactic use.
4. General Sales List medicines (GSL): includes many ectoparasiticides.

Medicated feedingstuffs

In addition there are further categories relating to medicated feedingstuffs (MFS). The incorporation of POMs (e.g. antibiotics) in the form of an MFS premix for addition to animal feedingstuffs by commercial compounders requires a veterinary prescription. The regulations do not affect owners of companion animals adding medicine to their animals' food. There are also medicated feedingstuff premixes that do not require a prescription (MFSX).

Feed additives, e.g. production enhancers, were previously considered to be veterinary medicines. In fact most production enhancers are antibiotics that are not used for therapeutic or prophylactic reasons. Under The Feedingstuffs (Zootechnical Products) Regulations 1999, these products are no longer classified as medicines but as 'zootechnical feed additives' (ZFA). Their use is controlled under EC legislation. Antibiotic enhancers include:

- Avilamycin e.g. Maxus, Elanco (ZFA),
- Bambermycin or flavophospholine, e.g. Flaveco, ECO (PML) and Flavomycin, Intervet (ZFA)
- Monensin, e.g. Ecox, ECO (PML) and Romensin, Elanco (ZFA)
- Salinomycin sodium, e.g. Bio-Cox, Alpharma (ZFA), Sal-Eco, ECO (PML) and Salocin, Intervet (ZFA).

Antibiotics as feed enhancers are restricted to those not used in human medicine.

Other examples of ZFA products are premixes containing the coccidiostat salinomycin (Sacox, Intervet, and Salinomix, Eurotec) given to broiler chickens. Prophylaxis of coccidiosis improves growth rate. Salinomycin is also given to pigs when it improves feed conversion rate (see chapter 11).

Market sector values

Involvement of pharmacists in this area of practice is limited and any colleagues intending to carry out such operations are recommended to consult the Veterinary Formulary. MFS prescriptions are valid for 3 months from date of issue and allow a 1-month supply.

The relative sizes of the markets in each category are shown in Figure 3.3.

It is likely that changes will be made in some of these arrangements as a result of the Dispensing Review (2000) chaired by Sir John Marsh.

Dispensing review

As part of an investigation into the costs of farming, the UK government announced a review of the arrangements for dispensing veterinary POMs in March 2000. Although primarily aimed at commercial animals, the review had implications for small-animal veterinary practices too. It was widely perceived that the *de facto* monopoly on dispensing was leading to overcharging by vets for medicines to supplement their inadequate consulting fees. Although it was open to vets to issue prescriptions for dispensing at pharmacies, they seldom did so.

The Review Group, chaired by Sir John Marsh, considered the reclassification of POMs to determine whether certain products should

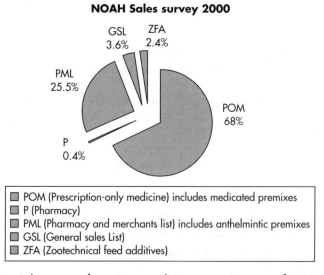

NOAH Sales survey 2000

GSL 3.6% ZFA 2.4%
PML 25.5%
POM 68%
P 0.4%

- POM (Prescription-only medicine) includes medicated premixes
- P (Pharmacy)
- PML (Pharmacy and merchants list) includes anthelmintic premixes
- GSL (General sales List)
- ZFA (Zootechnical feed additives)

Figure 3.3 Sales survey of veterinary medicine sectors (courtesy of NOAH).

be made more widely available and reviewed dispensing procedures with the possibility of requiring vets to issue prescriptions to be dispensed by pharmacists rather than selling medicines direct to their clients as at present.

After conducting wide-ranging consultations with interested parties, including the Royal Pharmaceutical Society of Great Britain (RPSGB), the report was published in May 2001 and concluded that veterinary surgeons should normally provide animal owners with a written prescription. It also recommended changes to the classification of POMs for animals.

The report stated that after a diagnosis and treatment decision has been made a written prescription should be provided, either at no charge or for a fee (that the Royal College of Veterinary Surgeons suggests should be no more than £2.50). Prescriptions could be dispensed by veterinary surgeons, pharmacists or, for some medicines, agricultural merchants. This would not apply to medicines given or used during surgery.Veterinary practices which have dispensaries were recommended to review their working practices so as to reduce costs. The independent review body said that there is a lack of transparency in the prices paid for animal medicines and many veterinarians are unaware of the cost of their dispensing services. The report's other main recommendation was that POMs prescribed for animals under a veterinarian's control should be reclassified into three subgroups:

- **POM (A)** Medicines administered only by veterinary surgeons or under their direct supervision.
- **POM (B)** Medicines sold or dispensed by veterinary surgeons after a clinical examination of the animal, or sold or dispensed by a pharmacy on prescription.
- **POM(C)** Medicines sold or supplied by veterinarians, pharmacists or competent agricultural merchants. A clinical examination of the animal would not be necessary. This would replace the existing PML category.

Parallel importing of veterinary medicines from the EU should be allowed, the review said, as well as the use of generic medicines developed for use in humans. In its evidence to the review, the RPSGB noted that specialised veterinary pharmacies were underdeveloped because there was currently little incentive for them. Individual pharmacists called for a number of products for pets to be moved to the pharmacy category. The report can be found in the publications section of the VMD's website (www.vmd.gov.uk).

A second review into the supply of veterinary medicines by the Competition Commission on behalf of the Office of Fair Trading yielded a report in spring 2003. The report confirmed the existence of a complex monopoly situation in the supply of prescription-only veterinary medicines within the UK, and offered nine remedies for consideration by the Secretary of State at the Department of Trade and Industry and a further 11 recommendations for the attention of the Secretary of State at the Department for Environment, Food, and Rural Affairs (DEFRA). Collectively, these measures would provide a much more transparent system of supply for veterinary POMs, with clients being charged a fair price and being in a position to choose whether they wished to have their prescriptions dispensed by a vet or a pharmacist. Other important recommendations included changes in licensing procedures, with medicines being placed in the lowest distribution classification consistent with their assessment of a product's safety, efficacy and quality. The creation of new classification categories was also recommended to allow specific categories of persons (such as agricultural merchants and saddlers as well as veterinary surgeons and pharmacists) to dispense certain veterinary medicines. At the time of writing the Office of Fair Trading has prepared draft legislation to implement the remedies; the recommendations are also being considered by DEFRA but there does not appear to be a timescale for their response.

Unlicensed veterinary medicines

If no product authorised for use in the UK exists for a condition in a particular species, in order to avoid unacceptable suffering, veterinary surgeons may exercise their clinical judgement by resorting to the 'cascade' for prescribing for animals under their care, whereby they select in this order:

- A medicinal product authorised for the same condition in another species or a different condition in the same species (off-label use), notwithstanding the possibility of differences in reaction between species and breeds mentioned below.
- A medicine authorised in the UK for human use. A veterinarian (or a person under his or her direction) may administer an authorised human medicine for use in a particular animal (ideally with the owner's consent). Pharmacists may obtain oral authorisation from a veterinarian for the supply of an authorised human medicine in the P or GSL categories but must obtain a prescription in the normal way for a POM. It is good practice for a record to be kept of oral authorisations.
- A medicine made up on a one-off basis – a 'veterinary special' – by a veterinary surgeon or other authorised person. Products such as Epsom salts or

light liquid paraffin are also considered as having been extemporaneously prepared if supplied by a veterinary surgeon for a medicinal purpose. Under normal conditions both of these products are freely available and would not normally be treated as veterinary medicines.

Reporting of adverse drug reactions

The importance of the reporting of suspected adverse reactions (SARs), including those involving vaccines and injectables, whether affecting the animal or the human administering the medication cannot be overemphasised. The report forms to be sent to the VMD are freely available. It is not always recognised that reports are expected and encouraged from pharmacists, as well as from veterinarians, farmers, animal owners and general practitioners (GPs) affording follow-up in cooperation with the marketing authorisation (MA) holder. Confidentiality is of course maintained. The yellow report form has one side for SARs affecting animals and the other for SARs affecting humans. Forms are included in *The Veterinary Formulary*, the Compendium of Data Sheets for Veterinary Products, and are also available from the VMD. Reports from pharmacists are included with those from doctors and represent about 5% of reports. The marketing authorisation holders are the biggest contributors at 55% followed by farmers at 16%, vets 7%, the public 6% and 'others' 7%. Pharmacists are in a strategic position to help in reporting for the benefit of patients, customers and pets, and for better recognition of their own professional role in healthcare.

Types of veterinary medicines

Once a diagnosis has been made and medication is considered necessary, appropriate safe and effective pharmacological drugs should be selected. Factors to be considered include:

- Dose and frequencies of administration.
- The optimal routes for delivery.
- The particular pharmaceutical forms to be used.
- Any public health or environmental implications and regulatory constraints.

Prophylactic medicines

These are designed to prevent disease and parasitic infestation and include:

- Endoparasiticides – prevent and treat infestations by parasites that invade the body, such as worms, flukes or coccidial protozoa.

- Ectoparasiticides – prevent and treat infestation by parasites that live on the outside of the animal, for example mites, ticks, fleas, flies.
- Endectocides – prevent and treat infestation of both types of parasite.
- Vaccines – prevent diseases caused by certain viral or bacterial infections.
- Antiseptics – prevent or minimise bacterial contamination.

Therapeutic medicines

These are designed to treat disease and include:

- Antibiotics – treat bacterial infection (covered in detail below).
- Hormones – treat reproductive problems.
- Anti-inflammatories.
- Sedatives.
- Cardiovascular drugs.
- Drugs acting on gastrointestinal tract.
- Immunological products.

Other medicines to help the veterinarian or the farmer

- Digestive enhancers – a very small group of specially approved antibiotics to help farm animals get the maximum benefit from their feed (see above).
- Anaesthetics – includes painkillers and euthanasia products (see chapter 1).
- Dietary supplements – these are medicines to treat or prevent specific dietary deficiencies, rather than nutritional supplements (see chapter 9).

General characteristics of veterinary medicines

Although veterinary medicines have broadly the same characteristics as human medicines in that their aim is to improve or maintain the health of the patient, veterinary formulations have certain added requirements, particularly with regard to safety. The safety requirements associated with the granting of a marketing authorisation make sure that a veterinary medicine can be used safely without causing harm to the animal being treated or to people giving the treatment and that in the case of farm animals it will be safe to eat the meat, milk, eggs or honey and that there will be no lasting effects to the environment.

Safety for humans

The following examples serve to illustrate different aspects of the potential risk to humans arising out of the administration of veterinary medicines.

Intrinsic toxicity

In September 2001, the VPC appraisal panel for human SARs to veterinary medicines published a report covering 1985–2000 (www.vpc.gov.uk). A large proportion of the reports relate to cat and dog owners and involve flea collars and small-animal spot-on products. Many of these problems could probably have been avoided if instructions for use had been adequately explained and followed.

Organophosphate sheep dips An example of intrinsic toxicity causing long-term problems for operators is the use of organophosphate sheep dips. Sheep suffer from external parasites, such as blowflies, or from keds, ticks, lice, and scab (see chapter 10). Sheep scab is a disease caused by a parasitic mite which lives on the skin surface. The feeding activities of the mite cause irritation and distress. This can result in stunting or severe loss of condition, loss of fleece, and death – especially of lambs. Sheep dips are considered to be vital in the fight against the devastating disease of sheep scab and are used widely by farmers who regard them as an effective and economical option. The latter is especially important in the current poor financial environment within the sheep industry. Protective clothing alone is not a practical method of preventing exposure to dipping solution for a farmer having to haul a heavy sheep in and out of dips, and the 'aerosol effect' of sheep shaking themselves dry after dipping means that the atmosphere is soon laden with the chemical.

The potential risk from handling these pesticides has been known for many years, with various precautions being recommended during use, including protective clothing. Improvements in packaging have also been implemented by manufacturers to minimise accidents. In 1995 the Health and Safety Executive, the Department of Health and the Ministry of Agriculture, Fisheries and Food jointly commissioned a major epidemiological study into the effects of long-term exposure to organophosphate sheep dips. Organophosphate compounds were initially developed as chemical warfare agents because of their action in inhibiting blood cholinesterase activity and interfering with neuromuscular transmission. Consequently, there had been much suspicion as to their possible adverse effect on farm workers.

The broad aim of the study was to investigate whether cumulative exposure to sheep dip organophosphates was related to clinically detectable measures of polyneuropathy. The study was carried out by The Institute of Occupational Medicine, Edinburgh, and the Institute of Neurological Sciences, Glasgow, in three phases and was published in

July 1999. It was the most comprehensive epidemiological study of ill health among a sample of sheep dippers in the UK. The study identified a definite link between sheep dipping and long-lasting nerve damage, depression and anxiety.

While acknowledging the importance of the report, NOAH supported continuing availability of organophosphate sheep dips pending moves to tighten safety measures. However on 1 September 2000, on the advice of the VPC, the UK government suspended the marketing authorisations for organophosphate sheep dips, pending satisfactory completion of plans being developed by manufacturers for closed systems for transferring organophosphate dip concentrate from the container to the dip bath. New organophosphate sheep dip products incorporating such closed-transfer systems received government approval, hence allowing a return of organophosphates to the market at the end of 2001. They continue to be available today, as do the safer synthetic pyrethroids and amidines.

It has been suggested recently that some farmers may have a genetic predisposition to the adverse health effects associated with exposure to organophosphates present in sheep dip. Exposure to organophosphates has acute effects on health, but evidence of chronic effects is unclear. An enzyme found in blood (paroxonase, also known as PON1) is responsible for breaking down diazinonoxon, the active metabolite of diazinon, which is an organophosphate used in sheep dip.

People who think they may be victims of organophosphate poisoning are, as a group, taking legal action against the manufacturers of the products. Court proceedings have been issued in nearly 100 cases. Most litigants are farmers and farm workers, although one is a truck driver who claimed that he was poisoned by leaking containers while making deliveries; another is a local sheep-dip inspector (see under 'dips' below for more information on dipping).

Toxoplasmosis vaccine Accidental self-injection or ingestion of living toxoplasmosis vaccine may cause disease in humans; prompt medical attention is required.

Drug residues – risk to the community from veterinary medicine residues The presence of veterinary drug residues is of increasing concern to human health. There are internationally set safety limits for residues of the majority of veterinary medicines in food. To monitor that these limits are being observed, the VMD manages two extensive surveillance programmes. One is statutory and helps fulfil the UK's obligations under EU law. The other is a non-statutory scheme that complements and supplements the statutory programme.

All constituents of residues are not equally toxic. Covalently bound residues are probably weakly toxic for consumers while compounds with more complex bonds may be extremely toxic, especially if they are repeatedly consumed. Some antibacterials, e.g. penicillin, tetracycline and sulfonamides, can produce allergenic responses in consumers of animal food products. A report by the Soil Association drew attention to the vast use of antibiotics in farming (Soil Association, 1998). It is claimed that the massive increase in the use of antibiotics in pig and poultry farming could be producing drug-resistant bacteria which can pass from animals to humans.

In the first of four reports entitled *Use and Misuse of Antibiotics in UK Agriculture* (Soil Association, 1998) the organic farming pressure group claimed that use of tetracyclines, one of the most popular antibiotics, has risen by 1500% in 30 years. Use of penicillins has increased by 600% over the same period. Many scientists claim that feeding antibiotics to animals at low levels over a long time fosters resistance that can be passed on to humans. It is suggested that the resistant bacteria can be picked up either by handling meat or eating it. Fears of such risks to human health have prompted the acceptance of a proposal from Sweden for a Europe-wide ban on four antibiotics used in animal feed. However, recently an independent group of scientists has concluded that the ban was not backed by sufficient scientific data.

The Soil Association is demanding much more. It is calling for a total ban on all non-medical uses of antibiotics in agriculture, and more careful monitoring by the government. It also accuses farmers of ignoring the fact that supposedly harmless food additives allowed under EU regulations all have some power to control disease. The development of drug-resistant bacteria could pose serious dangers for hospital patients who may have poor immune systems or who already have an infection for which drugs have become ineffective. There is a danger of an increase in drug-resistant *Salmonella* spp. caused by the use of therapeutic drugs in livestock production.

In fact antibiotic use in animals is not seen by many experts as a major contributor to human antibiotic resistance problems. The World Health Organization's Berlin Conference in November 1997 reported that the tragic growth of antibiotic resistance in human medicine was 'primarily' due to overuse and misuse in the practice of human medicine around the world, a view echoed by the House of Lords Select Committee on Science and Technology. Following this conference, and a further conference in Geneva in 1998, the World Veterinary Association, the International Federation of Agricultural Producers and the World Federation of Animal Health Industry have announced a new set of global principles to ensure responsible and prudent use of antibiotics in animals. The three organisations are committed to implement the principles in daily practice, so that antibiotics can be used to improve animal health and welfare without sacrificing human health. Some of the key basic principles are:

- Antibiotics are health management tools which are licensed to enhance good husbandry practice for the purposes of disease prevention, disease treatment and production enhancement. They are a complement to these good husbandry practices and should never be used to compensate for or mask farm and veterinary practices. Codes of good practice, quality assurance programmes and education programmes should promote the responsible and prudent use of antibiotics.
- Professional supervision, particularly by veterinarians, and record keeping are essential in the use and control of antibiotic products.
- Antibiotics used for therapy should be used for as short a duration as possible, but for as long as needed and at the appropriate dosage regimen. Attention should be paid to label instructions.

Farmers argue that the basic food for any domesticated farm animal can never reproduce exactly the varied diet its ancestors would have enjoyed in the wild, so supplements are needed. Pigs for instance are unable to produce the amino acids they need for growth from a purely cereal diet, so fish-meal and soya protein are added. Next comes the modern consumers' desire for lean meat. Meat produced naturally is marbled with fat. If cattle are fed growth hormones they add muscle quickly, rather like athletes do, without fat having time to develop. The result is lean steak. Antibiotic growth hormones were banned in the EU in 1986 but are still used in the USA and some other meat-exporting countries. Intensive farming can cause problems by keeping animals or birds in a confined space, thereby aiding the rapid spread of disease. This is another reason for the addition of antibiotics to farm diets.

Another example of a potentially harmful residue is tiabendazole. It was first marketed in 1961 as a veterinary anthelmintic and later as a human medicine and agricultural fungicide. Some benzimidazole anthelmintics have provided broad-band protection safely. However, parbendazole, which was introduced in 1967 for sheep, was thought to be associated with some teratogenic effects in humans. There is also ongoing discussion about the use of compounds exhibiting hormone-like activities, e.g. anabolic steroids.

Environmental safety

After the animal has been treated with a drug, the body metabolises the substance to some degree and then it is excreted, predominantly in the fecal matter. These fecal residues retain some of the biological activity of the drug, and investigation of the consequences of this characteristic forms an important part of the environmental risk assessment procedure.

According to NOAH there is no evidence that populations of dung beetles and flies are adversely affected by the use of internal parasiticides. Any specific effects (e.g. on insect larvae) are limited and the total effect on the rest of the population is claimed to be negligible.

There is another problem that is giving cause for concern, namely environmental contamination from waste sheep-dipping fluids. Ironically, while the newer pyrethroid dips are much safer for humans than organophosphates (see above) there has been clear evidence over a number of years that they pose a significant risk to the environment, typically being 100 times more toxic to many forms of aquatic life than are organophosphate dips. The 1980 Groundwater European Directive, stating that waste dip must be incinerated, or dumped at licensed land-fill sites, was passed into UK law in 1999. Farmers are required to seek permission from government agencies to dispose of waste dipping material on land. In order to reduce the amount of fluid involved it has been suggested that deep-plunge pools are replaced by dip showers or even pour-on formulations. Unfortunately, neither of these alternatives is considered to be as effective as full dipping.

Risk during administration

The risk of needle-stick injuries when giving injections to moving targets, as occurs when inoculating maybe 2000 sheep, is just one factor in favour of the development of pour-on formulations to treat systemic conditions such as those used to control endoparasites as well as ectoparasites (see below). The potential for topical administration to achieve a systemic effect is attractive, provided the issues of safety and efficacy in use can be reliably ascertained.

The reporting by a customer or patient of a needle-stick injury obviously needs prompt attention, especially as an accidental self-injection with an oil-based vaccine can cause not only severe pain but also ischaemic necrosis and loss of a digit. In such cases, reliable details of the formulation are essential for hospital notification and keeping the patient's GP and the veterinarian, if involved, informed and subsequently reporting information to the VMD. It is estimated that there is still serious under-reporting of such events in the UK.

Safety issues for animals

Toxicity

A number of adverse reactions are possible as a result of a drug's intrinsic toxicity, including the following:

- Allergies – nausea, vomiting or urticarial rash. Attenuated and inactivated vaccines contain protein material designed to promote an immune response. Occasionally they may cause a generalised hyposensitivity usually treated with adrenaline given subcutaneously. Ivermectin may cause allergies in horses. Hepatic changes have also been reported (examples are aspirin, griseofulvin (dogs), sulphonamides).
- Renal changes (non-steroidal anti-inflammatories, amphotericin, cephalosporins).
- Central nervous system effects (glucocorticoids, clindamycin).
- Dermatological – eczema, alopecia (coal tar shampoos, griseofulvin, prednisone).
- Ocular – a transient 'blue eye' may be produced by certain canine vaccines.

Interactions

Pharmacists will be well aware of the possibility of pharmacodynamic and pharmacokinetic interactions between orthodox medicines, orthodox and herbal medicines and herbal and herbal medicines, and should be just as vigilant with veterinary medicines. A comprehensive list of interactions may be found in the Veterinary Formulary.

Injury from administration method

The problems associated with reusing injection needles include blood-borne transmission of disease between animals and abscessing at the injection site caused by bacterial contamination of the needle. Local allergic responses to adjuvants or vehicles may also occur. Physical injury and/or infection may also result from incorrect use of intermammary tubes, balling guns and drenching equipment. In the latter case, operators should avoid using undue force or pushing the bolus too far down the back of the animal's throat as this could result in serious injury. Drenching (see below) may cause injury to the pharyngeal diverticulum if an operator uses drenching guns designed for other species. The risk of adverse reactions from topically applied creams and ointments that may be licked by cats and dogs makes it important that potentially toxic materials are not used in formulating these products unless appropriate precautions can be taken (see below).

Convenience of use

Medicines that come ready for administration, i.e. do not require premixing, are convenient to use and preclude any errors. With some unstable products, e.g. injections, this may not be possible.

Calculating the dose can be difficult particularly in the case of OTC veterinary products, e.g. worming tablets, where the dose is often given in terms of weight. Gone are the days when pet owners were helped to push their dog on to the pharmacy scales in order that the necessary calculation could be made. Weighing machines – at least the free ones! – are a thing of the past. Deciding on what is a small, medium or large dog can be tricky and can vary with manufacturer.

Storage requirements may necessitate a refrigerator; an oral route of administration rather than by injection is preferable to pet owners.

Palatability

Trying to feed animals unpalatable medicinal products, especially tablets, can be a nightmare. Some specialised manufacturers prepare flavoured dosage forms that animals will take readily. Cats like sardine and tuna flavours. Various flavours are available for other animals. Flavoured tapeworm tablets for cats and dogs (Johnson's) are available to mask the taste of dichlorophene.

Cost

Although cost is inevitably an important consideration in purchasing treatment for animals, it has rather different significance for pet owners than for owners of farm animals. Because of the emotional link with their animals pet owners are generally prepared, within reason, to accept that there is a price to pay for their pets' health, and that they have a responsibility to get Fido or Felix well. Farmers on the other hand, who it must be stressed also have their animals' welfare at heart, are running a business and need to take economic decisions in justifying a course of action when treating an animal. An example might be the farmer who has five animals suffering from long-standing mastitis in a dairy herd of 40–50. These animals' milk would affect the overall quality of the pooled milk and could lead to rejection under the Milk Proficiency Testing Scheme. A decision to cull the infected animals might be taken in the interests of overall profitability.

Efficacy

All medicines must do what they claim to do when used as instructed on the label. Extensive tests are carried out in the laboratory, in disease-challenge studies and in field trials, to make sure that the product will actually work in practical real-life situations against the specified disease in the named species of animal, at the dose rate, frequency and duration of treatment recommended, and by the route of administration specified. Because treating farm animals is a commercial decision, farmers will require to see medicines working in their environment, otherwise they will be unwilling to make funds available. Similarly, the speed of onset of action is vital.

These factors are particularly important when trying to immobilise a large animal, sometimes necessitating the use of a cocktail of drugs to achieve the desired effect.

Withdrawal period

Use of animal medicines in food-chain farm animals in the UK is strictly controlled by European law and requires observance of the withdrawal period (NOAH, 2001). This is the time which passes between the last dose given to the animal and the time when the level of residues in the tissues (muscle, liver, kidney, skin/fat) or products (milk, eggs, honey) falls below the maximum residue limit (MRL). Until the withdrawal period has elapsed, the animal or its products must not be used for human consumption.

For food-producing animals, studies are required to see how quickly residues of the medicine are eliminated from the animal. MRLs are established to set a maximum level of the substance(s) concerned that may remain in the animal without posing a risk to consumers of produce taken from it. Withdrawal periods (the time between administration of the medicine and slaughter or the taking of food produce, e.g. milk or eggs) are then set to ensure that any remaining residues are below the MRL. Huge safety margins are built into the system to ensure that consumers are not put at risk. If and when it proves to be necessary, in the light of experience, MRLs can be, and are, revised.

In some cases it may be possible for the farmer to consider methods of treatment that have different withdrawal periods and choose the one most appropriate for the circumstances prevailing at any given time.

Main chemical groups of veterinary medicines

There is a wide range of approved veterinary medicines available and many others that veterinarians can use from the human armamentarium if necessary. A full description of all these agents is beyond the scope of this chapter. Five therapeutic areas have been chosen as being of particular interest in veterinary pharmacy:

1.   Parasiticides.
2.   Antimicrobials.
3.   Rehydration and electrolyte balance products.
4.   Antiseptics and disinfectants.
5.   Vaccines.

The first four of these will be dealt with here and the remaining topic – vaccines – is covered in chapter 4.

Parasiticides

Many highly effective and selective parasiticides are available, but such compounds must be used correctly and judiciously to obtain a favourable clinical response and to minimise selection for anthelmintic resistance.

Characteristics of the ideal parasiticide are:

- They have a broad spectrum of activity against mature and immature parasites.
- They are easy to administer to a large number of animals.
- They are safe and are compatible with other medicinal agents.
- They do not cause allergic responses.
- They do not require long withholding periods because of residues.
- They are economical.
- They are easily available from convenient sources.

Endoparasiticides

There is a wide range of chemical groupings used to treat endoparasitic infestation involving roundworms (nematodes), tapeworms (cestodes), flukes (trematodes) and assorted other invaders.

Benzimadazoles The benzimadazoles are the largest chemical family used to treat endoparasitic diseases. The many variants are all based on the same chemical structure namely 1,2-diaminobenzene (see Formula 3.1).

Formula 3.1 1,2-diaminobenzene   Formula 3.2 Tiabendazole

The first derivative that satisfied the requirements for an anthelmintic was tiabendazole (see Formula 3.2). Newer benzimadazoles are characterised by novel substituents on the benzimadazole nucleus and replacement of the thiazole ring by methylcarbamate (see Formulae 3.3 and 3.4). Such modifications have produced a new generation of drugs with much slower rates of elimination, higher potencies, broader spectra and complex metabolic pathways.

Formula 3.3 Fenbendazole

Formula 3.4 Mebendazole

All the benzimadazoles act on parasites by interfering with the energy-generating metabolism. The benzimadazoles currently used in the UK are albendazole, febantel fenbendazole, mebendazole, netobimin, oxfendazole, oxibendazole, tiabendazole, thiophanate and triclabendazole. Both albendazole and triclabendazole are active against liver flukes. However, unlike all the other benzimadazoles, triclabendazole has no activity against roundworms.

A number of benzimadazoles including febantel (Bayverm, Bayer), used in such diverse species as horses, ruminants, pigs and pigeons, thiophanate (Nemafax 14, Merial), and netobimin (HapadexCattle/ Sheep Wormer, Schering-Plough) exist in the form of prodrugs, active because they are metabolised in the body to the biologically active benzimidazole carbamate nucleus.

Some variants of the benzimadazoles are teratogenic and, depending on the dose rate and species, are contraindicated in early pregnancy; these variants require withholding periods. They are more effective in ruminants and horses in which their rate of passage is slowed by the rumen or caecum. Residues of albendazole, oxfendazole, fenbendazole, febantel, netobimin and tiabendazole concentrate primarily in the liver in cattle and sheep, and persist longest in this tissue. Residues are more persistent for fenbendazole, oxfendazole, and febantel than for albendazole or tiabendazole. In dogs and cats, mebendazole is used for treatment of roundworms, hookworms and tapeworms. Fenbendazole has been used against tissue-dwelling larvae of *Toxocara canis* and *Ancylostoma caninum*.

Imidazothiazole   Levamisole is mainly used for gastrointestinal roundworms in ruminants and pigeons. It acts by interfering with parasitic nerve transmission causing muscular paralysis and expulsion.

Macrocyclic lactones (avermectins and milbemycins)   These are products, or chemical derivatives of the soil microorganisms *Streptomyces avermitilis* and *S. cyanogriseus*. Products containing them are labelled 3-AV. They interfere with parasitic nerve transmission by opening chloride channels in the postsynaptic membrane. The injectable and oral formulations of ivermectin, abamectin, doramectin and moxidectin are given to cattle and sheep at 0.2 mg/kg, whereas the pour-on formulation is used at 0.5 mg/kg. The different formulations have somewhat different spectra of activity, but all are effective against immature and adult stages of the most common gastrointestinal nematodes. The formula of ivermectin is shown in Formula 3.5 (on page 88).

Tetrahydropyrimidines, such as pyrantel (Pyratape P, Intervet and Strongid, Pfizer) and morantel (Exhelm, Pfizer) cause parasitic neuromuscular paralysis. A sustained-release ruminal bolus for use in cattle, which releases the morantel over 90 days, has been developed (Paratect, Pfizer). Products containing this chemical are labelled 2-LM. Pyrantel was first introduced as a broad-spectrum anthelmintic against gastrointestinal parasites of sheep, and subsequently has been used in cattle, horses, dogs and pigs. It is well absorbed by pigs and dogs, but less well by ruminants. Morantel is the methyl ester analogue of pyrantel and, in ruminants, it tends to be somewhat safer and more effective than pyrantel.

Formula 3.5 Ivermectin

Component B_{1a} R=CH$_2$CH$_3$
Component B_{1b} R=CH$_3$

Other chemical groupings mainly, but not exclusively, active against flukes in the UK are the salicylanilides (closantel, niclosamide) and substituted phenols (nitroxynil).

Ectoparasiticides

Restrictions are applied to many of the ectoparasiticides indicated for use in food-producing animals to ensure that unacceptable residues are not present in products intended for human consumption. These restrictions may require that animals are not slaughtered for up to 49 days after administration of the product or that the product is not used in animals producing milk for human consumption. Labels and data sheets on all products contain specific instructions on restrictions, including withdrawal periods, which must be adhered to. Chemical groups of ectoparasiticides are listed below.

Carbamates and organophosphates Carbamates and organophosphates share the same mechanism of action. They inhibit acetylcholinesterase, an enzyme that is normally responsible for acetylcholine (neurotransmitter) destruction. Applications of organophosphates or carbamates to insects produce spontaneous muscular contractions followed by paralysis. When these compounds are used for flea or tick control it should be determined before treatment if any other cholinesterase inhibitor has been used on the animal or in its environment. Organophosphates approved for use in the UK are:

- Azamethiphos (used for salmon infested with sea lice, *Lepeophtheirus salmonis* and *Caligus* spp.).

- Diazinon (dimpylate) used as a dip for a variety of ectoparasites on sheep, and as an impregnated collar for dogs (fleas and ticks) and cats (fleas).
- Fenthion used as a spot-on application for fleas on cats and dogs.
- Phosmet used against warble-fly larvae, lice and mites on cattle and mites and lice on pigs.

Approved carbamates include carbaryl and propoxur, both used for fleas on cats and dogs. Examples of other organophosphates available overseas are chlorpyrifos (Australia, New Zealand and USA), chlorfenvinphos (Australia and New Zealand), coumafos (Australia, New Zealand, USA), cythioate (Australia and New Zealand), dichlorvos (USA), malathion (Australia, New Zealand, USA), metrifonate (New Zealand) and phoxim (Eire). Bendiocarb is a carbamate used against lice and flies on cattle in Australia.

The related organochlorines have been withdrawn in many parts of the world because of concern regarding environmental persistence. However, the best known variant, lindane, continues to be available in the USA as a dip concentrate for dogs and a pressurised aerosol for a variety of domestic pets and farm animals.

Formamidines Amitraz is the only formamidine used as an ectoparasiticide. It acts by inhibiting monoamine oxidase, and offers a useful approach for treatment and control of ticks and mange mites on dogs.

Nitroguanidine The only compound in this category currently available for veterinary use is imidacloprid (Advantage, Bayer) applied as a spot-on against fleas on cats and dogs. Imidacloprid acts by binding to postsynaptic nicotinic acetylcholine receptors in insects.

Phenylpyrazoles This group of compounds has insecticidal and acaricidal activity. The only member of this group currently available for use in veterinary medicine is fipronil. Fipronil acts on the insect γ-aminobutyric acid (GABA) receptor by inhibiting GABA-regulated chloride flux into the nerve cell by binding at a site within the chloride channel of this receptor. Fipronil is readily absorbed into sebum and has prolonged residual activity on both dogs and cats.

Pyrethrins and pyrethroids These compounds disrupt sodium and potassium ion transport in nerve membranes, leading to paralysis. The action is extremely rapid, but paralysed insects can recover very quickly; the synergists piperonyl butoxide and N-octyl bicycloheptene dicarboxymide will interfere with the insect detoxification mechanism.

Natural pyrethrins are extracted from chrysanthemum flowers and are notable for their rapid but brief action and relative lack of toxicity in dogs and cats. Synthetic pyrethroids are pyrethrum-like compounds that generally have greater potency and residual effects. They include permethrin, fenvalerate and cypermethrin.

Microsomal enzyme systems of insects are often included as synergists in the formulations of topical preparations, particularly those containing pyrethrins and can prolong the activity.

Miscellaneous Benzyl benzoate is an inexpensive acaricide useful as an adjunct in the treatment of sarcoptic mange in dogs. It is toxic to cats. Sulfur is still used, although infrequently, in the form of lime-sulfur solution for the treatment of notoedric mange in cats. Various borate formulations are used as flea larval stomach poisons and desiccants in carpets. While the compounds listed above have documented insecticidal and acaricidal activity, treatment methods that use ultrasonic devices, brewer's yeast, garlic and dietary sulfur are completely unsubstantiated. Rotenone, obtained from derris and cube roots, is a naturally occurring insecticide that is occasionally used in Australia against lice and mites on sheep. D-Limonene and linolool are products extracted from fresh peels of citrus fruits. They have insecticidal activity that can be enhanced when synergised with piperonyl butoxide.

Insect growth regulators A number of insect growth regulators are used throughout the world, including the insect juvenile hormone analogues methoprene and fenoxycarb, the chitin synthesis inhibitors diflubenzuron and lufenuron, and cyromazine which prevents exuviation. The compounds may be applied topically on the target animal or administered orally; the inhibitors are released into the feces and thus reduce the generation of fecal-dwelling nuisance flies.

Insecticides may be used to provide environmental control of some insects by application to premises. The compounds used for this purpose include the organophosphates, pyrethrins and pyrethroids, amitraz and fenoxycarb. Carbamates, which act to inhibit insect acetylcholinesterase reversibly, are also used on premises and as topical insecticides in some countries. The insect pheromone (Z)-9-tricosene is incorporated into some products to attract insects to the site of insecticide application.

Repellents Dimethyl phthalate and synthetic pyrethroid permethrin have some repellent activity against fleas, ticks and mosquitoes, and are used mainly on horses and cattle. Citrus and herbal oils are sometimes included in insecticidal products to enhance repellent activity.

Antimicrobials

Antimicrobials are chosen on the basis of:

- A spectrum of activity appropriate to the condition being treated, i.e. against the bacterium, fungus or virus causing symptoms of the disease, and an ability to reach the site of infection at inhibitory concentrations.
- Species, breed of animal – some species metabolise antibiotics slower than others, e.g. cats are less able than other species to metabolise chloramphenicol. Penicillins should not be administered to small mammals.
- Age of animal. The ability to metabolise drugs will vary with age and this should be reflected in the dose and route of administration.
- Toxicity considerations. This refers to intrinsic toxicity within a particular species (see examples above) or toxicity associated with the site of infection. Renal impairment may cause drugs to appear more toxic than expected. Ideally, a selective toxicity is required to exploit the differences in structure and metabolism of pathogens and host cells without harming the animal.
- Antimicrobial policy. In order to prevent resistance it may be necessary to choose an antimicrobial according to a protocol produced by government veterinary advisers. Further concerns about the overuse of antibiotics may dictate the choice of drug.

The many groups of antimicrobials are described in the following alphabetical list and their modes of action are summarised in Table 3.1.

Table 3.1 Site of action of antibiotic drugs

Site of action	Antibiotic or group
Cell-wall synthesis	Bacitracin
	Penicillins
	Vancomycin
Protein synthesis	Aminoglycosides
	Chloramphenicol
	Fusidic acid
	Macrolides
	Sulphonamides
	Tetracyclines
Nucleic acid synthesis	Metronidazole
	Quinolones
	Rifampicin
	Trimethoprim

Aminoglycosides

Aminoglycosides include gentamicin, kanamycin, neomycin, strepto-mycin and tobramycin (human approved drug used in reptiles and exotic birds). Active against Gram-negative and some Gram-positive organisms, particularly in high pH environments and therefore useful for urinary tract infections. Side-effects include vestibular or auditory ototoxicity, neuromuscular blockade and nephrotoxicity; these effects may vary with the aminoglycoside and dose or interval used, but all members of the group are potentially toxic and should only be used for short periods of time. Neomycin and kanamycin may be toxic to aquatic invertebrates.

Spectinomycin (Spectam Scour Halt, Ceva) is not an aminoglyco-side but is related to streptomycin. It is used in calves, lambs and piglets.

Cephalosporins and cephamycins

Related to the penicillins (see Formula 3.6) these bactericidal drugs are suited to use in rabbits and rodents. Cephalosporins interfere with the action of cell-wall enzymes. The antibiotics are most stable and effective at a pH of 6–7.

Chloramphenicol and congeners

Chloramphenicol and its congeners inhibit microbial protein synthesis. It is a broad-spectrum antibiotic active against *Chlamydia* and *Rickettsia* spp. as well as most aerobes and anaerobes. Under European Directive 2377/90/EC chloramphenicol cannot be used in food-produc-ing animals. Horses metabolise the drug rapidly, thus its use in this species is limited; cats have problems with metabolism and thus treat-ment should be limited to a week. Chloramphenicol is a relatively stable compound and is unaffected by boiling, provided that a pH of 9 is not exceeded. A chloramphenicol ophthalmic product is available for instill-ing into feline or canine eyes or for subconjunctival injection (Chloromycetin V, Pharmacia & Upjohn). Chloramphenicol may be toxic to aquatic vertebrates.

Lincosamides

Lincosamides include clindamycin and lincomycin. They are closely related to the macrolides (see below). Lincomycin is active against

Gram-positive bacteria and *Mycoplasma* spp. It is incompletely absorbed from the gastrointestinal tract but absorption from an intra-muscular injection site is good. Nevertheless it is available as a con-stituent in a feed premix (MFS) for pigs and as an oral powder for addition to drinking water for poultry (Linco–Spectin, Pharmacia & Upjohn). Clindamycin is stronger acting than lincomycin. Side-effects include colitis in horses and small mammals. Clindamycin palmitate is used orally while clindamycin phosphate is given intramuscularly.

Macrolides

Macrolides include erythromycin, tilmicosin and tylosin. They work by interfering with protein synthesis in the invaders. Erythromycin has a spectrum of activity that is effective against *Streptococci, Staphylococci* and *Campylobacter* spp. Tylosin is active against *Mycoplasma* spp. and is also used to improve growth rate and feed conversion in pigs. Tilmicosin is used to treat pneumonia associated with *Pasteurella* in cattle and sheep. It is available as a subcutaneous injection (Micotil, Elanco). This drug is also available as a premix (MFS and POM) for addition to feed for the fattening of pigs (Pulmotil, Elanco). Macrolides are significantly more active at higher pH ranges of 7.8–8.

Penicillins

The penicillins are a large group of antibiotics based on a β-lactam structure (see Formula 3.6) that share many features, including chem-istry, mechanism of action, pharmacological properties, clinical effects and immunological characteristics. They have a 5-membered ring attached to a central common core while the closely related cephalosporins (see above) have a 6-membered ring.

Formula 3.6 Structures of penicillin (left) and cephalosporin (right)

Penicillins impair the development of bacterial cell walls and are active against both aerobic and anaerobic Gram-positive bacteria; with a few exceptions they are inactive against Gram-negative organisms at usual concentrations. Most penicillins in aqueous solution are rapidly absorbed from parenteral sites. Absorption is delayed when the inorganic penicillin salts are suspended in vegetable oil vehicles. The penicillins are rather unstable, being sensitive to heat, light, extremes in pH, heavy metals and oxidising and reducing agents. Also, they often deteriorate in aqueous solution and thus require reconstitution with a diluent just before injection.

Penicillin G, available in the UK as Crystapen (Schering-Plough) is inactivated by gastric acid so cannot be administered orally. Penicillin V tablets (human approved drug) and oral powder for addition to feed (Potencil, Vericore LP) and the longer acting procaine benzylpenicillin (various brands) are also available for veterinarians to prescribe. Several products exist that contain a mixture of the latter two narrow-spectrum penicillin variants (e.g. Duphapen LA, Fort Dodge and Norocillin, Norbrook). Procaine benzylpenicillin is used in the treatment of mastitis in non-lactating animals (dry cows). It is administered as an intramammary paste (Mylipen Dry Cow, Schering-Plough).

Flucloxacillin has a broader spectrum of antibacterial activity and may be administered to cats and dogs orally for penicillin-resistant staphylococcal infections. Cloxacillin and oxacillin are similar compounds and are used as ingredients in intramammary suspensions and ophthalmic preparations.

The broad-spectrum antibiotics – ampicillin and amoxicillin – are principally active against Gram-negative bacteria. Amoxicillin is administered by a variety of routes, all of which are appropriate for cats and dogs: intramuscular injection (cattle, sheep, pigs), subcutaneous injection and orally in drinking water or feedingstuffs (calves, pigs, piglets, poultry, pigeons).

Co-amoxiclav (amoxicillin with clavulanic acid), available in oral (tablets and powder for reconstitution) and intramuscular forms (Synulox, Pfizer), has a wider spectrum of activity. It is authorised for use in cattle, pigs, cats and dogs.

Piperacillin is active against anaerobic infections and is used in amphibians and reptiles.

Quinolones

The quinolones include nalidixic acid and are active against Gram-negative bacteria. They are thought to interfere with bacterial DNA replication. Substitution with a fluorine molecule in the quinolone ring markedly enhances activity against both Gram-negative and Gram-positive bacteria. The fluoroquinolone variants include difloxacin, marbofloxacin and enrofloxacin. Enrofloxacin (Baytril, Bayer) is used in a wide range of species from cattle and pigs to rabbits, rodents and exotic birds. Quinolones are commonly administered orally, although injectable forms of enrofloxacin are available. Ciprofloxacin is available as ophthalmic drops for superficial bacterial infections.

Sulphonamides and sulphonamide combinations

Sulphonamides are widely used in veterinary medicine because of their low cost and efficacy in treating some common bacterial diseases. They are derivatives of sulphanilamide. All have the same nucleus to which additions of functional groups or substitutions have been made (see Formula 3.7).

Formula 3.7 Sulphonamide

Sulphonamides block several bacterial complex enzyme systems, eventually causing suppression of protein synthesis, impairment of metabolic processes and inhibition of growth. They are active against a range of Gram-positive and Gram-negative bacteria. The synergistic action of sulphonamides with specific diaminopyrimidines, e.g. sulfadiazine with trimethoprim (Co-trimazine) has reinforced sulphonamide therapy (see Formula 3.8). The latter drug is widely used in the UK and overseas. It may cause salivation in cats, and tablets should be fed whole.

Formula 3.8 Trimethoprim

Tetracyclines

Tetracyclines are active against aerobic and anaerobic Gram-positive and Gram-negative bacteria, *Mycoplasma, Chlamydia* and *Rickettsia*. The tetracyclines are considered to be wide-spectrum antibacterials. The exact site involved in the antimicrobial activity of tetracyclines has not been clarified, but they are thought to inhibit protein synthesis. The core structure of tetracyclines is shown in Formula 3.9.

Formula 3.9 Tetracyclines

Chlortetracycline, doxycycline and oxytetracycline, and the lesser-used tetracyclines, are available in several dose forms and are used in many farm and companion animals, birds and poultry.

Tetracyclines seem to have an affinity for concentration in developing dentition and if given to pregnant bitches or queens, or to puppies or kittens, may cause defects or discolouration in the young animal's primary teeth. Horses under stress may develop colitis when given the drug. When given by intramuscular injection a local irritation may occur (depending on the vehicle used) and local anaesthetics may be included to reduce this discomfort.

Miscellaneous antimicrobial agents

Fusidic acid This is a steroidal antibiotic with action against Gram-positive bacteria.

Nitrofurans Nitrofurans are synthetic chemotherapeutic agents with a broad antimicrobial spectrum; they are active against both Gram-positive and Gram-negative bacteria and some protozoa. Nitrofurantoin is the only UK example; this drug cannot be used in food-producing animals.

Nitroimidazoles The 5-nitroimidazoles, of which metronidazole is a member, are a group of drugs that have both antiprotozoal and antibacterial activity. The precise mode of action is unclear but the drugs are thought to interfere with DNA structure. Metronidazole is available as tablets (human approved generic), an oral paste for horses (Metronex, Pharmacia & Upjohn), intravenous infusion (Torgyl, Merial) and intramuscular injection. The injectable version may be used for local irrigation of wounds.

Polymixin Polymyxin B and polymyxin E (colistin) (colistinmethate sodium) are the most commonly used drugs in this group of polypeptide antibiotics. They are administered topically (particularly for Gram-negative ocular infections) and orally for gastrointestinal problems.

Rifampicin Rifamycins interfere with the synthesis of RNA in microorganisms and have been used as extended-spectrum antibiotics for the treatment of intracellular infections. They may be combined with erythromycin in the treatment of pneumonia-like conditions in foals.

Tiamulin Tiamulin (Tiamutin, Leo) is active against Gram-positive bacteria, mycoplasmas and anaerobes, including *Treponema hyodysenteriae*. It is also clinically effective in the treatment of swine dysentery (see chapter 11) and mycoplasmal arthritis.

Vancomycin Vancomycin is a glycopeptide active against most Gram-positive bacteria but is not effective against Gram-negative cells because of their large size and poor penetrability. The drug is administered by injection into the abdominal sinus of lobsters against gaffkemia (red tail) a bacterial infection caused by *Aerococcus viridans*.

Combination antibiotics

Most combination products include a procaine penicillin and streptomycin as an injection or as an oral powder for addition to feed. Neomycin is also combined with procaine benzylpenicillin (Neopen, Intervet) and with streptomycin (Orojet, Fort Dodge). There is a premix for addition to pigs' feedingstuff containing chlortetracycline and procaine benzylpenicillin (Microfac HP, Vericore HP) and a premix and powder for addition to drinking water containing lincomycin and spectinomycin (Linco-Spectin, Pharmacia & Upjohn).

A product called Stomorgyl (Merial, Belgium) combines metronidazole with spramycin and is used in cats and dogs. Finally, there is a POM sulphonamide premix combination of sulfadimidine with tylosin (Tylasul, Elanco).

There are various combined antibacterial products used in the treatment of mastitis in non-lactating animals; these are administered by way of intramammary infusion or intramammary paste.

Bacteriophages

An entirely different approach to antibacterial treatment described by Professor S M Denyer at the British Pharmaceutical Conference in Manchester in 2002 employs bacteriophages to control infection. The method was originally advocated in the treatment of dysentery, typhoid and cholera between the World Wars but was then largely dropped with the advent of antibiotics. Bacteriophages are viruses that multiply and destroy bacteria. Investigations are underway to use bacteriophages to clear *Campylobacter* from broiler-house chickens instead of the use of feed-additive antibiotics.

Rehydration and electrolyte balance

Body fluids

Sixty per cent of an animal's body weight is water in which various solutes are dissolved. Of this almost 70% is intracellular; the balance is extracellular fluid (ECF) split between intravascular water (25%) and interstitial water in the supporting tissue (75%). The latter is affected during diarrhoea. The membranes separating these areas or 'compartments' are freely permeable to water, which moves under the force of osmotic pressure until the osmolality of each compartment is equal. When osmotically inactive water is added to one body compartment it is distributed evenly throughout all body water compartments. Plasma osmolality is a function of the ratio of body solute to body water; it is regulated by changes in water balance.

Dehydration may result from inadequate fluid intake or abnormally rapid fluid loss and electrolytes from the body. Water intake is derived primarily from three sources:

- Ingested water.
- Water contained in food.
- Water produced from oxidation of carbohydrates, proteins and fats.

Inadequate fluid uptake is most usually due to circumstances under which free access to water is denied. Water loss occurs in the urine and stool, as well as by way of evaporation from the skin and respiratory tract. Theses losses may also occur from the tissues during gastro-intestinal illnesses, especially those producing vomiting or diarrhoea, and as a result of blood loss or burns.

Alterations in plasma osmolality of as little as 1–2% are sensed by osmoreceptors in the hypothalamus. These receptors initiate mechanisms that affect water intake (increased thirst) and water excretion to return plasma osmolality to normal. If the animal is not drinking at all, through incapacity, or is not drinking enough to make up for fluid loss, clinical symptoms emerge (see Table 3.2).

A scouring calf may lose as much as 100 mL of water per kg body weight in 12 hours. The body attempts to conserve ECF, urine volume falls, blood urea levels rise and pH falls. Na^+, K^+ and HCO_3^- are lost. Ketones also accumulate.

Fluid therapy

Fluid therapy is used to replace intravascular volume (perfusion) and interstitial fluid volume (dehydration) or to correct electrolyte abnormalities (hypocalcaemia, hypokalaemia, hyper- or hypo-natraemia). Examples of the requirements for three conditions are shown in Table 3.3.

Formulating a fluid therapy plan for the critically ill small animal patient requires careful determination of the current fluid and electrolyte status. Once a need for fluids has been established it must be determined which fluid compartment(s) are involved and what components need to be supplemented or reduced in the fluids administered. The volume and rate of administration will be guided by pathological conditions.

Table 3.2 Clinical effects of changes in osmolality

Estimated percentage change in osmolality	Clinical effects
5	Dry oral mucous membranes but no panting
7	Dry oral mucous membranes, slight tachycardia and normal pulse pressure.
10	Dry oral mucous membranes, tachycardia and decreased pulse pressure.
12	Dry oral mucous membranes and significant signs of shock.

Table 3.3 Comparison between fluid therapy requirements for common conditions

	H^+	Na^+	Cl^-	K^+	HCO_3^-	Water volume	Possible treatment
Bowel obstruction	*	*			*	Decreased	Hartmann's solution + expander
Diarrhoea	*	*		(*) if long term	*	Decreased	Hartmann's solution
Vomiting	*	*	*	*		Decreased	Ringer's solution

The amount of fluid needed for replacement depends on the animal's status. The volume of fluid administered during the dehydration phase is based on an assessment of fluid needs for returning the animal's status to normal, replacing normal ongoing losses and replacing continuing abnormal losses.Oral hydration is usually sufficient for most cases of diarrhoea. Solutions contain sodium and glucose that help to facilitate water uptake. Citrates and bicarbonates may be included to correct any acidosis. Specific electrolyte imbalances may be addressed by adding the required ions to the rehydration fluid. For example, herbivores may become hypokalaemic when anorexic because their normal diet contains high concentrations of potassium.

Ringer's solution is commonly used for rehydration therapy. It is a clear colourless physiological solution of sodium chloride, potassium chloride and calcium chloride prepared with recently boiled pure water. The osmotic pressure of the solution is the same as that of blood serum. Ringer's solution is used for maintaining organs or tissues alive outside the animal or human body for limited periods.

There are a large number of commercially available oral rehydrating agents. In mild dehydration, subcutaneous fluids are also useful. Isotonic fluids should be used but no more than 2–5 mL/kg should be given at each injection site. The rate of subcutaneous fluid flow is usually governed by patient comfort. Generally, all subcutaneous fluids are reabsorbed within 6–8 hours. If fluids are still noted subcutaneously after this time, the use of intravenous fluids to re-establish peripheral perfusion should be considered.

In the severely dehydrated animal, ECF must be restored by parenteral plasma or infusion of sterile Ringer's solution; Compound Sodium Lactate Intravenous Infusion BP (Hartmann's solution) may be injected intravenously to treat dehydration. A plasma expander (dextran or gelatin) may be added if blood or plasma loss has been sustained through injury. In general, intravenous fluid administration is indicated in dogs and cats with 7% or greater dehydration.

The intraperitoneal route is quick and the fluids will generally be reabsorbed, thus increasing the circulating volume. However, there is the potential for bacterial peritonitis, perforating viscera and decreasing ventilation from impeding diaphragmatic excursion. Mild hypokalaemia in dogs may be treated through the inclusion of increased dietary fruit, vegetables and meat items high in potassium content.

Antiseptics and disinfectants

Although the bacterial origin of infection was unknown before Pasteur's work in Paris, and Lister's work at the Glasgow Royal Infirmary, antiseptics and disinfectants have been used empirically since the ancient Egyptians started embalming bodies. The decline in the spread of bubonic plague in Europe in the Middle Ages was partly aided by burning sulfur and aromatic substances, it has been suggested.

Various chemicals became available in the 19th century, and a solution of chlorinated lime was used by Semmelweiss in 1847 in Vienna for hand disinfection, thus reducing the incidence of fevers associated with childbirth. Antiseptic literally means 'against putrefaction' or 'prevention of sepsis' but the term is usually used to describe agents applied to living tissues in order to destroy or inhibit the growth of infectious microorganisms. Antiseptics and disinfectants are non-selective, anti-infective agents that are applied topically. Their activity ranges from destroying all microbes on the applied surface to simply reducing the number of microorganisms to within safe limits. The former are classified as bactericidal agents (they are usually applied to inanimate surfaces) and the latter as antiseptic or bacteriostatic agents. Bacteriostats prevent organisms from increasing in number, relying on the host-defence to cope with a static population; they may be less efficacious in immunocompromised patients. Sometimes the same compound may act as an antiseptic or as a disinfectant, depending on the drug concentration, conditions of exposure and number of organisms.

Requests from clients for advice as to what is available to treat their animals' minor cuts and abrasions can often be satisfied with an antiseptic product. In general, antiseptics are applied on tissues to suppress or prevent microbial infection. To achieve maximum efficiency, it is essential to use the proper concentration of the drug for the purpose intended. Most of these compounds exert their antimicrobial effect by denaturation of intracellular protein, alteration of cellular membranes (often through extraction of membrane lipids) or enzyme inhibition.

There is also a large market for the care of teats and udders to prevent the onset of mastitis in dairy animals. The skin surrounding the teats can serve as a reservoir for large numbers of environmental bacteria present in the milking parlour including *Streptococcus dysgalactiae*, *S. agalactiae* and *Staphylococcus aureus*. The observance of scrupulous hygiene protocols is vital to prevent onset of infection that can be debilitating to the animal and extremely costly financially to the farmer whose milk may be refused.

Before milking, teats should be initially cleaned with water to which a disinfectant has been added. Clean teats should then be dried with a disposable paper towel or muslin square. They may then be dipped with a fast-acting disinfectant solution and thoroughly dried before attaching the milking unit. After milking the teats should be coated with teat dip or spray to kill bacteria that may have been acquired during the milking process, and to prevent infection of any minor injuries sustained by the animal. Iodine products are useful for this purpose because they provide visible confirmation of coverage through staining. To minimise the ingress of bacteria after milking, animals should not be turned out until the teat canals have closed.

Antiseptics and disinfectants available

Ideal products should exhibit the following characteristics:

- They should have a broad spectrum and potent germicidal activity, with rapid onset and long-lasting effect.
- They should withstand environmental factors (e.g. pH, temperature, humidity) and must retain activity even in the presence of pus, necrotic tissue and other organic material.
- High lipid solubility and good dispersibility increase their effectiveness.
- Antiseptic preparations should not be toxic to the host (either through licking or dermatological reaction) and should not impair healing.

Available products include disinfectants for teats and udders, and antiseptics for general first aid (see also chapter 10).

Disinfectants for teats and udders   Disinfectants for teats and udders include cetrimide, chlorhexidine chlorine compounds, dodecyl benzene-sulfonic acid, glutaral iodine compounds, polyhexidine and compound products, e.g. chlorhexidine with cetrimide and benzalkonium chloride with chlorhexidine.

Antiseptics for general first aid   Commercially available preparations for minor cuts and abrasions include one or more of the following ingredients in spray, ointment and cream formulations: benzalkonium chloride, chlorocresol, chloroxylenol, cetrimide and povidone-iodine. There are also at least two wound dusting powders on the UK Market.

Table 3.4 lists some commonly used antiseptic compounds.

Table 3.4   Examples of common antiseptics

Antiseptic agents	Properties
Benzalkonium Chloride	A quaternary ammonium compound active against some Gram-positive bacteria and other microbes but not bacterial spores
Cetrimide	Broad spectrum May be inactivated by soaps, blood, pus, protein, rubber and fabrics
Chlorhexidine	Broad spectrum Most active at slightly alkaline conditions Inactivated by soap Less irritating than some other compounds
Chlorocresol Chloroxylenol	Phenolic compounds with low toxicity and irritancy Reduced activity in presence of blood and pus
Crystal violet	Bacteriostatic, especially against Gram-positive organisms Some inhibitory activity against fungi and yeasts
Dodecyl benzene-sulphonic acid	Antibacterial: not active against spores
Glutaraldehyde (Glutaral)	Active against Gram-positive and Gram-negative bacteria
Hydrogen peroxide	Readily cleanses wound, releasing oxygen in direct contact to wound Short acting Effects reduced in presence of blood, pus and organic matter

(continued)

Table 3.4 *Continued*

Antiseptic agents	Properties
Magenta	Effective against Gram-positive bacteria and some fungi
Providone-iodine	An aqueous complex of povidone and iodine. Similar to iodine, with broad spectrum. Povidone-iodine does not sting or stain.
Tea tree oil	Non-irritant herbal skin antiseptic Thought to be active in presence of pus

Vaccines

To discuss immunological preparations for animals requires much more than a paragraph or two. The reader is referred to chapter 4 which deals with the topic in detail.

Types of presentation

Injections

Injection is generally via intravenous, intramuscular, or subcutaneous routes. The route chosen may affect the effectiveness of the medicament:

- For the intravenous route aqueous solutions are preferable; these lead immediately to predictably high blood levels with a rapid onset of action. Irritating and non-isotonic solutions can be injected intravenously if administered slowly and carefully.
- The intramuscular route can be used for aqueous or oleaginous suspensions, solutions and other depot preparations. Absorption occurs either through the blood stream or via lymphatics and is usually fairly rapid except for long-acting preparations. Moderately irritating preparations can be injected intramuscularly, but tissue reaction and necrosis may become evident with time. The duration of drug action is longer than for intravenous injection but normally a little shorter than for subcutaneous administration; however, this is not always predictable. A disadvantage of the intramuscular route is the possibility of improper deposition in nerves, blood vessels, fat or between muscle bundles in connective tissue sheaths.
- The advantages of the subcutaneous route are similar to those of the intramuscular route, although irritant preparations and oily vehicles should be avoided due to possible undesirable reactions. The rate of absorption from subcutaneous injection sites may be unpredictable and depends on several

factors. The most important of these is blood flow, and the presence of vaso-constrictors or vasodilators can substantially alter rates of absorption. Usually, the rate of absorption is slightly slower than from intramuscular sites.

Precautions must be taken to avoid contamination with bacteria, dirt and animal hair during the injection process. The area where the needle is to be introduced should be clipped and swabbed with a suitable anti-septic agent. For many injections in small animals the vet will grasp a fold of skin at the back of the neck and insert the needle into the middle of this fold. Intrathecal injections are often used during euthanasia (see chapter 1). Amphotericin B can also be administered to cage and aviary birds by this route.

For on-the-farm herd inoculations Sterimatic Ltd of Stroud, England supplies an automatic, needle-cleaning system that can be attached to any standard, multidose, disposable syringe, as well as adapters for use with metal syringes. The system gives added safety to the user, reducing the risk of scratch and needle-stick injuries, and auto-matically cleans the needle between every injection. Other injection routes include epidural, intraperitoneal and intrathecal. Subconjunctival injections of the antibiotic kanamycin (Kannasyn, Sanofi) can be used in cattle to treat some Gram-negative bacterial eye infections.

'Projectile syringes' or darts are fired from a blowpipe, crossbow or gun and are useful for immobilising wild animals. Dart guns are con-trolled under the Firearms Act in the UK. Immobilon, a veterinary anaesthetic based on the compound etorphine, is used in dart guns to immobilise wild animals. It was discovered and developed in the research and development laboratories of Reckitt and Colman and is now distributed by C-Vet VP.

Accidental self-injection with Immobilon requires immediate reme-dial action – nalaxone should be injected immediately. The veterinary antidote diprenorphine hydrochloride (Revivon, C-Vet) may also be used in humans in extreme emergency.

Intramammaries

These preparations are used to treat clinical and subclinical mastitis in cows. A sterile infusion is introduced into the infected quarter using a syringe. An appropriate administration protocol is as follows:

1. Wash the teats and udder thoroughly with warm water containing a suitable dairy antiseptic.
2. Dry the teats and udder thoroughly.

3. Using alcohol pads provided, scrub clean each teat end to be treated, using a separate pad for each teat.
4. Warm the syringe to body temperature.
5. Choose the desired insertion length (full or partial) and insert tip into the teat canal.
6. Instil entire contents of one syringe into the quarter.
7. Massage the udder after treatment to distribute the product throughout the quarters.
8. Treat all of the teats with a suitable teat dip (see above).

Intramammaries are also available in a paste formulation.

Oral liquids

'Drenching' refers to the practice of administering liquid medicines to animals. The process, using a species-specific gun, must be carried out slowly for there is a risk of pneumonia if the liquid 'goes down the wrong way'. Some products may be provided as oral powders for reconstitution as solutions or suspensions or for addition to drinking water.

Liquids for oral or ocular use

Multidose containers (dropper bottles) or single-dose vials are available for ear or eye treatments.

Oral solid-dose forms

Bolus

A bolus is a medicine in a paste form presented in a cylindrical mass (approximately 5 cm long and 1 cm in diameter) given orally. A slow-release variant is used to administer anthelmintics or trace elements. Cosecure boluses (Telsol) are designed to supplement the diet of grazing cattle with the nutritionally essential minerals copper, cobalt and selenium for up to 6 months. They are made from a special kind of soluble glass and as a result share some of the properties of common glass; therefore they are susceptible to sudden changes in temperature. The rumen of a cow or sheep is approximately 40 °C and it is important that the bolus that enters this environment is not significantly colder than this.

Cattle wormers, e.g. fenbendazole (Panacur, Intervet) are available as boluses and are classified PML. Schering-Plough have a ruminal bolus (Autoworm) comprising a number of tablets of oxfendazole that are released at 3-week intervals and act against gastrointestinal roundworms, lungworms and tapeworms.The boluses are given orally often using a Cosecure oesophageal balling gun which delivers the bolus directly to the top of the gullet. The balling gun should be used to place the bolus on the very back of the tongue, the animal will then swallow the bolus itself. The mouth should be held closed and observed for a short time to ensure that the animal has swallowed the bolus.

Bullets

Bullets are administered to cattle and sheep using a special dosing gun and are used as a means of providing the animal with a supply of magnesium or cobalt over a period of around 85 days. The bullets are costly and may not be retained but they are still used where other methods are deemed inappropriate. Magnesium bullets are about 5 cm in diameter, 15 cm long and weigh about 250 g. They need to be installed at least a week before the high-risk period starts. The release rate is 2 g/day, which is only a marginal supplement of doubtful efficiency. The requirement of a cow producing 20 L of milk is 15 g/day (a recommended daily allowance takes into account the requirement and the availability of magnesium from feeds). Magnesium bullets may not give sufficient protection when magnesium absorption is being affected by high dietary potassium.

Capsules

Veterinary capsules provide a convenient way of dispensing powder formulae. For example fenbendazole 8 mg capsules (Panacur, Intervet) are used to dose pigeons against roundworms. A range of different sizes of capsule accommodate the needs of different species of animals. Table 3.5 gives examples of this.

The capsules may be delivered in large animals with the aid of a gun similar to the balling gun described above.

The use of gelatin capsules to administer liquids orally is more convenient than drenching, increases compliance and is safer. Further, both the trauma of intubation and the risk of aspiration pneumonitis are eliminated. Capsule presentations may also be used as pessaries.

Granules and pellets

Granules and pellets provide a convenient method for administration of wormers, e.g. fenbendazole to cats and dogs and horses. PML wormers are also given as pellets for cattle and pigs (Panacur 1.5%, Intervet).

Table 3.5 Capacities of veterinary capsules and examples of species treated

Approx average capacity of capsule	Animals
14 g	Goat (70 kg) Dog (30 kg)
6 g	Goat (45 kg) Dog (25 kg)
8 g	Goat (25 kg) Dog (20 kg)
4 g	Cow, calf, horses, deer, goats (20 kg) Dogs (5 kg)
2.5 g	As for 4 g capsules + ostrich, pigs

Oral paste and gels

Fenbendazole is administered as an oral paste (PML) in horses (Panacur Equine, Intervet); Sherley's Worming Cream (piperazine citrate 250 mg/g) is an oral paste (GSL) administered to kittens and puppies over 2 weeks of age with the aid of an appropriately calibrated applicator. There are also oral gels available.

Tablets/pills

Commercial animal medicines may be available in only one tablet size. Giving that tablet to a small dog or to a horse can pose problems. The tablet may be too large to give to the dog, and an excessive number of tablets may need to be given to the horse! Other dose forms are available for large animals, e.g. paste or pellets.

An interesting letter to the *Pharmaceutical Journal* in March 1996 by Mr Graham Weeks, then living in Greenford, Middlesex, recalls his early experience in a pharmacy in Thirsk where one of his clients was James Heriot. The celebrated veterinarian presented prescriptions for large aniseed flavoured pills known as 'horse balls'. These were apparently dispatched to Newmarket, Ireland and France.

Topical

Dips

Sheep dips are veterinary medicines rather than pesticides, which relate to crop-protection products. They are used to protect sheep against external parasites. The majority of formulations contain organophosphate active ingredients. Sheep dogs may also be dipped although this now seldom happens in the UK. In the USA, however, there is a dip containing 4.85% chlorpyrifos (Dursban (Davis, Vedco)), an organophosphate, marketed for the treatment of fleas, ticks and mites on dogs.

Until 1989, the UK law required compulsory dipping twice a year in an effort to eradicate scab, a notifiable disease. In 1989 and 1990, only one dip was required. The effectiveness of dipping was brought into question by numerous pressure groups. It was claimed that the mean annual incidence of scab in the five double-dipping years (1984–88) was not significantly different from that in any other five consecutive years or from the whole period since sheep scab was introduced in 1972. In 1992, dipping for scab ceased to be compulsory and the disease became no longer notifiable (sheep scab remains a notifiable disease in Northern Ireland). The Ministry of Agriculture, Fisheries and Food (MAFF), now superseded by DEFRA, announced that it would not hesitate to prosecute those who did not deal promptly and satisfactorily with an outbreak of scab in their flocks. MAFF complained that the sheep industry had failed to cooperate with the mandatory dipping policy. The industry in turn accused MAFF of failing to police compulsory dipping. Human safety considerations from contact with organophosphate sheep dips has been discussed earlier in this chapter. It is illegal to sell organophosphate sheep dips unless the buyer has the support of a certificate. Therefore, anybody who buys organophosphate sheep dip must have a certificate of competence in the safe use of sheep dips or satisfy the distributor selling the dip that they are the employer of, or acting on behalf of, somebody who has the certificate. Dips should be stored in original containers, out of reach of children and animals, and not mixed with other concentrates or washes unless directed to do so by the manufacturer.

Ear tags

Ear tags impregnated with cypermethrin are used against biting and nuisance flies on cattle.

Foam

An innovative preparation containing permethrin for the treatment of flea infestation in cats is marketed as a foam (Defencat, Virbac). It is applied to the cat as a ball of foam, approximately 8 cm in circumference. Another ectoparasiticide for treating fleas is offered as a mousse (Flea Killing Mousse, Bob Martin).

Pour-ons and spot-ons

Systemic parasiticides may be administered as a pour-on when liquid is poured along the dorsal midline of the animal or as a 'spot-on' when a small amount of liquid is applied to an area on the head or back. An example of the former is doramectin (Dectomax, Pfizer) used against both ecto- and endoparasites in cattle and of the latter, the cat and dog ectoparasiticide prescription-only drug fenthion (Tiguvon, Bayer). One or more drops of ivermectin 1% solution may be placed on the neck of birds to treat wheezing and breathing difficulty caused by tracheal mites in canaries and finches or gapeworm in larger birds. Active material is absorbed through the skin and passes into the circulation and then into the ectoparasite.

The treatment is purchased as a ready-to-use formulation and does not require dip tanks, spray races or hand-held, pressurised spray equipment. Instead, oil-based formulations are provided in sachets or bottles for pouring over the back of the animal, normally from the base of the neck to the tail. Concentrates of *cis* and *trans* isomer mixtures of permethrin are the most popular constituent, with various oils acting as a 'spreader'. Physical characteristics (such as a hairy fleece) and animal behaviour (such as licking the application site) may limit the effectiveness of the product in some circumstances. Little is therefore known about potential effects on user health and the surrounding environment of permethrin and other pyrethroids used in pour-on and dip formulations. Inevitably, their misuse, including poor user safety and disposal practices, particularly in developing countries of the world (where they are used widely to control the tsetse fly), is likely to have some detrimental effect.

Dusting powders

Several ectoparasiticides exist as dusting powders. Examples include a pigeon louse powder containing pyrethrins (Harkers), and a flea powder containing permethrins (Sinclair). Dusting powders for environmental control are also available; these should not be used on animals.

Ointments and creams

Ointments and creams are often extremely effective as there is immediate contact between drug and the area to be treated. The vehicle is important because:

- It affects the degree of skin hydration.
- It may have a mild anti-inflammatory effect.
- It may facilitate absorption of the drug through the skin.

The skin area to be treated should be clipped and any hair, fur or debris removed from the surface using an appropriate antiseptic. In order to try and reduce the tendency for cats and dogs to lick off any topical medication it should be applied before feeding or exercise or the animal should be fitted with a restraint. Constant licking will also exacerbate the wound or lesion. The most widely used version of this is known as an Elizabethan collar. It is usually made of cardboard in the shape of a lamp shade that is attached to the animal's collar and fits over its head, so preventing access to the affected parts.

Gel

Gels are semi-solid solutions that are easy to apply and wash off. An example is pirlamycin gel which is a product formulated for the treatment of clinical and subclinical mastitis in lactating cattle. It has been proven effective against *Staphylococcus* species such as *Staph. aureus* and *Streptococcus* spp. such as *S. agalactiae*, *S. dysgalactiae* and *S. uberis*.

Liniments and embrocations

These are oily preparations designed to be rubbed into the tissue and often include potentially toxic constituents (e.g. aconite, belladonna and chloroform liniment), so should be stored and used with care. Liniments are used to treat a range of soft-tissue injuries, strains and sprains.

Shampoo

Shampoos help to clean the skin and remove dirt and dermatological debris. They are formulated carefully so as not to cause any localised allergic or dermatological reactions. They are particularly indicated for the treatment of seborrhoeic conditions (e.g. salicylic acid, selenium sulfide, coal tar) and for skin disinfection (e.g. chlorhexidine). Although antiparasitic shampoos exist, they offer little residual control if the parasite is still in the environment, since the lather is rinsed off after a short while. This is an important factor in flea control. A shampoo containing chlorhexidine 2% and miconazole 2% (Malaseb, Leo) is the treatment of choice in *Malassezia pachydermatis* infection.

Lotions

Lotions are used for minor skin infections and abrasions or as skin cleansers and antiseptics. An example is Vetzyme Vetinary Antiseptic Lotion (Seven Seas). Antifungal lotions (e.g. may be used to treat ringworm in rodents (e.g. gerbils)).

Pessaries and suppositories

Pessaries are used mainly for uterine treatments and for introduction to the teat canals of the mammary gland. Suppositories are used to reduce inflammation or irritation of the rectal mucous membrane or as an aperient.

Sprays and aerosols

Aerosol sprays (e.g. benzalkonium or iodine) provide pharmaceutically elegant formulations for dermatological preparations and being in sealed containers do not leak (assuming the valve is operating correctly). Spray presentations are used widely for ectoparasitic treatment, e.g. an aerosol spray containing piperonyl butoxide 1% and pyrethrins 0.2% (Anti-Mite & insect Spray, Johnson's) is used against lice and mites in pigeons and cage birds; 10% fenvalerate is used on cattle (Deosan, Fort Dodge). The noise from propellant escaping when the button is pressed may frighten some pets. Amitraz solution can be sprayed all over a pig's skin and in the ears to control mange.

Sprays also provide a convenient presentation for the environmental control of ectoparasites, e.g. 0.25% permethrin and 0.1% pyrethrins (Secto Household Flea Spray). Amitraz is available in the UK as a solution concentrate for dilution and application as a buildings spray (Taktic, Intervet).

Some factors affecting the efficacy of veterinary medicines
(see also chapter 8)

Pharmacological

The chemical structure of the active drug and the formulation will both affect the pharmacological properties of the drug being used.

Pathogenic

Wolfhounds are at particular risk from the use of barbiturate anaesthetics because they may have health problems which will make them even more susceptible. These include heart disorders such as dilated cardiomyopathy and arrhythmias.

Physiological

Species

Species that are physiologically similar tend to have similar drug reactions and the same dose regimes can often be used for a particular drug. Thus, dose regimens recommended for dogs can be used for cats. Extrapolating human dose regimes to dogs may not be so reliable because they are often based on body weight; animal doses based on the same body weight calculation may be inappropriate. So while aspirin may be given to a human at doses of 10 mg/kg of body weight every 6 hours, with a cat, the same dose (10 mg/kg) would be given every 48 hours.

There are some examples of species-specific reactions to drugs. Cats are more sensitive than dogs to the adverse side-effects of a variety of drugs (e.g. some analgesics and antiarrhythmics), and extra precautions must be taken when these drugs are used. Aspirin in high doses gives a cat hepatitis, gastric irritation and respiratory problems. Cats also have extreme trouble dealing with paracetamol. Amongst zoo animals it is well known that giraffes are difficult to immobilise and anaesthetise, making hoof trimming a problem. A cocktail of drugs is used together with various management.

Breed

Differences in drug outcome amongst different breeds of the same species are not well documented. One example can be described in dogs. Wolfhounds can have a problem with the barbiturate anaesthetics. This is because their ratio of bone to body weight is high. Further, large breeds require less anaesthetic per kilogram of body weight generally than smaller breeds because of the difference in their metabolic rate. When calculating the amount of anaesthetic to give, surface area should be used as the indication, not body weight. There are charts available for converting size and body weight to surface area in order to calculate the correct amount of anaesthetic required.

Age

Changes in pharmacodynamic and pharmacokinetic mechanisms, accompanied by a reduction in body weight with age (sometimes by up to 30%), result in changes in the pathways by which drugs are metabolised. This necessitates adjustment of treatment.

Route of administration

Differences in the route of administration have a profound effect on the speed of onset of action. In some cases drugs may only be active by one specific route – usually injection – but also as a topical for local effect.

Technique of administration

The confidence with which animals are given medicines may well affect the efficacy, particularly if the tablet or capsule is not swallowed or oral dose forms are spilt due to a lack of dexterity on the part of the owner.

References

NOAH (2001). *Withdrawal Periods for Veterinary Products 2001–2002*, 10th edn. Enfield: National Office of Animal Health.
NOAH (2004). *Compendium of Data Sheets for Veterinary Products 2001–2002*. Enfield: National Office of Animal Health.
Soil Association (1998). *Use and Misuse of Antibiotics in UK Agriculture*. Bristol.

Further reading

Aiello SE, ed. (2000). *The Merck Veterinary Manual*, 8th edn. Rahway: Merck and Co.
Bishop Y, ed. (2001). *The Veterinary Formulary*, 5th edn. London: Pharmaceutical Press.
Boden E, ed. (2001). *Black's Veterinary Dictionary*, 20th edn. London: A & C Black.
Booth NH, McDonald LE, eds. (1988). *Veterinary Pharmacology and Therapeutics*, 6th edn. Iowa: Iowa State University Press.
Pattison I (1984). *The British Veterinary Profession 179–194*. London: Allen.
Porter R (1997). *The Greatest Benefit to Mankind*. London: Harper Collins.

Useful address/website

National Office of Animal Health (NOAH), 3 Crossfield Chambers, Gladbeck Way, Enfield, EN2 7HF, UK. Tel: +44 (0)20 8367 3131 (http://www.noah.co.uk/index.htm).

The website includes the NOAH (2001) publication given in References, above.

4

Veterinary vaccines

Lucy Whitfield

History of vaccines

A type of vaccination was used as early as the 11th century by the Chinese in an attempt to protect people against smallpox, as it was noted that individuals who recovered from the disease were immune to further infections. Practitioners deliberately transferred some virus from an infected patient to a healthy patient by scarifying the skin. Unfortunately, this is likely to have resulted in the deaths of as many patients as it saved. This practice of 'variolation' was later refined so that only milder cases were used as a source of virus and the survival rate in deliberately infected patients was improved.

At the end of the 18th century, the physician Edward Jenner observed that milkmaids did not suffer from smallpox, while those around them did. Jenner observed that cows were affected by a similar skin disease, cowpox, which was also contracted by the milkmaids but which appeared to protect them from the related human virus, smallpox. Jenner proved his theory by deliberately infecting a boy with cowpox, then subsequently attempting to infect him with smallpox virus. This provided a much safer alternative to the variolation technique using the actual human pathogen.

Vaccination was further developed by Louis Pasteur in the 1870s, when he showed that injection of old cultures (possibly containing dead bacteria) of 'fowl cholera' into chickens protected them against later exposure to live virulent cultures of the organism. Currently, there are several hundred vaccines licensed for veterinary use in the European Union (EU) and over 2000 are licensed in the USA.

Why use vaccines?

Vaccines are used in the control of human and animal diseases following the old adage that 'prevention is better than cure'. Why is it important to prevent disease?

Any disease that causes illness in an animal will compromise its welfare. 'Freedom from pain, injury or disease' is one of the five freedoms set out by the Farm Animal Welfare Council and used as a measure of an animal's wellbeing. Control and eradication of major infectious diseases has led to great improvements in animal welfare.

Infectious diseases may cause economic loss in terms of death of the animal (especially the more susceptible young or old individuals in the group) through the loss of production during the acute illness or due to sequelae of disease that last for the animal's lifetime.

Vaccines may be used in a programme to eradicate disease from a population of animals. In immunising and protecting the susceptible population, the disease organism is no longer able to spread through and remain amongst that species, so may die out after a period of time. The ease of achieving eradication depends on the characteristics of the infectious organism and the effectiveness of the vaccine and the vaccination programme.

Increasing consumer pressure against the use of therapeutics, such as antibiotics, to treat disease has encouraged research into methods of disease prevention, rather than clinical or prophylactic treatment of disease. However, some 'organic' systems also restrict the use of vaccines, which can reduce the options for disease prevention.

The immune system

The immune system allows an individual to combat the large variety of infectious agents that exist in the environment. The immune system can be divided by function into the innate system and the adaptive system. The innate system consists of physical and biochemical defences against invading organisms, such as the intact skin, lysozyme (in secretions such as tears) complement, and phagocytic white blood cells which engulf and destroy foreign particles.

Complement is a cascade series of enzymes that are triggered by microorganisms; it binds to the cell membrane of the pathogen and causes cell lysis. The complement system also attracts phagocytic white blood cells to the site and contributes to the local inflammatory response.

Some invading organisms have developed methods of evading destruction by the phagocytic cells, or fail to activate the complement system. The body's phagocytic cells have non-specific receptors that allow them to attach to and engulf foreign organisms, but some organisms can evade this 'recognition' system. The adaptive immune system has evolved to work in combination with the innate system to identify and present invading organisms for destruction.

The adaptive immune system counteracts invading organisms by producing a specific molecule (antibody) to attach to their surface, which activates the complement cascade and phagocytes. These antibodies, produced by the B-lymphocytes of the adaptive immune system, act to 'visualise' infectious agents, marking them for attachment by phagocytes. Phagocytes have receptors for the 'constant end' of the antibody molecule, so will recognise antibody-coated, or opsonised, micro-organisms more readily, leading to rapid phagocytosis and destruction.

Antibodies

Antibodies are a group of specialised proteins that exist in the blood and tissue fluids of mammals. Each antibody is specific for and can bind to a particular infectious organism; the body is able to make millions of varieties of antibodies to attach to the huge number of possible invading organisms. Some organisms, such as bacteria, may be very large, so the antibody may bind to a particular place or 'antigen' on the cell surface.

The antibody molecule has two functional regions: the 'variable end' binds to the antigen and the 'constant end' to host tissues such as phagocytic cells. Antibodies, or immunoglobulins (IgG), can be grouped into one of several classes, which have slightly different structures and may be predominantly associated with different regions of the body. IgG is the most abundant class of antibody and is the major circulating immunoglobulin. IgA is secreted from the epithelium of the intestinal and upper respiratory tracts and occurs in secretions such as milk and tears. It is involved in defences at the external body surfaces. IgE is important in some parasitic infections and in allergy.

Each antibody is produced by a particular line of white blood cells (B-lymphocytes) each of which is programmed to make only one antibody, according to the specific receptor placed on its cell surface. When a particular antigen binds to the receptor, the cell is triggered to multiply and mature into both antibody-producing cells and 'memory' cells. This is clonal expansion (Figure 4.1).

The memory cells remain in the body, acting as part of the immunological 'surveillance'. When the cells are again stimulated by the antigen, they proliferate in the 'secondary response' which allows the subsequent immune reaction to be much faster and larger, usually enabling the eradication of the organism before disease results.

It is this ability to mount an amnestic (immunological memory) response that is the rationale behind vaccination: production of the memory cells in response to an antigen (from disease or vaccine) results in long-lasting immunity following the initial challenge, so that when

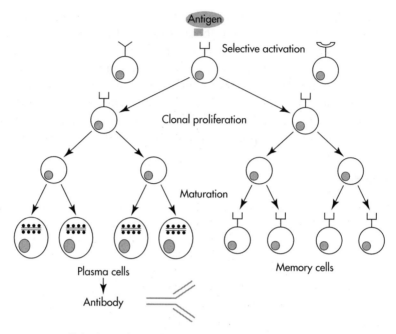

Figure 4.1 Cellular basis for antibody production and memory.

the disease organism is encountered, the secondary response is triggered immediately and the organism can be eliminated quickly with minimal effect on the host.

Principle of vaccination

Vaccination takes advantage of the specificity and memory characteristics of the adaptive immune response; the immune system produces a much faster and stronger response the second or subsequent time that it encounters a pathogen or antigen.

In the natural state, the animal's immune system produces antibodies to the diseases that it encounters (assuming that the animal survives the encounter!). However, there is a time lag between infection and the production of antibodies following clonal selection, expansion and maturation of the B-lymphocytes. Production of a neutralising antibody to a new pathogen takes several days and the disease can do much harm during this time.

In a vaccine, the antigens associated with the disease-causing organism or its virulence factors are given to the animal but are altered in some way in order to render them harmless to the animal but still recognisable to its immune system. In this way, the animal is able to produce immunity to the pathogen but does not suffer the ill effects of the disease itself.

Vaccination with the antigen(s) results in selection of the appropriate B-lymphocytes, leading to a primary antibody response and production of memory cells. On encountering the disease organism the next time, the B memory cells are stimulated and the immune system is able to produce a swift and effective response to infection, eradicating the organism before debilitating disease results. Figure 4.2 represents a typical antibody response following vaccination with an inactivated vaccine.

In order to design a good vaccine, there are a few factors that must be understood and taken into account: the vaccine should include the antigen(s) most involved in producing the appropriate protective antibody and the correct part of the immune response must be stimulated at the site of microbial invasion. The vaccine produced must be safe.

Vaccination should be distinguished from 'passive protection' of the animal by the administration of an antiserum. Antiserum contains specific preformed antibodies that were produced in another animal or in culture. It is administered to the non-immune patient to provide temporary protection against disease challenge such as in a young animal or one that has not been vaccinated. Antibodies have a finite lifespan in the circulation, usually only a few weeks, so the protection provided is short-lived but it may be useful in a crisis situation. Antisera are much more expensive to produce than vaccines and there may be inherent risks to the patient in administering a product produced in another animal.

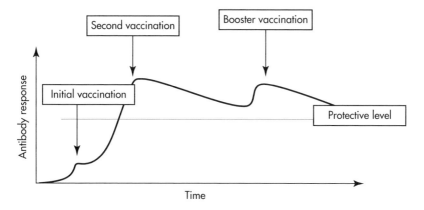

Figure 4.2 Typical antibody response following vaccination using an inactivated vaccine.

What is a vaccine?

A vaccine basically consists of the disease-causing organism or parts of the organism (antigens) that are relevant in producing neutralising antibodies. These are presented in such a way as to be harmless to the animal and in a form which helps the immune system to recognise them and produce an appropriate response.

Constituents of a vaccine

Antigen

This is a molecule that is recognised by the immune system and to which antibodies are produced. A disease-causing organism, such as a bacterium, may have many different antigens on its surface. Parts of organisms (subunits) or virulence factors, such as toxins, may be antigenic.

Adjuvant

A substance that helps present the antigens to the immune system in an easily recognisable form and which improves the quality and size of the immune response. The exact mode of action for all adjuvants is not known. They may act by providing a slowly released depot of antigen, allowing its easier uptake by lymphocytes, by causing retention of lymphocytes in the regional lymph nodes or direct effects on the B- and T-lymphocytes. Some adjuvants are thought to act in a manner analogous to detergents in dispersing the antigen.

Adjuvants have been produced from metallic salts, such as aluminium hydroxide, and plant extracts, such as Quil A (quillaia), derived from the soapbark tree. Other adjuvants contain antigens as oil-in-water or water-in-oil emulsions, or in immune-stimulating complexes (ISCOMs).

Diluent

This is the liquid that makes up the remainder of the vaccine to enable it to be administered in a reasonable dose volume.

Preservative

Some vaccines contain preservatives. However, since vaccines are prepared and should be used under sterile conditions, use of preservatives in vaccines is generally being phased out.

Types of vaccines

Vaccines can be divided into two types: live ('attenuated') and inactivated ('killed'). The difference in formulation is important, as the two have slightly different characteristics, so both the effect on the immune system and dosage regimes may differ.

Live vaccines

These contain an organism that is attenuated but still capable of limited reproduction in the body. This ability to replicate is carefully controlled so that no, or only very mild, clinical signs result from its multiplication in healthy animals. However, live vaccines may be less suitable for debilitated animals with poor nutritional status or suffering intercurrent disease. Advances in live-vaccine technology have produced safer and more effective live-viral vaccines for a range of animals; research is continuing to improve these further. There are various methods of producing a live attenuated vaccine, some examples of which follow.

Cross-protection from a related organism

The organism may be closely related to the pathogen, so the resulting antibodies will also protect against the disease ('cross-protection'). An example of this was the use of cowpox virus in protection against smallpox in man, or the current use of Shope fibroma virus in the vaccination of rabbits against myxomatosis.

Passage

The organism may be grown in tissue culture through many cycles of cell infection, such that the virus obtained from the final culture is less virulent than the original isolate. Antigenically, the vaccine organism resembles the pathogen but its potential to cause disease is much reduced.

Pathogen strain

A strain of pathogen may be chosen that is not fully able to replicate in the host. For example, a respiratory virus may grow optimally at 38 °C but not at the slightly lower temperature of the nasal passages. When this strain of virus is administered into the nose in an intranasal vaccine, sufficient viral replication occurs to stimulate the local immune response, but not enough to produce overwhelming infection. Immunity is stimulated at the site where natural infection would occur and is therefore very effective against subsequent challenge. Some cattle respiratory vaccines work in this way.

Gene deletion

The genome of pathogens can be artificially manipulated such that they lack a gene necessary for rapid replication in the host while retaining their antigenic characteristics.

Inactivated vaccines

A measured amount of antigen is presented to the immune system in a dose of vaccine and there is no multiplication within the host following vaccination. Two doses of inactivated vaccine are usually required in the primary course in order to stimulate sufficient antibody response. Subsequent 'booster' vaccinations may be required to maintain antibody levels; the interval between these varies according to the vaccine type. Inactivated vaccines may be less immunogenic than live vaccines, so require an adjuvant to produce a protective immune response. Inactivated vaccines are efficient in stimulating humoral (antibody) immunity but less so in stimulating cell-mediated immunity.

The inactivated pathogen retains its 'appearance', or antigenicity, with regard to the immune system, but is no longer able to replicate or produce the associated virulence factors which cause disease. The antibodies produced by the body in response to the inactivated organism given in the vaccine will be able to recognise and bind to the live pathogen. Bacterial vaccines are commonly inactivated. They are produced by growing the organism in culture and killing the cells before purification and formulation of the vaccine.

Improving the specificity of vaccines

In some cases, the harmful part of the infection is due to toxins produced by the organism, rather than simply the infection itself. Examples of this occur in *Clostridium perfringens* infection of ruminants, where some species of these bacteria may live as harmless commensals in the gut lumen. The disease process results from the various extracellular bacterial toxins entering the circulation when the animal becomes compromised.

Isolated bacterial toxins can be inactivated by modification and included in a vaccine in the form of toxoids, which remain antigenically similar to the harmful toxin but have none of its effects. Toxoid vaccines are a safe means of stimulating the appropriate neutralising immune response.

Some vaccines contain only certain parts of the organism. Research has identified the subunits of the organism that are most relevant in producing a protective immune response. These are separated, purified and included in the vaccine, without the need to include the remainder of the organism. For example, the antigens may be surface molecules, pili, or synthetic peptides.

This method of preparing vaccines has several advantages:

- The immune system only has to respond to a limited number of antigens, concentrating its response and reducing the likelihood of unwanted adverse reactions.
- It may be possible to produce the organism subunits in culture, resulting in a purer vaccine.

The antigens associated with organisms may vary according to the environmental or culture conditions in which they are grown. Hence, organisms produced *in vitro* may express different antigens to those expressed by organisms isolated from an infected animal. These differences must be taken into account in culture of organisms for vaccine production, as the absent antigens may be important in producing an effective immune response. The efficacy of a vaccine that does not include these antigens would be reduced. For example, Gram-negative bacteria grown *in vivo* or in iron-restricted culture produce surface proteins that are involved in iron uptake; those growing in culture where iron is freely available do not. Antibodies produced against these iron-regulated proteins are very effective in neutralising the infective organism; if these antigens are not included in the vaccine it will be much less efficient at producing a protective response in the vaccinated animal.

In some cases the relevant antigens are not produced by the pathogen until infection is established; in these instances it is not possible to protect the host as effectively by use of an inactivated vaccine. This may be the case for bacterial 'virulence factors' such as endotoxins. However, it is now possible to produce many of these toxins *in vitro* and to include the inactivated toxin or its antigenic subunits in the vaccine. An example of this is enteric *Escherichia coli* vaccines where toxin subunits are included in an inactivated vaccine. The characteristics of live and inactivated vaccines are summarised in Table 4.1.

Table 4.1 Characteristics of live and inactivated vaccines

Live	Inactivated
Organism replicates in host	No replication
Immunity rapidly produced	Onset of protection relatively slow
Usually stimulates cell-mediated immunity also	Usually stimulates humoral immunity
Local administration possible	Adjuvant usually needed
Generally good immune response stimulated	Immune response may be shorter-lasting
Chance that organism could revert to virulence	Organism unable to multiply or revert to virulence
Risk of contamination with another live organism	Risk of contamination minimal

Homeopathic nosodes

Nosodes are homeopathic remedies used to 'immunise' the body against a specific disease. They are prepared by specialised pharmacies, and some homeopathic veterinarians, from a pathological specimen, such as blood, pus or secretions; tissue such as a tumour may also be used. The sample is then 'potentised' by serial dilutions to produce the nosode for that condition (see chapter 5).

The major difference between a nosode and a conventional vaccine is that nosodes contain an extremely small (if any) quantity of physical substance. The mechanism of action of nosodes is not understood but it is thought to be the 'energy' pattern, rather than the substance that is effective in a homeopathic remedy.

There is no set dose programme for nosodes, rather the protocols of administration are produced for individual cases. Nosodes are available for some companion animal diseases, such as kennel cough, and have been used against mastitis in cattle. There is limited evidence of effectiveness from trials (see chapter 5) and conventional vaccination should generally be recommended.

Improving the immune response to vaccines

Microbial antigens vary in their expression depending on their growth conditions; not all of the antigens expressed are necessarily important in terms of producing an effective immune response. It is therefore important to identify the relevant antigens and the method of producing vaccines that contain them.

Route of administration

The aim of a vaccine is to produce an appropriate immune response to protect the animal against disease. Different pathogens enter the body by different routes, so it may be useful to produce the immune response at the site of entry of the organism. For example, respiratory pathogens generally multiply in the epithelium of the upper respiratory tract. Stimulating local IgA antibody at this site will provide relevant protection against infection at the site where it is needed. A modified live respiratory virus vaccine may therefore be formulated for intranasal administration.

Adjuvants

Antigens, by definition, will produce an immune response but may not elicit sufficient effect to be used alone. The mode of action for all adjuvants is not entirely understood but some may act as carriers, which improve the immune response to an antigen, or have direct actions on lymphocytes. As vaccines become more refined and include subunits rather than the whole organism, their relative antigenicity may be reduced, therefore adjuvants are required to augment the immune response.

As previously noted, adjuvants commonly used in veterinary vaccines are metallic salts such as aluminium hydroxide, plant derivatives, or oil emulsions. The type of antigen used may be selected to maximise the type of immune response required (whether mainly humoral or cell-mediated).

The animal's response to particular adjuvants must also be considered. Granulomas at the site of injection may be seen as unacceptable in pet animals, so vaccines containing adjuvant may not be appropriate in these circumstances. In food-producing animals the effect of any injection-site reaction on carcass quality must be considered; in these circumstances the intramuscular route of administration may best be avoided. The effect on the consumer of the adjuvant must also be considered and adjuvants must be shown to be safe.

Vaccination regimes

The vaccination programme must be designed to produce greatest immunity in those animals at greatest risk. This requires some knowledge both of the disease process and of the husbandry and biology of the animals in question. Vaccination and husbandry systems should be optimised to gain the full potential from the vaccine.

The protection afforded by the animal's immune system and its antibody levels is relative to the challenge from the pathogenic organism to which it is exposed. Even where an animal has a high level of circulating antibody, a massive challenge from a virulent organism may overwhelm the host's defences and the animal will succumb to disease. Similarly, if the animal's ability to mount an immune response is compromised due to poor nutrition, old age or concurrent disease, a lower pathogen challenge may still result in disease in a vaccinated animal.

Protection of neonates against pathogens encountered early in life will require transfer of immunity from the dam, as there is not sufficient time for the young to produce their own protective immune response prior to disease challenge. Protection of very young animals requires that the dam is vaccinated and has high levels of circulating antibody in her bloodstream that may be transferred to the offspring. The amount of antibody transferred prenatally depends upon the placentation type of the species. In primates, there is very good antibody transfer from dam to fetus; in ruminant species, there is no significant transfer to the offspring *in utero*. The degree of transfer in species such as dogs lies in between these two.

In ruminants and pigs, antibody from the dam's circulation is secreted into the udder and especially concentrated in the first milk (colostrum) produced shortly before parturition. The newborn of these species depend on ingestion of sufficient colostrum in early life in order to ensure that sufficient antibodies are transferred to protect it in the first weeks after birth. Good husbandry of the animals to ensure adequate colostrum intake in the newborn is therefore as important as the vaccination programme itself.

The vaccination course for the dam should be timed to produce the maximum circulating antibody response just prior to transfer to the offspring. Where there is prenatal antibody transfer, the dam may be vaccinated before mating; where antibody is secreted into colostrum, peak levels should be reached a few weeks prior to expected parturition date. Vaccination during pregnancy is not always possible where live vaccines are used. This is because there may be a risk to the non-immune developing fetus. Hence, when using these vaccines, primary or booster vaccinations for the dam are carried out before mating. Inactivated vaccines can generally be given to the pregnant animal.

Generally, a course of two vaccinations is required in order to produce a satisfactory immune response with an inactivated vaccine, depending on the adjuvant that is used. Further booster doses may be required at intervals to maintain antibody levels. The interval between vaccinations may vary according to the vaccine type, pathogen host species, or predicted challenge to which the animal may be exposed. Typically, booster vaccinations for veterinary vaccines are required once or twice annually.

A single vaccination with a live vaccine may be sufficient to elicit the antibody and memory cell response in the animal. Booster doses may be needed less frequently than with inactivated vaccines but, again, the interval depends on vaccine type, pathogen, host and expected challenge. Typically, booster doses are required one or more years apart.

Problems with vaccines

Failure of protection

A vaccinated animal may contract the disease against which it was apparently vaccinated. Vaccines may protect the animal against the clinical signs of disease but it may still become infected by the organism. This can occur for a variety of reasons such as failure of passive transfer or general poor health. Even where the animal has good circulating levels of antibody, an overwhelmingly large challenge with the pathogen may overcome the capacity of the immune system to neutralise the infection.

Poor nutritional status, especially with regard to trace elements and vitamins, old age or other stresses may reduce the animal's ability to mount a rapid protective immune response to the invading organism. It is important that animals are in good health when vaccinated in order to maximise their response.

Cortisol is an endogenous steroid hormone produced as part of an animal's response to stress. Chronic stresses, such as pain, poor environmental conditions or bullying may lead to continual cortisol production; this causes suppression of the immune system.

Failure of passive transfer of immunity, especially where this depends on the newborn animal suckling sufficient colostrum, is a common cause of poor immunity in young farm animals. There is a relatively short period (6–12 hours) after birth when the gut of the neonate is able to take up antibody from the mother's colostrum, hence adequate intake in these first hours is essential for protection in the first weeks of life.

Changes in the disease organism

Some pathogens may alter with time in an effort to evade the immune system's antibody defences. Some viruses, such as influenza, have particularly changeable outer proteins. The haemagglutinin and neuraminidase outer proteins may change slightly over time (antigenic drift) or become markedly different (antigenic shift). Vaccines that do not contain the most recent version of the virus will be less able to protect against new infections. Influenza virus vaccines produced for equines must therefore be reviewed frequently and kept up to date in order to contain the most relevant antigens. A phylogenetic tree can be constructed to show the changes that have occurred in the virus over several years (see Figure 4.3).

Risks from vaccination

There is relatively little intrinsic risk to the animal given an inactivated vaccine, except that the adjuvant may provoke a sterile local reaction at

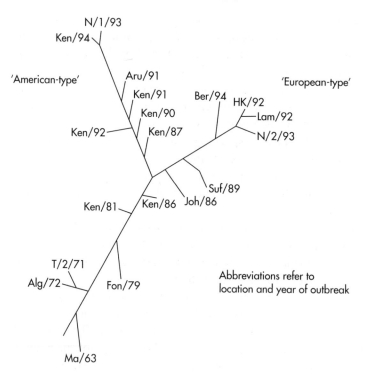

Figure 4.3 Phylogenetic tree constructed from equine influenza A (H3N8) HA1 amino acid sequences. (Adapted, with permission of Dr J Mumford, Animal Health Trust, Newmarket.)

the site of injection, causing swelling or a firm lump. These adjuvant reactions generally resolve over a few weeks but the siting of injections may be important where they are given in companion animals, close to anatomically sensitive areas, or near to the higher value cuts of meat in slaughter animals.

Vaccines are produced and packaged in aseptic conditions in order to prevent possible contamination with organisms from the environment. All injectable vaccines should be administered taking sterile precautions, as commensal skin bacteria or other contaminants may be inadvertently introduced. Injection of contaminated vaccine may result in sepsis at the site of injection or even endotoxic shock and death.

It is possible that the attenuated virus in live vaccines may revert to virulence, either by spontaneous mutation or by recombination with 'wild type' virus while replicating. Both events are very rare, the latter requiring that the same cell is infected with vaccine and natural virus at the same time. Prevention of reversion to virulence is one of the parameters examined when considering the safety of live vaccines.

Since the pathogen used in vaccine production may originally have been isolated from animal tissue, vaccines are also checked for possible contamination with any pathogens known to cause disease in the species for which they are intended. This is especially important where live vaccines are produced. Risk of contamination may be lower where genetically engineered subunit vaccines are produced in culture.

There is concern that vaccines may produce adverse effects in some animals through overstimulation of the immune response, especially following repeated administration. This may be more likely in companion animals, such as pet cats and dogs, as they tend to live longer and may receive more vaccinations in their lifetime than farm species. Awareness of immune-related diseases has become greater in recent years and these are now diagnosed in these species more frequently.

The incidence of immune-mediated disease is rare in all species, which increases the difficulty of performing epidemiological studies to investigate the concerns regarding any link with vaccination. However, current investigations into animals with immune-related disease, comparing them with the contemporary population, has not found any link between vaccination and triggering these conditions. When vaccines are given it is important to weigh the benefits of protection from debilitating or lethal diseases against the possibility of adverse effects for the vaccinated animal.

As research continues into vaccine design and efficacy and disease epidemiology, it may be possible to tailor effective vaccination programmes for the individual animal, using this research in combination with knowledge of the animal's history and likely risk profile.

Vaccines as medicinal products

In the UK, 'veterinary medicinal products', including veterinary vaccines and other medicines, are primarily classified into one of four groups: General Sales List (GSL), Pharmacy Medicines (P), Pharmacy and Merchants List (PML) and Prescription Only Medicines (POM). Veterinary vaccines are classified into the PML, POM or P categories, depending on the type and constituents of the vaccine and the species for which it is intended. Products classified as PML may be supplied by a veterinary surgeon for animals under his care or in pharmacies under the supervision of a pharmacist. They may also be supplied by an agricultural merchant registered with the Royal Pharmaceutical Society of Great Britain (RPSGB) or the Department of Agriculture Northern Ireland (DANI). Products classified as POM may only be supplied by a veterinary surgeon for animals under his care or by a pharmacist on a veterinary surgeon's prescription.

Vaccines are produced and manufactured under carefully controlled conditions to good manufacturing practice regulations. Safety, quality and efficacy must be proven before a marketing authorisation can be granted for a vaccine. A further check is kept on the vaccine's safety and efficacy in the target animal by postmarketing surveillance and periodic reporting of any suspected adverse reactions to the responsible authority where the vaccine is registered.

Careful handling and storage of vaccines is essential in order that they retain their potency. Vaccines are produced under sterile conditions, although once the product container is broached, sterility can no longer be assured. It is important that the end user takes aseptic precautions when withdrawing vaccine doses from the container and in administering vaccines by injection routes. This is particularly important where vaccines are presented in multidose containers such as for use in farmed species.

Some adjuvants, such as metallic salts (where antigen is adsorbed onto the molecule) or ISCOMs (see p. 120), depend on their physical structure or characteristics for their function. Vaccines may therefore be inactivated by physical changes that affect this structure. For example, the crystals formed when a liquid vaccine is inadvertently frozen may disrupt the antigen–adjuvant relationship and destroy its ability to elicit an immune response. The manufacturer's instructions on storage should always be strictly followed and there should be a system in place for monitoring the temperature of the rooms or refrigerators used to keep vaccines.

New developments in vaccine technology

The increasingly high cost of pharmaceuticals' development and the desire to move away from therapeutic use of antibiotics has prompted more research into vaccines. Novel immunological techniques may be developed by small biotechnology companies, either alone or in partnership with established global companies. The new technologies aim to overcome some of the adverse effects sometimes encountered with older vaccines containing high levels of antigen or adjuvants that provoke a local reaction at the injection site.

Subunit vaccines

Study of the pathogen may reveal its most important parts with respect to producing neutralising antibodies in the animal. The DNA sequence which codes for these subunits can be identified and then multiplied in culture; the resulting antigens can then be extracted for use in the vaccine. The feline leukaemia vaccines currently available for cats are subunit products.

'Gene-deleted' vaccines

Deletion of a specific sequence of DNA from the genome of the pathogen is used to reduce the pathogenicity of the organism while retaining its antigenicity and ability to replicate in the host. This technique is especially useful for bacterial pathogens, such as *Salmonella typhimurium*, and has been used to develop vaccines for poultry and cattle.

Deletion of a specific section of DNA, or gene, that codes for an antigen enables the vaccinated animal to be distinguished from one that was infected by the natural infection. This may be important where a disease-eradication programme is in place and vaccination is used to protect individuals during the eradication. This ability to distinguish vaccinated and naturally infected animals may also be useful in the control of some disease outbreaks. Vaccination is used to reduce the population of susceptible animals which can become infected and perpetuate the disease, while retaining the ability to track the pattern of natural infection. These 'marker' vaccines are available, for example, for immunisation of cattle against the respiratory disease infectious bovine rhinotracheitis.

Disabled infectious single cycle (DISC)-virus

A single gene that controls viral replication is removed from the genome. The virus is able to infect a cell but only replicate once. This produces sufficient virus to stimulate the immune response but cannot reach the levels that would cause disease in the host. A whole-virus vaccine is produced which has a safety profile similar to that of subunit vaccines, while eliciting a full immune response in the animal.

Vector vaccines

The protective antigen is inserted into a modified virus or bacterium that is harmless but can infect the host species. This has the advantage that the antigen is delivered into the target species without the need for an adjuvant. However, it is important that the virus chosen to contain the antigen does not cause disease in the target animal. Further, it must be specific for the target animal and not spread to other species. Equine herpes virus-1 is currently under investigation as a possible vector virus for use in vaccination of horses.

Other technologies

Inclusion of antigen genes into plant DNA may allow vaccination against enteric pathogens as the animal eats the plant. This would have welfare benefits for the animal in reducing morbidity associated with handling the animal and injectable vaccination. However, this is technically difficult to achieve and there are currently public concerns about the genetic modification of growing plants.

DNA itself may be used to elicit an antibody response in the animal, while reducing the risks of vaccination associated with use of live vectors. DNA is relatively robust, so production and storage of the vaccine may be made simpler, reducing costs. However, the delivery system into the cell is more difficult with this method and research is still at a relatively early stage.

The future for vaccines?

In farmed species, emphasis is moving away from therapeutic or prophylactic use of antimicrobials. 'Food safety' vaccines are likely to be used to protect animals (and therefore the consumer) against zoonotic pathogens such as *Salmonella* and *Campylobacter*.

For companion animals, investigations continue into the individual requirements for vaccinations for each animal and the limits of duration of immunity that can be produced by vaccinations given throughout life.

Vaccines have a significant role to play in keeping animals free from disease and safeguarding their welfare, so are likely to become increasingly important in the future.

Further reading

Roitt I M, Delves P J (1998). *Roitt's Essential Immunology*, 5th edn. Oxford: Blackwell Science.

Peters A, ed. (1993). *Vaccines for Veterinary Applications*. Oxford: Butterworth Heinemann.

National Office of Animal Health (2002–2003). *Compendium of Data Sheets for Veterinary Products*. Enfield: National Office of Animal Health.

National Institute of Allergy and Infectious Diseases (1998). *Understanding Vaccines*. US Dept of Health and Human Services. National Institutes of Health Publication no. 98–4219 (available from
http://www.niaid.nih.gov/publications/vaccine/pdf/undvacc.pdf).

Useful website

British Society for Immunology website at http://www.immunology.org

5

Complementary and alternative therapies

Francis Hunter and Steven B Kayne

Most complementary therapies that have been used for humans have also been tried on animals. This chapter outlines the most common disciplines in use in some detail and gives less comprehensive descriptions of others. The three complementary therapies that are most widely used on animals are acupuncture, herbal medicine and homeopathy, but for convenience the various treatments discussed in this chapter are presented in alphabetical order.

Terminology

The word 'complementary' is favoured by health professionals in preference to 'alternative' because most of the therapies can be used to good effect in conjunction with conventional or other non-conventional treatment if desired, rather than alone as implied by the term alternative. However, research has shown that there is a tendency for consumers to buy remedies over the counter instead of orthodox medicine, i.e. in an alternative way. Thus there is now a move towards the North American terminology of complementary and alternative medicine (CAM). This term will be used in this chapter.

CAM and veterinary medicine – legal status

The Veterinary Surgeon's Act 1966 states, subject to a number of exceptions, that only registered members of the Royal College of Veterinary Surgeons (RCVS) can practise veterinary surgery in the UK.

Veterinary surgery is defined as:

> '... encompassing the art and science of veterinary surgery and medicine which includes the diagnosis of diseases and injuries in animals, tests performed on animals for diagnostic purposes, advice based upon a diagnosis ...'

The exceptions include:

- Veterinary students and veterinary nurses – governed by various amendments to the Veterinary Surgeons Act.
- Farriers – whilst farriers have their own Farriers Registration Acts they are also governed by the Veterinary Surgeons Act and are not allowed to perform acts of veterinary surgery.

The other exceptions (including CAM) are governed by an order that was introduced to amend the Veterinary Surgeons Act to take such legitimate therapies into account. As far as complementary therapies are concerned, this order refers to four categories:

- Manipulative therapies. This covers only physiotherapy, osteopathy and chiropractic and allows these therapies where a vet has diagnosed the condition and decided that this treatment would be appropriate.
- Animal behaviourism. Behavioural treatment is exempt, unless medication is used where permission must again be sought from the vet.
- Faith healing. According to the RCVS *Guide to Professional Conduct*, faith healers have their own code of practice which indicates that permission must be sought from a vet before healing is given by the 'laying on of hands'.
- Other complementary therapies.

According to the RCVS:

> 'It is illegal, in terms of the Veterinary Surgeons Act 1966, for lay practitioners, however qualified in the human field, to treat animals. At the same time it is incumbent on veterinary surgeons offering any complementary therapy to ensure that they are adequately trained in its application.'

Thus, apart from the manipulative therapies, behavioural treatment and faith healing, all other forms of complementary therapy are illegal in the treatment of animals in the UK when practised by non-vets.

Acupuncture

Introduction

Veterinary acupuncture is one part of traditional Chinese medicine (the other being Chinese herbal medicine) and can be traced back over 3000 years, having developed from observations made by veterinarians in ancient China. They discovered that pain could be relieved by applying digital pressure to particular places on animals' bodies and this technique, known as acupressure, is still practised today. In Europe the first veterinary schools taught acupuncture until early in the 19th century, but with the advance of veterinary medicine it was gradually dropped from the curriculum. Veterinary acupuncture has enjoyed a resurgence during the last 30–40 years in parallel with its increased medical use.

Theory

This philosophy of Chinese medicine is very different from that of Western medicine, but it is important to realise that it is just as rational and produces excellent results at considerably less expense!

Yin and Yang

Chinese acupuncture is based on the observation that everything in the world is in a state of perpetual change. Additionally, this change is in a state of balance, which in turn leads to the concept of Yin and Yang. The theory of Yin and Yang maintains that everything has two aspects and these are at the same time both opposite and interdependent. The ancient Chinese symbolised water as Yin and is anything that is dim, cold, hypoactive, static and substantive, while fire is Yang and is bright, hot, hyperactive, moving and non-substantive. The properties of Yin and Yang are not absolute but relative and neither can exist in isolation. These two opposites are in constant motion, not stationary, and in terms of the circadian rhythm Yin is night and Yang is day. It follows that as night (Yin) fades it becomes day (Yang) and as Yang fades it becomes Yin. Yin and Yang are therefore both changing into each other and at the same time balancing each other. Two other terms are often referred to in Chinese medicine, 'Xu' and 'Shi', in connection with illness and disease. Xu in its broadest sense means a deficiency and Shi an excess. These in turn are related to the basic principle of Yin and Yang.

The organs

In the concept of Chinese medicine there are 14 main meridians or channels linking the organs. The organs of the body are divided into two systems: the Zang (solid) and Fu (hollow) organs. The Zang organs are the heart, liver, spleen, lung, kidney and pericardium. These are only representations of the various organs when related to Western medicine and therefore the heart controls the circulation of the blood and keeps the 'mind' in good order by supplying the brain with oxygen, thus regulating normal mentality, memory and sleep; the liver stores blood and governs the 'free flowing' of blood and 'Qi' (see below) through the body. The spleen regulates the digestive process, the lung is connected to skin disease and the kidney with the genital rather than the urinary system. The Fu organs are very similar in their function to the organs of the same name in Western medicine. They are the small intestine, the gall bladder, the stomach, the large intestine and the urinary bladder.

Qi

Qi, pronounced 'chi', is a form of energy. It is a fundamental concept of Chinese thought and does not have a corresponding ideal in Western medicine. Qi relates to the manifestation of any invisible force. The growth of a plant, the movement of a leg or arm or even a heavy thunderstorm can be called Qi. Qi, together with blood and body fluids, sustains the vital activities and also nourishes the body, keeping the various organs and tissues in good working order. It follows therefore that a dead body or organ has no Qi. If the internal balance of Yin and Yang is upset then the vital energy or Qi, which 'travels' along the meridians, is also disturbed. This is then corrected by inserting needles in the appropriate place to restore normal Qi. Pathogens are often seen as being related to the elements; heat corresponds to infection and cold to longstanding or chronic conditions. Wind indicates the changeability of symptoms, such as twitchings and spasms and symptoms that wander about the body, while damp is 'sticky' and 'greasy' and is illustrated by conditions such as indigestion.

Diagnosis

Two important aids to diagnosis in traditional Chinese medicine are the tongue and the pulse. The outer thin, red edge to the tongue and also the colour and nature of the coating of the tongue are significant in making a diagnosis. An experienced Chinese physician is able to recognise 12 different pulses at the wrist, corresponding to 12 of the 14 main meridians.

Law of the five elements

It is also necessary to mention the law of the five elements, which completes the philosophy of traditional Chinese medicine. This is an intricate and interesting subject in itself and too complex to expand upon in this chapter. It comprises the five elements: fire, earth, metal (which is air in the Western tradition), water and wood, and their influence on each other in promotion and control.

Veterinary application of acupuncture

Acupuncture may be carried out on any species but in practice is used most often on dogs and horses and to some extent on other large animals and cats (see Figures 5.1 and 5.2).

The various points on the channels (meridians) may be used to control pain and it is now thought that activating different and predetermined points, depending on the condition being treated, releases endorphins and other natural body chemicals. 'Needling', as the insertion of the acupuncture needles is often called, produces at the acupuncture point a warm, tingling effect in humans, which presumably also occurs in animals. Interestingly, although the Chinese did not know it, the electrical resistance of the skin is lower over an acupuncture point than it is over the rest of the skin and therefore the various points can be located electrically.

Initially it is usual to carry out three to four sessions of about 20–30 minutes, a week apart. If there is no improvement in that time it is unlikely that acupuncture is going to help the patient. Animals with chronic problems that respond to treatment are likely to need 'top-up' sessions at different time intervals varying from 3–4 weeks to 2–3 months or longer depending on the results achieved.

Animals suffering from acute conditions possibly need daily treatment for a few days to begin with. Electroacupuncture, which involves passing a low current down some of the needles, thus stimulating the whole channel, has become quite popular and is effective. In addition to the recognised points it can also be effective to stimulate tender spots known as Ah shi points.

Ear acupuncture is another fascinating aspect of this type of therapy, although it is not much used in animals. The human ear resembles the unborn baby lying upside down in the womb with the lobe corresponding to the head and the top of the pinna the hands and feet. This association between the ear and the rest of the body has been verified (see Case study 5.1).

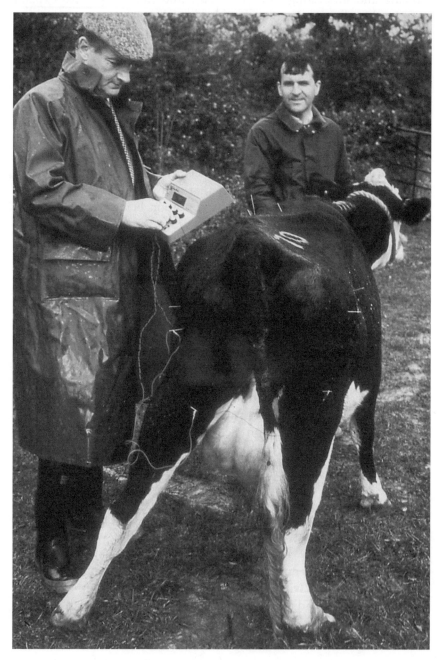

Figure 5.1 Application of acupuncture on a cow. (Courtesy of F Hunter.)

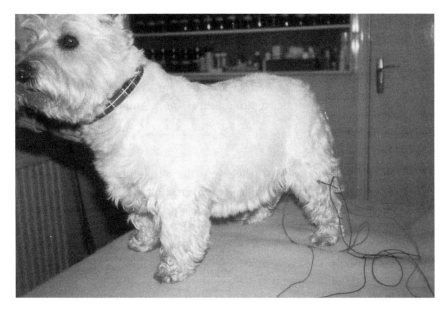

Figure 5.2   Application of acupuncture on a dog. (Courtesy of F Hunter.)

   CASE STUDY

Case study 5.1
A labrador dog, although only 6.5 years old, was presented with chronic and painful arthritis and rheumatism. All conventional treatment caused vomiting and other side-effects. Over the next 7 years the dog had more than 100 sessions of acupuncture, to which it responded extremely well. The dog eventually died at 13 years of age from kidney failure.

Aromatherapy

Introduction

Aromatherapy, the use of aromatic or essential oils, as a form of treatment has existed for hundreds of years. When Tutankhamun's tomb was opened in 1922 many scent pots were discovered showing that frankincense and myrrh were used by the Egyptians as long ago as 1300 BC. The Greeks used plant oils to heal wounds and the early Romans also relied on essential oils to assist healing. In Britain, records show that plant essences were employed as medicines in the Middle Ages and were also popular in the 18th and 19th centuries. They began to go out of favour in the last century as modern, more powerful and faster-acting drugs were developed. In recent years, however, aromatherapy has seen a revival and has become once again a useful and popular form of therapy.

Essential oils

The essences (essential oils), rather than the whole plant, are utilised in the preparation of different oils. There are around 400 different oils available and about 80 of these are frequently used. The oils are extracted from different parts of the plant. For instance, ginger and angelica come from the roots; bay and marjoram from the leaves; lavender and origanum from the flowering tops; nutmeg and parsley from the seeds; camphor and frankincense from the bark; and lemongrass and peppermint from the whole plant. Each oil has a complex structure and the components are made up from different constituents such as acids (cinnamon), aldehydes (citronella), alcohols (menthol) and phenols (thymol). They have an intricate composition which makes it impossible to reproduce them in the laboratory. Eucalyptus, for example, contains around 250 different constituents. There are various methods of extracting the oils, depending on their source, and these include distillation and solvent extraction. Different oils require diluting in different ways and with various carriers such as grape oil, sweet almond oil, olive oil and wheatgerm oil. The oils all have antiseptic properties; in addition some have analgesic, antibacterial, or diuretic properties.

Use of aromatherapy

Aromatherapy can be used in four main ways:

1. The oils can be applied locally to wounds as healing agents. For example, lavender oil.
2. The oils can be massaged into the skin to relieve the discomfort and/or pain of sprains and strains and also to generally relax the patient. In addition they can be used in baths or as compresses, for example wintergreen oil.
3. They can be employed as inhalants to relieve and prevent chronic chest and respiratory problems, for example eucalyptus oil.
4. They can be used as mouthwashes or taken internally in the same way as herbal medicine. Examples include: mouthwash, lemon or tea tree oil. Orally: carrot seed oil for liver disorders, and garlic oil to assist in combating infection.

Aromatherapy in veterinary practice

Aromatherapy can be used on any animal but in practice it is probably most commonly used on dogs and horses.

Chiropractic

Introduction

Chiropractors, with the skill of their hands, endeavour to correct and improve disorders of the spine and also those in joints and muscles. Misalignments of the spine can cause pain in other parts of the body and not just in the spine itself. The pain may manifest itself in the shoulder, arm, hip or leg, possibly bringing on conditions such as lumbago and sciatica. Chiropractic is in some ways similar to osteopathy but makes more use of X-rays and conventional methods of diagnosis. Most chiropractors have their own X-ray apparatus. The art of chiropractic was developed by a Canadian, Dr Daniel David Palmer in 1895, who cured deafness in a patient, following a slight accident, by manipulating the bones (vertebrae) in the neck. The techniques of chiropractic in fact go right back to Ancient Egypt where manipulative treatments were described in early manuscripts. They were also used in early times by the Hindus and Chinese.

Using chiropractic

Chiropractors usually work by rotating the upper spine in one direction and the lower in the other. This partially locks the joint and then the practitioner with the use of his hand exerts slight pressure on the affected joint, followed by a sharp thrust to the vertebra. This helps to restore normal movement in the joint. The procedure should not be painful if done skilfully.

Veterinary application of chiropractic

Chiropractors are mostly involved in treating working horses, racing greyhounds and pet animals. Chiropractic has been used more extensively in recent years for treating ongoing, often chronic, conditions of the neck and back, which are causing pain either in the spine itself or in other parts of the body.

Flower remedy therapy

Introduction

Flower remedies fall in between herbalism and homeopathy not really belonging to either therapy. There is a wide range of flower remedies of which the variant known as Bach flower remedies are the most widely used in the UK. Bach flower remedies (pronounced 'Batch') were discovered by the medical practitioner Dr Edward Bach, who was born in September 1886. He qualified in 1913 and in 1919 was appointed to the Royal London Homeopathic Hospital as a pathologist and bacteriologist. In 1930 he moved to Wales where he studied in detail plants and wild flowers. His work led to the discovery of 19 remedies. A further 19 were developed when he moved to Sotwell near Wallingford in Oxfordshire and set up the 'Bach Centre' in his home 'Mount Vernon', which still exists today. Of these remedies, 37 are derived from plants, trees or bushes (most, but not all indigenous to the British Isles); the 38th is prepared from pure spring water. The remedies do not work on physical symptoms but act on states of mind that are out of balance.

Preparation

Bach flower remedies divide into two categories according to their method of preparation, which take place in three stages: (1) making of the mother tincture, (2) making up the stock bottle, and (3) making up the treatment bottle.

Stage 1

The 'sun' method is used for flowers blooming in the late spring and summer when the sun is at its hottest. The different flowers for each remedy should be picked at about 9.00 am, because the sun is gaining in power during the 3 hours before 9.00 am. The picked flower heads are then placed in a sterilised bowl of pure water and left in the hot sun for 3 hours. At the end of this time the flower heads are removed without touching the liquid with the fingers (a stalk of the chosen flower is often used). The mother tincture consists of a 30 mL bottle half filled with brandy (grape alcohol is now used as the preservative) and half with the flower liquid.

The 'boiling' method is used for flowers, bushes, plants and the twigs of trees, which bloom early in the year before there is much sunshine. The gathered leaves and twigs are boiled for half an hour in bottled mineral or pure spring water. After cooling, the material is taken out (as above in the sun method) and the resultant liquid is filtered to remove any sediment. The mother tincture is then made up in a 30 mL bottle half filled with grape alcohol, as in the sun method.

Stage 2

The stock bottle is prepared by adding two drops of mother tincture to a sterilised 30 mL bottle filled with grape alcohol. The remedies may be used singly or in combination.

Stage 3

To make a treatment bottle two drops of each remedy are placed in a sterilised 30 mL bottle of pure water with a little grape alcohol added as a preservative.

The veterinary use of Bach flower remedies

These are used by some practitioners to deal with emotional problems in all species, but particularly in highly bred, sensitive, horses and dogs. The most popular remedy used in many veterinary practices is the 'rescue or recovery remedy'. Rescue remedy is a combination of five remedies: (1) cherry plum for general fear (not being able to cope with 'shows', etc.); (2) clematis for unconsciousness and 'detached' sensations; (3) impatiens for nervous irritation, anger and agitation; (4) rock rose for sheer terror and panic; and (5) star-of-Bethlehem for the after-effects of shock and/or trauma. It is very useful for treating shock after any accident or injury – for reviving weakly and 'fading' calves, lambs and puppies – and also pre- and postoperatively.

Herbalism

Introduction

Herbal medicine must be one of the oldest forms of therapy to be used in humans and animals. Today about 80% or more of the world's population still base their medicine on the use of extracts from plants, and many modern drugs were originally developed from plants. The Chinese had extensive pharmacopoeias in 3000 BC. Herbal medicine in early times was very much linked with myth, magic and even religion. The growth of the use of herbal remedies coincided with the development of printing presses by William Caxton in the 15th century. Before that time books on herbal medicines were written laboriously by hand, making them often difficult to access by the relatively few people who could read. It was Nicholas Culpeper's *The English Physician Enlarged* published in 1649 and *The Complete Herbal* published in 1653 that really established herbal medicine and made it widely available. Advances in navigation also played a part in spreading herbal remedies, as the knowledge of the medicinal use of herbs in different parts of the world could be integrated and combined. The use of herbal medicine was at its height in the early 1800s when Henry Potter set up his firm in London and produced his *Potter's Cyclopaedia of Botanical Drugs and Preparations*. Herbal medicine was largely superseded by the scientifically based drugs developed during the late 19th and 20th centuries.

Problems with herbal remedies

Worries about the side-effects of many modern medicines have led to herbal medicine becoming more widely used, the popular belief being that they are a safer option. However, this assumption is far from true and some herbal remedies have proved to be dangerous for a variety of reasons. Some herbs, e.g. *Symphytum* (knitbone) and *Aristolochia* have been withdrawn from sale because of intrinsic toxicity, while warnings about interactions with concurrent use of others (e.g. St John's wort) have been circulated. Another problem with herbal medicine is that it is difficult to standardise the various plants.

Classification

Herbal medicines may be classified into three main groups according to their action on the patient:

1. Herbs, such as senna, which invoke the body to produce a response, in this case purgation.
2. Herbs like hawthorn that act as supportive agents and balance organ systems, such as the circulatory system, aiding blood flow and pressure.
3. Plants such as dandelion that help to rid the body of toxins and can be beneficial in cases of arthritis and dermatitis.

Herbs often produce their best effects when several are combined and skill is required to select the correct mixture.

Herbal medicines can be further divided into groups according to their specific action, bearing in mind that many have more than one effect on the body:

- Anti-inflammatory properties acting on arthritic joints, chronic bowel conditions, e.g. colitis, and some skin conditions.
- Antimicrobial properties assisting the body's immune system to fight infections. Garlic, echinacea and myrrh all produce this effect.
- Herbal diuretics: dandelion and buchu act upon the kidneys in cases of renal failure and also promote the production of urine and the excretion of waste products and toxins.
- Expectorant herbs: these usually affect the respiratory system. Some act by irritating the mucosa lining the respiratory tract and others like marsh mallow and liquorice have a soothing action, while elderflower and garlic combine both functions.
- Hepatics: gentian for instance helps to increase the flow of bile and other digestive juices, and berberis can be useful for treating chronic liver conditions.
- Nervines: as the name suggests nervines act on the nervous system and a mixture of skullcap and valerian is widely used as a sedative in veterinary practice.
- Other groups include anticatarrhal herbs such as elder for sinusitis, antilithics like parsley to help to prevent and remove urinary gravel and even small bladder stones; astringents to assist wound healing; demulcents containing mucilage have a soothing action in chronic cases of bronchitis, cystitis and digestive conditions; and vulneraries like marigold or burdock which assist wounds to heal both externally and internally.

Herbal applications in veterinary practice

Herbal medicine is quite widely used in practice and is an expanding discipline, especially in the companion animal field. It is necessary to take great care when using it for farm animals, because of the danger of residues and the possible tainting of meat, milk and eggs.

Topical preparations, particularly ointments, are useful in sprains and strains and in the treatment of bruising where arnica is effective.

Because of the possibility of toxic side-effects or poisoning from incorrect dosing, it is important that herbs used singly or in combination should be prescribed by experienced practitioners.

Homeopathy

Introduction

Homeopathy is probably the most widely applied form of the complementary therapies used in veterinary practice. The word homeopathy comes from two Greek words: 'homeos' meaning like and 'pathos' meaning suffering. The main principle of homeopathic medicine 'Similia similibus curantur' translated as 'Let likes be cured by likes' goes back to the time of Hippocrates. However, the founder of modern homeopathy was Samuel Christian Hahnemann, a German physician, philosopher and linguist who lived from 1755 to 1843. He discovered the concept of homeopathy when translating a materia medica by the Scottish physician William Cullen from English into German. Hahnemann disagreed with a theory in Cullen's writing and set about trying to prove this difference of opinion by experimenting on himself. Initially he made himself ill by taking doses of cinchona bark (quinine). He found that the drug produced symptoms very similar to those of marsh fever (as malaria was called at that time). He then relieved the condition by taking minute doses of the same substance that caused his discomfort.

Source material

A homeopathic medicine can be made from any natural source – animal, vegetable or mineral – and also from synthetic substances. Examples include:

- Animal: *Apis mellifica* (honeybee), lachesis (from snake venom), sepia (from the ink of the cuttlefish).
- Vegetable: belladonna (deadly nightshade), pulsatilla (windflower).
- Mineral: silicea (sand or granite), phosphorus, mercury.
- Isopathics: A miscellaneous group of source materials including tautopathic remedies (prepared from drugs and toxic chemicals, such as pesticides, and used to counter any ill- or side-effects caused by these substances), allergodes (prepared from allergens for example grass pollens or animal fur) and nosodes ((Greek nosos – disease) prepared from diseased tissues, organisms or the products of disease (pus for instance) and sarcodes which are prepared from healthy tissue (bacterial cultures or natural secretions)). Nosodes and sarcodes are sometimes administered prophylactically by veterinary surgeons and are inaccurately referred to as 'vaccines'. They are not vaccines in the accepted orthodox terminology and should not be labelled as such (see chapter 4).

About 60% of homeopathic medicines are made from plants, many of which are highly toxic. Homeopathy should not be confused with herbalism which is quite different. Herbalism uses many different plants with curative properties in material amounts. This means that there must be no measurable residues or odours remaining in milk for example, after treatment. Homeopathic medicine on the other hand uses minute amounts of a substance to promote healing and leaves very little or no residue at all.

Mode of action

The exact way in which homeopathic remedies work is still not fully understood but it seems that there is a form of 'energy' produced in the making of a homeopathic medicine (see below), which sets up a reaction in the patient that in turn brings about relief from symptoms. Consequently the number of times that a medicine is taken is significant, but the size of the dose is not important. In fact it is the same for an elephant, a person or a mouse.

Preparation of remedies

Starting solution

The raw material must first be converted into a soluble form. Solids that are naturally insoluble are first made into 'colloidal' states by 'trituration' and dilution with lactose powder until the third dilution is reached. Trituration involves grinding 1 part of the raw material with 99 parts of pure lactose, using a pestle and mortar, to produce the 1c potency. This is then diluted further (see below) to obtain the 3c potency. The resultant product is then dissolved in a water/alcohol mixture. For some higher potencies a saturated solution is needed to prepare the remedy.

Mother tincture

Vegetable material is first infused in a mixture of alcohol and pure water for varying lengths of time, depending upon the nature of the source material (roots, leaves, buds), and in accordance with the instructions laid down in a homeopathic pharmacopoeia. In the UK, the German pharmacopoeia is used widely for this purpose. The filtrate that results from the infusion is called a mother tincture.

Potentisation

The mother tincture (or the triturate 3c solution) is then diluted and shaken in a special way, known as succussion, to make the various potencies or strengths. One drop of the mother tincture is mixed with 99 drops of an alcohol/water solvent and succussed usually with the aid of a mechanical agitator, although some pharmacies still carry out the process manually. The resulting solution is said to be at the first potency, designated as '1c'. One drop of this potency is then mixed with a further 99 drops of water and succussed to form the second potency 2c. This process is repeated until the various potencies that are in common use are produced. There is another scale known as decimal or 'x' in which the dilution process is on a 1 + 9 parts of diluent scale.

The difficult concept to accept is that the more the preparation is diluted and succussed the greater its power, strength or potency becomes. Dilution without succussion does not produce the same effect. It seems that it is the succussion at each stage of dilution, which results in the production of the energy, that achieves the desired effect and cures or relieves the disease or condition suffered by the patient. The other concept that has to be accepted, if the principles of homeopathy themselves are valid, is that after a certain dilution (Avagadro's limit) is reached there is no active molecule of the original substance detectable by analysis; only an 'imprint' or 'energy' remains in the diluent.

Dose form

There is a whole range of oral and topical formulations. While many animal owners do not have difficulties in administering tablets or pills, granules (that can be added to food as well as placed on the tongue) and liquid forms (that can be placed in the drinking water facilitating re-dosing by the animal) are particularly popular.

Legal classification of remedies

Almost all homeopathic remedies are classified as general sales list (GSL) in the UK and may be sold without restriction in a wide range of retail outlets. Exceptions include very low potencies of traditional poisons (e.g. aconite and belladonna) that would have little if no use in homoeopathy, and certain formulations, such as eye drops and injections, that are presently unlicensed. It is appropriate to exert some voluntary control when certain nosodes are being used as veterinary 'vaccines' (see above) without veterinary supervision. Homeopathic veterinary remedies may be registered under the European Directive in the same way as human medicines are, but so far no manufacturer has chosen to do so. Ranges of homeopathic medicines labelled for veterinary use are sold.

Uses of homeopathy

Homeopathic treatment may be divided into four main categories:

1. First aid: there are a number of useful remedies for treating simple wounds, accidents and conditions, such as coughs, colds, sore throats etc. (arnica is extremely effective for treating bruising, stiffness and pain following a minor trauma).

2. Organ or system prescribing: certain remedies have an affinity with particular organs in the body. For instance *Crataegus* (hawthorn) acts on the heart and circulatory system, *Chelidonium* (celandine) on the liver and *Berberis vulgaris* (berberry) on the kidneys and urinary system.

3. Pathological prescribing: some medicines have a beneficial effect in different specific diseases and conditions. For instance *Cocculus* (Indian cockle) helps to prevent travel sickness and jet lag, *Colocynth* (bitter cucumber) is often very effective in treating the symptoms of colic and *Arsenicum album* (white arsenic) is excellent for treating vomiting and diarrhoea.

4. Constitutional prescribing: in these cases a remedy is selected to match as nearly as possible a whole range of the patient's symptoms, both mental and physical. There is usually some empathy between the remedy and the patient's character or appearance. For example, patients with a phosphorus constitution very often have red hair and 'fly off the handle' (i.e. explode) spontaneously. The chosen medicine affects all the systems of the body and the mind. The symptoms in such cases can be both subjective and objective and the treatment is therefore 'holistic' in nature. *Lycopodium* (club moss) and *Pulsatilla* (the windflower) are other examples of constitutional medicines.

Veterinary applications of homeopathy

Homeopathy is a very versatile form of treatment and may be used to good effect on any species of animal. Horses as a species, for instance, appear to respond particularly well to homeopathic treatment. Traditionally, homeopathic medicines have been given orally and are thought to be absorbed through the mucous membrane of the mouth. Some work almost at once and have hardly had time to enter the blood stream – aconite in cases of acute shock for instance. They also work well given by subcutaneous injection and *per vaginum* in cattle with reproductive problems for example. On the farm the medicines can be used for mass medication of the flock or herd by placing the medicine in the drinking water. Mastitis and ringworm may be treated in this way.

Chronic conditions, such as arthritis or rheumatism and sinusitis and coughs, will often improve following treatment. There are no detectable residues in milk or eggs, so farm animals can be treated safely. Mastitis can be treated or prevented in milking cows by the use of nosodes (see above). Dogs, cats, birds, fish and the more unusual animals, such as tortoises and lizards, all have responded to homeopathic treatment.

It is also possible to use constitutional prescribing in animals (see Case study 5.2).

 CASE STUDY

Case study 5.2

- A riding horse that had been lame on and off for 8–9 months appeared to have a deep-seated infection in the foot. A course of treatment with the remedy silica (sand or quartz) induced a deep abscess to 'point' to the surface, burst and discharge pus and then heal over, so that the animal became sound again.
- A dog with sinusitis, a constant nasal discharge and cough over a period of 2–3 years, was referred for treatment after a visit to a veterinary teaching hospital had produced a poor response. Constitutional prescribing of the remedy pulsatilla gradually improved the condition over a 3-month course of treatment.
- A parrot with persistent enteritis and diarrhoea failed to respond to conventional medicine, but cleared up in 3–4 weeks after treatment with mercurius (liquid mercury).

It is safe to use homeopathy at a first aid level for animals. It is important to realise that if there is no noticeable improvement after a few hours, or if the animal is perceived to be in distress, that professional assistance should be sought.

Veterinary homeopathy and the pharmacist

There is an increasing demand from the public for homeopathic medicines to treat animals. Under the Veterinary Surgeons Act 1966, diagnosis and treatment of animals is restricted to veterinarians and owners and this applies to homeopathy too. An illustration of the potential problems that can occur is provided by pharmacists' involvement in supplying borax to farmers during a foot-and-mouth disease epidemic (see Box 5.1).

Box 5.1   Homeopathic borax and foot-and-mouth disease

In the first quarter of 2001 the UK was in the grip of a major epidemic of foot-and-mouth disease with hundreds of thousands of animals being slaughtered throughout the country. The disease started at a pig farm in north-east England and spread quickly throughout the country. Farmers desperate to provide protection for their animals from foot-and-mouth disease turned to homeopathy for help, placing extreme pressure on many pharmacies to supply them with the appropriate remedy. Demand for the remedy – borax 30c – increased rapidly as the knowledge of its existence spread amongst the farming community. There was some anecdotal evidence of its beneficial use during the last foot-and-mouth epidemic to hit the UK in the 1960s but the Faculty of Homeopathy, the governing body for medical and veterinary homeopathy, felt that this was insufficient to claim its effectiveness in preventing the disease.

The eradication scheme being followed by the government relied on a wholly susceptible animal population in order to be able to detect the disease signs promptly. According to Chris Day, Veterinary Dean to the Faculty, the danger of using any potentially prophylactic medicine was that, if it had been effective, it may have rendered the animals unsusceptible. This could theoretically have resulted in animals being able to harbour the virus and to shed it while remaining symptom-free themselves. It is recommended that pharmacists direct enquiries for homeopathic borax to a suitably qualified veterinary surgeon.

Massage

Massage can be used on its own or in conjunction with oils as in aromatherapy or together with herbal medicine. Massage relaxes tense and injured muscles and increases the flow of both blood and lymph to the affected tissues. It can also assist in the healing of pulled, sprained or strained ligaments and tendons. In addition, damaged joints may benefit from massage. When used with essential oils, liniments and lotions it can help to reduce stress-related symptoms and pain.

Massage is best carried out using the whole palm of each hand, not only the fingers, although the pads of both fingers and thumbs are useful for some movements.

There are three basic strokes:

1.   Effleurage: these are long, smooth strokes and it is recommended that they are used at the beginning and end of a session, also between other movements.

The pressure may be variable and deep pressure is used to assist in directing the blood as it flows back to the heart. Lighter, gliding strokes are used when massaging away from the heart and over other parts of the body.

2. Kneading: this involves using the palms, the lengths of the fingers and/or the pads of both fingers and thumbs. Kneading helps to break down tense muscles that are in spasm and also to stimulate the circulation to an affected area. Both hands are used alternately and rhythmically and one hand or the other is constantly in contact with the skin producing the kneading effect. Knuckling is a variation of kneading and the fingers are turned in allowing the knuckles to be used. It may be employed to good effect in the region of the chest and neck.

3. Friction: friction strokes are used to reach deep muscle tissue and this involves using the heel of the hands and/or the finger and thumb pads. Knotted muscles and pain nodules can be broken down by firm thumb pressure. The movements may be circular to promote maximum pressure over an area. It is advisable not to use friction when there is sciatic pain as this can irritate the nerve further.

Veterinary application of massage

Massage may be used to benefit any species of animal. In practice it is used most widely on animals that are used for performance. This includes racehorses, show jumpers, point-to-pointers, racing greyhounds and working and agility dogs. In acute cases massage may be carried out 2–3 times daily and once the condition has improved the sessions can be gradually reduced to every 2 or 3 days and then to weekly as required.

A practitioner trained to work on animals or somebody who has received specific training for a given set of circumstances should carry out massage on animals.

Osteopathy

Introduction

Osteopathy was pioneered in the USA by Dr Andrew Still in the 1880s and 90s. He became disillusioned with the form of medicine practised at that time and began with the premise that the skeleton was not just the physical framework to which muscles and other tissues were attached, but that it was also concerned with the normal functions of life, as well as being a protective covering for the brain and spinal cord. Dr Still named this form of therapy osteopathy from the Greek words 'osteon' meaning bone and 'pathos' meaning disease. He believed that disease represented an upset of the balance of the biochemistry, psychology and structure of the body. Dr Still soon demonstrated that many diseases were related to disorders of the spine and that non-bony conditions were improved by the manipulation of different parts of the body. This is a system of therapy that uses the manipulation of the spine and other parts of the body to restore the patient to a state of natural health. In addition, it is a holistic form of treatment that involves the detailed history-taking of the case and careful observation of the stance and movement of the animal to be treated.

Method of treatment

Osteopathy involves gentle manipulation of the various joints in the body, in addition to the spinal column, and easing tension that has built up in the surrounding muscles, ligaments and tendons. The 'cracking' and 'popping' noises often heard during a session of osteopathy are nothing to do with joints going in and out of place as is commonly thought. Joints contain lubrication in the form of synovial fluid which is under a partial vacuum. This means that the pressure in the joint capsule is slightly lower than the surrounding atmospheric pressure. As manipulation takes place the surfaces of the joints are separated a little and the pressure in the joint capsule is disturbed slightly. This allows thousands of very tiny bubbles of gas (carbon dioxide) to come out of solution causing the 'cracking' sound. This can be likened to the 'fizzing' sound when the top of a bottle of sparkling drink is opened after shaking it.

Veterinary application of osteopathy

Osteopathy is used mainly to treat injuries in 'working' animals, such as racehorses, greyhounds and other dogs used for sporting purposes. It can also be used to good effect in other animals with back and disc lesions including slipped discs. Osteopathy should only be carried out by trained practitioners.

Physiotherapy

Introduction

Physiotherapists play an essential role in helping people and animals achieve and maintain healthy and functioning bodies. Using exercise, manual and electrotherapeutic techniques they assess, treat and prevent a vast range of injuries and bodily dysfunction.

Veterinary application of physiotherapy

Physiotherapy on animals is a growing discipline. Sir Charles Strong was the first chartered physiotherapist to initiate a group working on animals in 1939. An association of Animal Complementary Therapists was officially formed in 1985, and recognised by the Royal College of Veterinary Surgeons, for fully qualified members to treat animals referred by a veterinary surgeon.

Examination

Before treatment can start it is necessary to examine the animal carefully by observation and assessment, taking note of skeletal and soft tissue symmetry and any discernible asymmetry. When examining horses prior to physiotherapy it is important to view them from above. Hence, it is necessary to stand on a box or chair to get a good perspective. If the animal is not too lame it is a good idea to watch the animal walk, trot and moving freely, to see if the action is smooth and symmetrical. When treating horses that are ridden it is important to examine the saddle carefully and also watch the horse in action with a rider on its back. A poor-fitting saddle can affect the spinal reflexes and also cause painful bruising of the soft tissues beneath it.

Any response or reaction to palpation indicating painful areas and tissues is important in assessing the treatment necessary for each patient.

Treatment

There are three main types of therapy for animals:

1. Manual therapy may include mobilisation and manipulation techniques and also a certain amount of traction.
2. Electrotherapy techniques may include laser, ultrasound or neuromuscular stimulation.
3. Hydrotherapy has gained popularity in recent years and is used for both horses (mainly racehorses and other event animals) and working dogs, and often for pets too. The pools in which the animals are immersed are often monitored by both under- and over-water cameras. In many cases it is necessary for the therapist to get into the pool with the animal. The pool should always be maintained at a temperature of 25–30 °C. Hydrotherapy is a part of physiotherapy and is best used alongside it, rather than on its own.

Uses

- Horses – spinal-related malfunctions such as an asymmetrical pelvis causing pain on movement, tendon and/or ligament strains and lesions. It is also useful to treat degenerative joint lesions with inflammatory changes.
- Dogs – lumbar spondylosis, hip dysplasia, knee injuries and other related inflammatory problems.
- Physiotherapy can be useful in all species both pre- and postoperatively, thus reducing dependence on drugs and other anti-inflammatory medicines.

Physiotherapy should only be carried out on animals by a qualified animal physiotherapist.

Radionics

Introduction

Radionics is concerned with the patterns of energy that exist within the body in both health and disease. It is therefore connected with the other forms of healing that utilise energy as their means of action. These include acupuncture, homeopathy, gem therapy and reflexology. Work in the field of quantum physics and mechanics has established that all living beings consist of and are surrounded by electromagnetic and other force fields, which vary with the condition of the individual, and which can be influenced by the application of other patterns of energy. Radionics utilises the discipline of radiesthesia which uses a pendulum as an aid to diagnosis. It has the advantage of being non-intrusive and the information gained is then subject to the clinical judgement of the practitioner. The term derives from Latin and Greek and literally translates as 'perceiving the emission of rays'.

Veterinary application of radionics

Radionics can be used on any species of animal but requires a skilled practitioner.

The editors acknowledge the assistance of John Saxton MRCVS VetFFHom in contributing this section (personal communication, 2002).

Concluding remarks

Almost every type of complementary treatment that has been used on humans, including faith healing, has been tried on animals. Some have been more successful than others and have become both feasible and useful forms of therapy. Such types of treatment are particularly useful when conventional medicine has evoked little or no response. Another reason for using CAM is in chronic, long-standing conditions where the animal has suffered side-effects from the prolonged use of ordinary drugs, or is likely to do so.

Further reading

Couzens T (1999). Bach flower remedies and the treatment of behaviour problems. *Br Holist Vet J* 1: 25–30.

Couzens T (1999). Herbal medicine: using plant based medicines in veterinary practice *Br Holist Vet J* 1: 15–18.

Hamilton D (1999). *Homeopathic Care for Cats and Dogs*. Berkeley: North Atlantic Books.

Hopkins C (1996). *Principles of Aromatherapy*. Wellingborough: Thorsons.

Hunter F (1988). *Homeopathic First Aid Treatment for Pets*. Wellingborough: Thorsons.

Hunter F (2002). *Everyday Homeopathy for Animals*. Beaconsfield: Beaconsfield Publishers.

Hunter F, Kayne S B (1997). *People are Pets*. London: British Homeopathic Association.

Ingraham C (2002). Equine aromatherapy notes. *Br Holist Vet J* 1: 25–39.

Kayne S B (1997). *Homeopathic Pharmacy. An Introduction and Handbook*. Edinburgh: Churchill Livingstone.

Kayne S B (2002). *Complementary Therapies for Pharmacists*. London: Pharmaceutical Press.

Lewith GT, Lewith NR (1983). Modern Chinese Acupuncture. Wellingborough: Thorsons.

Mann F (2000). *Acupuncture*, 2nd edn. London: Pan Books (William Heinemann Books Ltd).

Martin J (2000). Animal physiotherapy: in touch. *J Organis Chart Physiother Priv Pract* 3: 20–24.

Price S (1991). *Aromatherapy for Common Ailments*. London: Gaia Books.

Standler S (1989). *New Ways to Health – A Guide to Osteopathy*. London: The Hamlyn Publishing Group.

Saxton J (1999). Pure energy medicine – radionics and pranamonics. *Br Holist Vet J* 1: 14–16.

Stanway A (1986). *Alternative Medicine – A Guide to Natural Therapies*. London: Chancellor Press.

Weeks N, Victor Bullen V (1990). *Bach Flower Remedies*. Saffron Walden: CW Daniel.

6

Legal requirements for the sale and supply of veterinary medicinal products

Gordon Appelbe

The primary source for the control and distribution of veterinary medicinal products is that of the European Union (EU), the primary source being the Treaty of Rome and the legislation made under it. This legislation is in four forms:

1. Regulations. These have direct effect and are binding on all member states and individuals.
2. Directives. These are binding as to their objectives but leave to member states the method of implementation, which is either legislative or administrative.
3. Decisions. These are binding on those to whom they are addressed and are usually in administrative form.
4. Recommendations. These are self-evident.

Most of the current UK law which applies to the sale or supply of veterinary products derives from European legislation in the form of directives and is implemented by regulations under the Medicines Act 1968 or the Animal Health and Welfare Act 1984. The current European law, which was consolidated in November 2001, is to be found in Directive 2001/82/EC. Certain amendments have been proposed in a subsequent consultation document and will eventually be implemented in UK regulations. Certain European definitions are laid down and include those of: (1) a 'proprietary medicinal product', and (2) a 'veterinary medicinal product'. Proprietary medicinal product means any ready prepared medicinal product placed on the market under a special name and in a special pack. A veterinary medical product means:

1. Any substance or combination of substances presented for treating or preventing disease in animals, or
2. Any substance or combination of substances which may be administered to animals with a view to making a medical diagnosis or to restoring, correcting or modifying physiological functions in animals.

Classes of veterinary medicinal products

All medicinal products, whether for administration to animals or humans, fall into one of four categories, namely:

1.   General sale list medicines (GSL)
2.   Pharmacy only medicines (P)
3.   Pharmacy and merchant supplies medicines (PML) (previously termed pharmacy merchant list)
4.   Prescription-only medicines (POM).

General sale list medicines (GSLs)

The medicinal products permitted for general sale as veterinary medicines are set out in Schedule 1 to the 1984 regulations as follows:

1.   Those listed in Table A (substances for internal and external use) or Table B (substances for external use only). Where a product contains an ingredient which is listed in either of these two tables it must comply with specifications in the table as to maximum strength (ms), maximum dose (md), maximum daily dose (mdd), use, pharmaceutical form or route of administration and be labelled accordingly.
2.   Excipients.
3.   Substances of animal origin (including extracts of such substances) used in the UK as a human or animal food.
4.   Substances of vegetable origin (including extracts and residues of such substances) used in the UK as a human or animal food.
5.   Grit in veterinary drugs for birds.

Retail pack sizes of certain products

Limits are imposed on the pack sizes of certain GSL products when they are sold or supplied by retail from businesses other than pharmacies. If sold outside the limits laid down, the medicinal products concerned are classed as Ps or POMs.

For veterinary drugs the quantities permitted in individual containers or packages are listed in Table 6.1.

Packs containing more than these quantities may only be sold or supplied from pharmacies and must be labelled P.

Products not to be on general sale

The GSL Order relating to veterinary medicinal products specifies that certain classes of products are not permitted to be on general sale.

Table 6.1 Quantities permitted in individual containers or packages for veterinary drugs

Drug	Permitted quantity
Aminonitrothiazole	100 mL of solution or 50 capsules
Aspirin	25 tablets or 25 sachets of powder
Bromhexine hydrochloride	20 g
Paracetamol	25 tablets
Phenylephrine hydrochloride	15 mL
Potassium chlorate	30 mL

They are:

1. Medicinal products for veterinary medicines promoted, recommended, or marketed:

    -   For use as eye drops or eye ointments.
    -   For administration by parenteral injection.
    -   For use as anthelmintics, except veterinary drugs consisting or containing dichlorophen, diethylcarbamazine citrate, piperazine adipate, piperazine calcium adipate, piperazine citrate, piperazine dihydrochloride, piperazine hydrate or piperazine phosphate.

2. Veterinary medicines promoted, recommended or marketed:
    -   For the internal treatment of ringworms.

Pharmacy only medicines (P)

Medicinal products, which are not included in a GSL, shall not be sold, offered or exposed for sale by retail, or supplied in circumstances corresponding to retail sale by any person in the course of a business carried on by him/her unless:

-   That person is, in respect of that business, a person lawfully conducting a retail pharmacy business.
-   The product is sold, offered or exposed for sale, or supplied on premises which are a registered pharmacy.
-   That person or, if the transaction is carried out on his/her behalf by another person, then that other person is, or acts under the supervision of, a pharmacist.

It should be noted that a retail pharmacy business must be under the personal control of a pharmacist so far as it concerns the sale of medicinal products including products on a GSL.

Pharmacy medicine defined

There is no legal definition of a pharmacy medicine. As such there is no definitive list of pharmacy medicines, as the total in the class cannot be determined. It comprises all those medicines which are not POMs or on a GSL and includes all medicines made in a pharmacy for retail sale under the exemptions from licensing granted to retail pharmacists.

Some GSL medicines, when presented in packs exceeding specified quantities, may only be sold or supplied from pharmacies and are designated as P medicines although there is no legal requirement for supervision by a pharmacist.

Exemptions for pharmacists

Subject to the work being done by or under the supervision of a pharmacist, no licence of any kind is required for any of the following activities being carried out in a registered pharmacy:

1. Preparing or dispensing a medicinal product in accordance with a prescription given by a practitioner, or preparing a stock of medicinal products for this purpose. The stock of medicinal products may be procured from a manufacturer holding the appropriate special licence. In respect of vaccines, sera and plasma for administration to animals, the exemption from licensing for pharmacists is subject to the same limitation which applies to veterinarians. The exemption for veterinarians from licensing is in respect of vaccines for administration to an animal (other than poultry) provided it is an autogenous vaccine.

2. Preparing or dispensing a medicinal product in accordance with a specification furnished by the person to whom the product is to be sold for administration to an animal or herd under his/her control, or preparing a stock of medicinal product for these purposes.

3. Preparing a medicinal product or a stock of medicinal products, not to the order of another person, but with a view to retail sale or supply, provided that the sale or supply is made from the registered pharmacy where it was prepared and the product is not the subject of an advertisement. In this connection, 'advertisement' does not include words appearing on the product or its container or package, or the display of the product itself, but does include a show-card.

4. Assembling a medicinal product. When medicinal products are assembled in a registered pharmacy for retail sale or supply they may not be the subject of any advertisement and may only be sold or supplied at the registered pharmacy where they are assembled or at some other registered pharmacy forming part of the same retail pharmacy business.

Prescription-only medicines (POMs)

Prescriptions

A prescription for a POM must comply with requirements set out below. In addition, it must carry a declaration by the veterinarian stating that the medicine is prescribed for an animal or herd under his/her care.

A Prescription Only Medicine may only be sold or supplied in accordance with a prescription given by a veterinary surgeon or veterinary practitioner. To meet that requirement, certain conditions must be satisfied.

The prescription:

(a)   Shall be signed in ink with his/her own name by the veterinarian giving it;

(b)   shall, without prejudice to subparagraph (a), be written in ink or otherwise so as to be indelible;

(c)   shall contain the following particulars:
  (i)   the address of the veterinarian giving it
  (ii)   the appropriate date (see below)
  (iii) such particulars as indicate that the practitioner giving it is a veterinary surgeon or a veterinary practitioner and
  (iv)   where the practitioner giving it is a veterinary surgeon or a veterinary practitioner, the name and address of the person to whom the POM is to be delivered and a declaration that it is for an animal or herd under his/her care.

(d)   shall not be dispensed after the end of the period of 6 months from the appropriate date, unless it is a repeatable prescription in which case it shall not be dispensed for the first time after the end of that period nor otherwise than in accordance with the direction contained in the repeatable prescription;

(e)   in the case of a repeatable prescription that does not specify the number of times it may be dispensed, shall not be dispensed on more than two occasions unless it is a prescription for oral contraceptives in which case it may be dispensed six times before the end of the period of 6 months from the appropriate date.

Where a prescription given by a veterinarian does not fulfil a required condition, the sale or supply is not rendered unlawful if the person making the sale or supply, having exercised all due diligence, believes on reasonable grounds that that condition is fulfilled in relation to that sale or supply. Similarly, the sale or supply is not rendered unlawful if made against a forged prescription provided the pharmacist has exercised all due diligence and believes on reasonable grounds that the prescription is genuine.

Pharmacy and merchant medicines (PML)

Certain veterinary medicinal products known as PML medicines which are not on a GSL may be sold by:

1. Holders of marketing authorisations.
2. Veterinarians and pharmacists. When sold in a pharmacy the sales must be supervised by a pharmacist.
3. A specially authorised person, that is a person specially authorised either by a direction of the licensing authority to assemble the veterinary drug otherwise than in accordance with the manufacturer's licence or by the marketing authorisation to sell the medicine under the alternative name specified in the authorisation.
4. By certain categories of dealers.

Two classes of dealers are described in the regulations: (1) agricultural merchants, and (2) saddlers.

Agricultural merchants

Agricultural merchants may sell any veterinary medicinal products listed by the minister subject to certain conditions (see below).

An agricultural merchant means a person who carries on a business involving in whole or in part the sale of agricultural requisites, being things used for soil cultivation or keeping of animals for production of food or game, equipment for collecting produce from animals kept for production of food, things for the maintenance of that equipment, and protective clothing.

It should be noted that a pharmacist who conducts a retail business from premises other than from a pharmacy is classed as an agricultural merchant and must comply with the relevant regulations.

Saddlers

Saddlers may sell any veterinary medicinal product listed by the minister which is a horse wormer, dog wormer or cat wormer.

A saddler means a person carrying on a business involving in whole or in part the sale of saddlery requisites, being products and equipment and things for the maintenance of that equipment, for keeping of horses or ponies, and including human clothing for that purpose.

The sale of listed veterinary medicinal products and wormers by merchants and saddlers is subject to certain conditions.

Registration requirements

Registration requirements are set out in an order made under the Medicines Act 1968, as amended by the Animal Health and Welfare Act 1984. The register is maintained by the Royal Pharmaceutical Society of Great Britain (RPSGB), which is also responsible for inspection and enforcement. In Northern Ireland, the register is kept by the Department of Health and Social Services for Northern Ireland.

An agricultural merchant or saddler is subject to conditions in respect of inclusion and retention on the register, namely s/he must:

1. Register his/her name and details of all premises where s/he sells or stores veterinary medicinal products.
2. Give details for each premises of the name and qualifications of a person nominated to be a suitably qualified person for the premises.
3. Pay the appropriate fee for each set of premises.
4. Pay a retention fee annually in respect of each premises and notify any change in particulars as soon as possible. Failure to pay the retention fees leads to removal from the register and the payment of higher fees to have the premises restored to the register.
5. Be a fit and proper person to sell such veterinary drugs.

In addition:

6. All premises used for sale or storage must be suitable for the purpose, and premises to be used for sale, which may include a stall of a permanent nature at a market or agricultural showground, must be capable of being closed so as to exclude the public. Any alteration to premises which affect their suitability must be notified to the registration authority.
7. Any proposed permanent change to the suitably qualified person nominated must be notified to the registration authority.

Conditions of sale

The conditions which must be complied with by an agricultural merchant or a saddler are that:

1. The premises at which sales of veterinary drugs are made must be occupied by him/her and under his/her control at all times when the premises are open for business, and s/he must store those products in a part of the premises partitioned off or otherwise separated from the rest of the premises and to which the public have no access.
2. The suitably qualified person nominated and notified or, in his/her temporary absence, an alternative suitably qualified person, shall authorise each sale of veterinary drugs.

3. Only exempted veterinary drugs listed by the minister may be sold.
4. Each veterinary drug sold must be in the container in which it was made up for sale by the manufacturer or assembler, which has not been opened since then, and must bear the manufacturer's label, which has not been altered, and not be sold after the date of expiry indicated on its label.
5. The sale is not by self-service methods.
6. If the product is a cat wormer, a dog wormer, or a horse wormer, the sale is to a person whom s/he knows or has reasonable cause to believe has in his/her charge a cat if it is a cat wormer, a dog if it is a dog wormer or a horse or pony if it is a horse wormer and will use the product for the treatment of the animal concerned.
7. S/he must keep records (see below).

Additional conditions to be complied with by an agricultural merchant are:

8. If the product is *not* a cat wormer, dog wormer, or horse wormer, the sale is to a person whom s/he knows or has reasonable cause to believe has animals under his/her control for the purpose of, and in the course of, carrying on a business either as his/her sole business activity or as a part of his/her business activities. N.B. This does not extend to a business wholly or mainly concerned with sales to the owners of pet animals. The keeping of animals as pets or the keeping of poultry, etc. for the sole use of the owner or his/her family or to give away is not 'carrying on a business'.
9. If the product is an organophosphate sheep dip or if the product is a sheep dip, not intended for export, the sale is made to a person whom the seller knows, or has reasonable cause to believe, is the holder, or the employer of or a person acting on behalf of the holder, of a Certificate of Competence, and the agricultural merchant keeps a record of the certificate number for 3 years from the date of the sale.

Certificate of competence

Certificate of Competence means a Certificate of Competence in the Safe Use of Sheep Dips issued by the National Proficiency Tests Council or by that Council and the Department of Agriculture in Northern Ireland showing that parts 1 and 2 of the assessment have been satisfactorily completed.

Code of good practice

There is a code of good practice for the sale and supply of animal medicines prepared by the Animal Medicines Training Regulatory Authority (AMTRA) which sets out the standards which agricultural merchants and saddlers dealing with animal medicines are expected to meet. The

code has no legal status but supplements the principal legal requirements with other provisions relating to personnel, sale and storage
arrangements and standards of premises.

Record keeping for veterinary products

General records for retail sales or supplies

Any person who sells veterinary medicinal products by retail intended
for administration to animals whose flesh or products are intended for
human consumption and in respect of which a withdrawal period must
be observed must keep a record.

Similarly any person who sells any other veterinary medicinal
products by retail intended for administration to such animals, unless
the products are on a GSL, must keep records.

For each incoming and outgoing transaction a record must be kept
of the:

1.   Date of transaction
2.   Name of the product sold
3.   Manufacturer's batch number
4.   Quantity sold or received
5.   Name and address of supplier or recipient
6.   Name and address of the prescribing veterinarian (where relevant) and a copy
     of the prescription.

In addition a detailed audit of all transactions must be carried out and
recorded, at least once a year, and reconciliation carried out between
incoming and outgoing stock.

Records for dispensed medicines

Every person lawfully conducting a retail pharmacy business is required
to keep a record in respect of every sale or supply of a POM. The entry
must be made on the day the sale or supply takes place or, if that is not
reasonably practicable, on the following day.

Additional particulars to be recorded in the case of a sale or supply
of a POM in pursuance of a prescription are:

1.   The date on which the medicine was sold or supplied.
     The name, quantity and, except where it is apparent from the name, the phar-
     maceutical form and strength of the medicine
2.   The date on the prescription and the name and address of the veterinarian
     giving it

3.   The name and address of the person for whose animal the medicine was prescribed.

For second and subsequent supplies made on a repeat prescription it is sufficient to record the date of supply and a reference to the entry in the register relating to the first supply.

The Prescription Only Record must be preserved by the owner of the retail pharmacy business for a period of 3 years from the date of the last entry in the record. The prescription must be retained for 2 years from the date on which the POM was sold or supplied, or, for a repeat prescription, the date on which the medicine was supplied for the last time.

All records must be durable but may be kept by electronic means. They must be kept for 3 years and be made available on request to any person having a duty of enforcement. The RPSGB has the duty to enforce concurrently with the ministers in England and Scotland and the National Assembly for Wales.

Labelling requirements for animal medicines

A 'container', in relation to a medicinal product, means the bottle, jar, box, packet or other receptacle which contains it, or is to contain it, not being a capsule, cachet or other article in which the product is or is to be administered; and where any such receptacle is or is to be contained in another such receptacle, includes the inner receptacle but not the outer.

It should be noted that a capsule, cachet or other article in which a medicinal product is to be administered is not normally a container, but if the capsule, etc, is not to be administered, then it is a container.

A 'package', in relation to any medicinal products, means any box, packet or other article in which one or more containers of the products are to be enclosed, and where any such box, package or other article is or is to be itself enclosed in one or more other boxes, packets or other articles, includes each of the boxes, packets or other articles in question.

In effect, the inner receptacle which actually contains the medicinal products is a container, every outer receptacle is a package.

Labelling of dispensed medicines

The standard labelling requirements do not apply to dispensed medicines.

A 'dispensed relevant medicinal product' means a relevant medicinal product prepared or dispensed in accordance with a prescription given by a practitioner.

The container of a dispensed relevant medicinal product must be labelled to show the following particulars:

1. The name of the person having possession or control of the animal or herd and address of the premises where the animal or herd is kept.
2. The name and address of the person who sells or supplies the relevant medicinal product.
3. The date of dispensing and
4. Where the product has been prescribed by a veterinarian such of the following particulars as s/he may request:
   - The name of the product or its common name
   - Directions for use of the product
   - Precautions relating to the use of the product or
   - Where a pharmacist, in the exercise of his/her professional skill and judgement, is of the opinion that any of such particulars are inappropriate and has taken all reasonable steps to consult with the veterinarian and has been unable to do so, particulars of a same kind as those requested by the practitioner which the pharmacist considers appropriate
   - The words 'Keep out of the reach of children' or words of direction bearing a similar meaning;
   - The phrase 'For external use only' (within a rectangle) if the product is for topical use, e.g. an embrocation, liniment, lotion, liquid antiseptic or other liquid preparation or gel and is for external use only.
   - The words 'For animal treatment only' unless the package or container is so small it is not practical to do so.
   - A container need not be labelled if it is enclosed in a package which is labelled with the required particulars.

Labelling of animal medicines

Animal medicines which possessed product licences prior to 1 January 1995 are subject to the same general and standard labelling requirements as medicinal products for human use.

All medicinal products for animal use obtaining new marketing authorisations or having their licences renewed have to comply with the provisions of the Marketing Authorisations for Veterinary Medicinal Products Regulations 1994. These regulations implement EC Council Directives.

The new regulations require the following information to appear in legible characters on the containers and outer packages:

- The name of the veterinary medicinal product and the quantity.
- A statement of the active ingredients expressed qualitatively and quantitatively per dosage unit or according to the form of administration for a given

volume or weight, using the international non-proprietary name or where none exists the usual non-proprietary name.
- Manufacturer's batch number.
- Marketing authorisation number.
- Name and address or registered business address of the person responsible for marketing and of the manufacturer if different.
- The species of animal for which the product is intended together with the method and route of administration.
- The withdrawal period, even if nil, in the case of products administered to food-producing animals.
- The expiry date in plain language.
- Special storage precautions, if any.
- Contraindications, warnings and special precautions for disposal of unused product or waste material.
- Any special precautions relating to use or other particulars essential for safety or health protection.
- The words 'For animal treatment only'.
- The words 'Store out of the reach of children'.
- The indications 'POM', 'P', 'PML', or 'GSL' in a box in which there is no other written material.
- Any other statements or particulars required by the marketing authorisation.

Labelling small containers for animal medicinal products

For containers such as ampoules the information required is:
- The name of the veterinary medicinal product.
- Quantity of the active ingredients.
- Manufacturer's batch number.
- Route of administration.
- The expiry date in plain language.
- The words 'For animal treatment only'.

Labelling of sales by agricultural merchants and saddlers

Exempted veterinary drugs must be labelled in accordance with the principal labelling regulations as amended.

The containers and the immediately enclosed package of an exempted veterinary drug, when sold or supplied by retail, must be labelled according to the five points listed below:

1. 'PML' (Schs. 1 and 2) or 'POM' (Sch. 3), as appropriate. The letters must be in capitals within which there shall be no other matter of any kind. N.B. For wholesale transactions the letters need only appear on the immediately enclosing package.

2. If containing hexachlorophene and for oral administration for the prevention or treatment of liver fluke disease in cattle, with a warning that it is not for use in lactating cattle, and also, if for liver fluke disease in sheep or cattle, with a warning that protective clothing must be worn when the product is being administered.

3. If containing aloxiprin, with the words 'Unsuitable for cats' and 'Contains an aspirin derivative'.

4. If containing aspirin, with the words 'Unsuitable for cats' and 'Contains aspirin' ('Contains aspirin' may be omitted where the word 'aspirin' is included in the name of the product).

5. If containing salicylamide, with the words 'Unsuitable for cats'.

In points 3, 4 and 5 the special 'Unsuitable for cats' wording must be within a rectangle within which there shall be no other matter.

Veterinary surgeons

The restrictions on retail sale or supply do not apply to the sale, offer for sale or supply of any medicinal product by a veterinary surgeon or practitioner for administration by him/her or under his/her direction to an animal or herd under his/her care. Furthermore, the restrictions on retail sale or supply do not apply to any person who sells any medicinal product to a veterinary surgeon or practitioner.

The Veterinary Surgeons Act 1966 is the principal statute dealing with the management of the veterinary profession in relation to registration, education and professional conduct.

'Veterinary surgery' means the art and science of veterinary surgery and medicine and includes: the diagnosis of diseases in, and injuries to, animals including tests performed on animals for diagnostic purposes; the giving of advice based upon such diagnosis; the medical or surgical treatment of animals; and the performance of surgical operations on animals.

Restrictions on practice as veterinary surgeons and use of titles

According to the Veterinary Surgeons Act 1966 no one may practise, or hold themselves out as practising, or being prepared to practise, veterinary surgery unless they are registered as a veterinary surgeon or are in the supplementary register as a veterinary practitioner. It is an offence for an unregistered person to use the titles 'veterinary surgeon' or 'veterinary practitioner' or any name, title, addition or description implying that s/he is qualified to practise veterinary surgery.

The Act provides some limited exceptions for students of veterinary surgery, for medical practitioners and dentists in certain circumstances, and for the carrying out of minor treatment in terms of exemption orders made under the Act. Examples include orders allowing treatment by physiotherapists at veterinarians' request, blood sampling for the brucellosis eradication scheme, vaccinations of poultry against certain diseases and use of epidural anaesthesia.

Exemption is also provided for the following treatments and operations to be given or carried out by unqualified persons:

- Any minor medical treatment given to an animal by its owner, by another member of a household of which the owner is a member, or by a person in the employment of the owner.
- Anything given, otherwise than for the reward, to an animal used in agriculture, as defined in the Agriculture Act 1947, by the owner of the animal or by a person engaged or employed in caring for animals so used.
- The rendering in an emergency of first aid for the purpose of saving life or relieving pain.
- The performance by any person aged 18 or more of any of the following operations:
  (a) castration of a male animal or caponising of an animal, whether by chemical means or otherwise (except the castration of a horse, pony, ass or mule; of a bull, boar or goat which has reached the age of 2 months; or of a ram which has reached the age of 3 months; the spaying of a cat or dog)
  (b) the docking of the tail of a lamb
  (c) the amputation of the dew claws of a dog before its eyes are open
  (d) the disbudding of a calf subject to certain conditions.
- Any medical treatment or minor surgery (not involving entry into the body cavity) to a companion animal by a veterinary nurse provided the animal is under the care of a veterinary surgeon, the treatment is carried out under his/her direction, and the veterinary surgeon is the employer, or acting on behalf of the employer, of the nurse.
- Any medical treatment or any minor surgery (not involving entry into the body cavity) to any animal by a veterinary nurse if the following conditions are complied with:
  (a) the animal is for the time being under the care of a veterinarian and any treatment or minor surgery is carried out under his supervision
  (b) the veterinarian is the employer or acting on behalf of the employer of the veterinary nurse
  (c) the veterinarian directing the treatment or minor surgery is satisfied that the veterinary nurse is qualified to carry out the treatment or surgery.

Legislation

Acts, regulations and orders governing the supply of veterinary medicines include:

- The Medicines (Labelling) Regulations 1976 SI No.1726 as amended.
- The Medicines (Veterinary Drugs) (General Sale List) Order 1984 SI No.768 as amended.
- The Medicines (Leaflets for Veterinary Drugs) Regulations 1983 SI No.1727.
- The Medicines (Veterinary Drugs) (Prescription Only) Order 1991 SI No.1392 as amended by SI 1991 No.2568.
- The Marketing Authorisations for Veterinary Medicinal Products 1994 SI No.3142.
- The Medicines (Exemptions for Merchants in Veterinary Drugs) Order 1998 SI No.1044.
- The Retailers' Records for Veterinary Medicinal Products Regulations 2000 SI No.7.
- Veterinary Surgeons Act 1966.
- Veterinary Surgeons (Schedule 3 Amendment) Order 1991.

Advisory booklets

The following advisory booklets are recommended:

- Medicines Act Veterinary Information Services (MAVIS) advisory leaflets: Veterinary Medicines Directorate.
- Animal Medicines European Licensing Information and Advice (AMELIA) advisory booklets: Veterinary Medicines Directorate.

Useful address/website

Animal Medicines Training Regulatory Authority (AMTRA)
8 Parsons Hill, Hollesley, Woodbridge, Suffolk IP12 3RB, UK
Tel: +44 (0)1394 411010
Website: www.amtra.org.uk

7

Business and financial aspects of veterinary pharmacy

Andrew Cairns

Veterinary pharmacy offers pharmacists an opportunity to supply into both the companion animal (pet) market and the large animal (commercial or food-producing) market. These two markets differ in their characteristics and need to be approached using different techniques for promotion and marketing.

The markets

Over half the homes in the UK have at least one pet and the current petcare market is worth around £1.7 billion (2001 figures) and is rising by approximately 10% annually (Pedigree Petfoods). The wellbeing of the pet is usually the first priority for owners, but the cost of animal care is also an important issue.

For the purposes of this chapter horses will be considered to be companion animals although in Europe they are often considered as food-producing animals.

The market place for food-producing animals, mainly cattle, sheep and pigs in the UK, is quite different from the pet market both in the financial resource needed to service it and the pharmacoeconomic input that it requires. Farmers are in business to make money, so most medicine purchases are inspected from the point of view of cost effectiveness.

The similarities between the two markets are in the legal classification of the medicines and in the pharmacy skills required, which include medicines management, advice on drug interactions and withdrawal periods, the last mentioned being particularly important when supplying medicines for use in food-producing animals. Maximum residue limits (MRLs) therefore are an important consideration for medicines going into the food chain.

Differences between the commercial and companion animal markets are illustrated here against four different sets of criteria:

1. Some pharmacies are less suitably positioned geographically than others to enter the commercial animal market. A pharmacy, correctly structured, can service an area of 30 miles' radius or much more in certain circumstances. It is self-evident that a city centre pharmacy will have further to travel to service farming customers than a market town or rural practice. Supply of medicines for companion animals, on the other hand, normally suits most pharmacies, whether urban or rural.

2. Selling and marketing techniques are different too, the commercial market relying heavily on carrying information and advice out to the farmer, the selling often being carried out in the farmyard. The pet side, where the contact with the animal owner is usually in the pharmacy premises, is more dependent on merchandising and display skills and product-focused training for the point-of-sale staff operating in the pharmacy. Mail order of pigeon and horse products is carried out very effectively by some specialist pharmacies where legally appropriate.

3. Significantly, selling to farmers is mainly credit trade with resultant cash-flow pressure. It is also likely to involve much greater turnover volumes, which demands good financial planning. Pet medicine sales, in contrast, fit the normal pharmacy-trading pattern of cash through the till when the sale is made. A good pet section may turnover £10 000–£20 000 per year whereas a commercial animal pharmacy needs turnover many times that to be viable.

4. In the commercial animal market, the fact that medicines leave residues that may enter the food chain creates a focus, as already stated, on withdrawal times and MRLs. Accurate, responsible and safe use of the medicine is important, something of which pharmacists are acutely aware. So, immediately, it becomes clear that we have an important professional role to play. For the companion animal the constraint on residues is not a controlling factor. The wellbeing of the pet itself and the safety of the person who handles the medicine are of more direct concern (see chapter 3).

These characteristics are summarised in Table 7.1.

Table 7.1 Charactersitics of companion animal and commercial animal markets

Companion	Commercial
• Suits most pharmacies	• Located near farms
• Pharmacy-based sales	• Farm-based contact
• Cash in the till	• Credit trade
• No food-chain implications	• Food-chain implications

Accessing the market

The markets for both companion and large animal medicine sales will be considered under the following headings:

- Market assessment – macro and micro
- Sourcing products
- Product selection and familiarisation
- Selling profitably.

Veterinary pharmacy offers pharmacists an opportunity to supply into both the companion animal market and the large animal market, although the two markets differ particularly from the marketing and financial points of view.

Market assessment – segmenting the market

A useful way of assessing at the market is by 'segment'. Most markets comprise a number of segments. Market segments are groups of buyers or customer types with similar needs or behaviour, e.g. dairy farmers or sheep farmers.

The competition for business from these buyers may be from one or more sellers in each segment. The dynamics and size of each segment may vary, sometimes quite quickly, over time.

The market may be considered as a box that may be divided up into different segments, by straight lines (see Figure 7.1).

- A market segment may have only one meaningful competitor (D) as shown in Figure 7.1, e.g. the only supplier of veterinary medicines to sheep farmers in a certain postcode area except for the farmer's veterinary surgeon.
- There may be two competitors (A and B) as shown in the second sector, e.g. there are two dairy engineers in addition to your own pharmacy that sells hygiene chemicals into the dairy farmer sector.
- There may be three or more competitors attacking the same sector – shown in Figure 7.1 as competitors A, B and C. In this situation a pharmacy would be under severe price pressure and might think seriously about withdrawing from this sector and direct energies elsewhere.
- To complicate matters, buyers often switch between brands and enter or leave the market for a variety of reasons. Further, the market segments can be expanding or contracting.

Clearly, a small business will find it difficult to quantify this on an ongoing basis. The pharmacist has, rather, to develop a feel for the local market and may benefit by considering the principles involved.

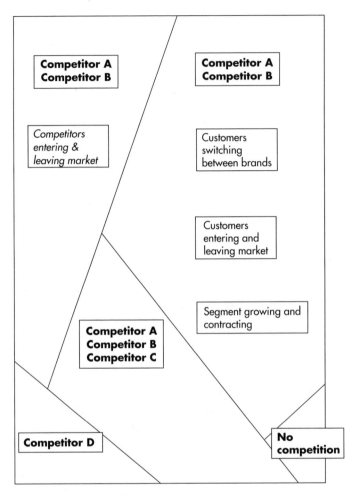

Figure 7.1 Dynamics of market competition.

There is also another possibility for a market segment as represented by the segment at the bottom right of the diagram. That is where there is no competitor, e.g. where there are no other pharmacists selling into the sector. Pharmacists are able to break bulk for farmers if they so request, a service that they find very useful and that provides added value.

A useful concept to consider is that of the product life cycle – a simplified version of the Boston Matrix (Figure 7.2).

From start to finish products go through the same cycle but spend differing amounts of time in each stage. We are faced with buying decisions daily and the way in which these decisions are taken are assisted by understanding where a product may be in its life cycle.

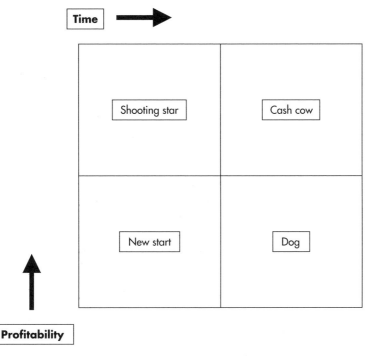

Figure 7.2   The product life cycle as Boston Matrix.

- A 'new start' product involves promotional expense and may not yield profits for some time.
- A 'shooting star' represents a very profitable product that reaches its potential in a short space of time.
- A 'cash cow' product is one that has become established and is maintaining a prolonged and profitable life in the marketplace.
- A 'dog' has lost its momentum (or has never gained any since a 'new start' can become a 'dog' without rising above the horizontal line in the chart) and costs more to promote or maintain than it yields.

The companion animal market

Market assessment and starting up a pet section

- Look at the competition – is it the pet shop, the supermarket, the vet or a combination? That information will help you to direct your sales emphasis.
- Assess the local catchment population – we know that two in five households have a cat or a dog. It is then possible to calculate what the available market value is since a pet-owning household spends an average of £35 per year on

pet medicines, although demography will have some affect on the average spend. How much of that market can you get? Initially it depends how many people already use your pharmacy. If you do your job well you may get more than 50% of your existing customers' pet business. Added to this, as your reputation grows you will attract new customers from your catchment area. Advertising and mailing will accelerate this. In a town of 30 000 population with a catchment of about 80 000 population my own pharmacy is turning over £15 000/year in one non-town-centre pharmacy. This level of trade was reached over a period of about 2 years. The average gross margin on the sales is currently over 30%.

- Train the staff – The National Pharmaceutical Association (NPA) has useful material and the Royal Pharmaceutical Society of Great Britain (RPSGB) Veterinary Pharmacists' Group a number of well-produced leaflets on horses, cats, dogs and pigeons. Manufacturers who sell direct to pharmacies, or one of the more efficient short line specialist wholesalers, often provide training. Pharmacists may consider the RPSGB Diploma in Veterinary Pharmacy, an excellent modularised course tailored specially to the requirements of practising pharmacists

Product selection and familiarisation

Decide on the range required by talking to:

- Certain manufacturers – Sherley's, Bob Martin's, Intervet, Bayer, Novartis and others. Full contact information is in the National Office of Animal Health (NOAH) Data Sheet Compendium published annually.
- Certain wholesalers – Vetchem (via NPA information department), Battle Hayward & Bower, Trilanco, a pet shop wholesaler, or ask your drug wholesaler. Full line national wholesalers should be asked for supplies of pet medicines to encourage them to stock full ranges.
- Other veterinary pharmacists (via the Veterinary Pharmacists' Group secretary at the RPSGB, London).
- *The Veterinary Formulary* is extremely good as a source of information on veterinary drugs and prescribing (if rather expensive). Also useful is the NOAH Compendium mentioned above.

Keep a comprehensive range of products to include:

- Wormers
- Flea products
- Nutritional supplements
- Grooming products
- Sundries – leads, cat litter etc.

Products for companion animals are described fully under species headings in Part 4 of this book.

Figure 7.3 shows part of a 2.5 m run of pet products, including horse products. It shows how a pharmacy only medicine (P)/pharmacy and merchant supplies medicines (PML) cabinet can be housed in a pet section.

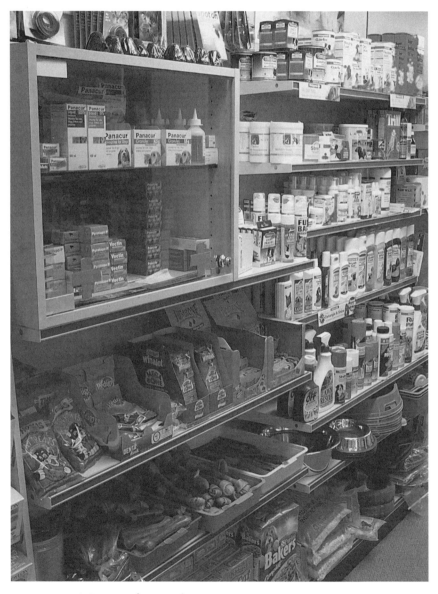

Figure 7.3 2.5 m run of pet products.

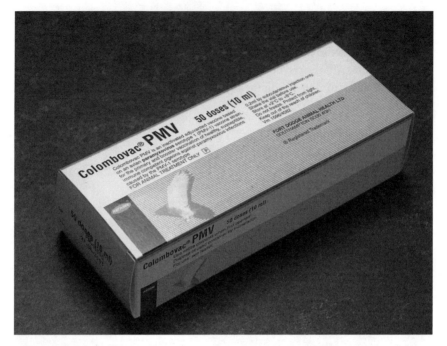

Figure 7.4 Colombovac pigeon vaccine.

Selling profitably

- Emphasise the PML and P only products – for example, Colombovac, a paramyxovirus vaccine for pigeons (see Figure 7. 4), presently classified P, has no other high street supply point other than the pharmacy. Build your ancillary range round these target lines. Many are high-value products and, with the exception of some horse wormers, are not price sensitive.
- Direct your staff training towards the added value in the pharmacy service and the optimal efficacy of products being offered rather than allowing choice to be based solely on price.
- Displace products that are proving less adequate in terms of stock turnover and profit margin. Initially allocate space of about a 1 m run of shelving as a minimum to get started.

Commercial animals

Accessing the market

Markets should be categorised or segmented. One has to decide which market in which interest is highest. Undertaking some sort of market-research programme will be useful in making this assessment.

The Department for Environment, Food, and Rural Affairs (DEFRA) (previously the Ministry of Agriculture Fisheries and Food (MAFF)) resources give a wide picture but local research is also possible. Mark off your trading area in increasingly wider circles and calculate the livestock and cereal data for each. A database can collate the figures – numbers of sheep, cattle, pigs; hectares of wheat, barley or silage crop. Visit farms for the information or use the telephone, which has become increasingly accepted.

One should remember that the British catering entrepreneur Charles Forte began his business activities by counting the number of people passing his street corner in London!

Having estimated the livestock type and numbers, these will have to be matched firstly with the product groups and then with the products themselves.

Typically, a farmer will spend the following on non-prescription medicines for his animals per year:

- Dairy cow   £10.50
- Sheep   £3.00
- Beef   £5.50

Based on the overall stock-density figures you calculate for your area it is a relatively simple matter to calculate the approximate value of the market you intend to service. As a broad guide, medicines will probably turn out to be about 50% of total sales generated. How much of the market you get will depend on factors such as:

- Competition
- Site of pharmacy
- Farm calling
- Level of training
- Marketing.

You have day-to-day control over the last three items. The energy and resources that you apply to the whole exercise will govern the speed with which the business is gained.

Sourcing – product selection and familiarisation

The NOAH Data Sheet Compendium is invaluable as a quick reference for information on proprietary products. *The Veterinary Formulary* has an excellent cross-reference facility linking generic names to proprietary equivalents.

Sourcing of products can initially be difficult. It is probably good advice to make contact with a practising veterinary pharmacist who is already in the market that you intend to enter. Until you build your volume of stock it may be necessary to buy from a pharmacist who has a wholesale dealer's licence or from one of the veterinary medicines wholesalers such as Battle Hayward & Bower or Trilanco. Following the 2003 report by the Competition Commission on the supply of veterinary medicines in the UK, a number of veterinary wholesalers are now prepared to supply pharmacies. Most manufacturers will sell direct to distributors who can handle sufficient quantities of products.

Selection of product groups to be handled can require more careful thought in the commercial animal market. Handling, storage and distribution become challenging logistics issues.

Examples of product groups to be considered are:

- Anthelmintics
- Vaccines
- Sheep dips and pour-ons
- Mineral supplements
- Trace element formulations
- Disinfectants
- Dairy hygiene and mastitis control
- Crop protection products
- Fly control
- Silage additives and grass seed.

Figure 7.5 shows a pharmacy shelving run housing a typical selection of medicines and ancillary products. Oral drenches have to be housed, in this case, on the bottom shelf because the volume of the containers is often 5 or 10 L.

Dairy hygiene products need heavy handling facilities. Figure 7.6 shows a racking run housing dairy hygiene and mastitis control products (mostly 20 L drums). An order assembly table is situated in front of the racking. This scale of handling is unlikely to be needed in the early years of developing the large-animal business.

Selling profitably – the business plan

Having decided on the goal, for example to achieve 50% of the market in your trading area within 10 years, you have to lay down specific rules for achieving the goal. These rules lead into the business plan. You may decide to employ a salesperson from day one. It is useful to be aware that the breakeven point for each salesperson will almost certainly be well over £100 000 at 25% gross margin, but that should be considered

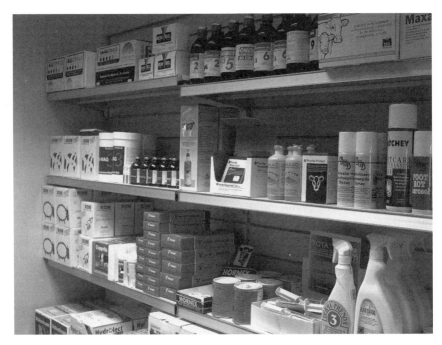

Figure 7.5 Selection of large-animal products.

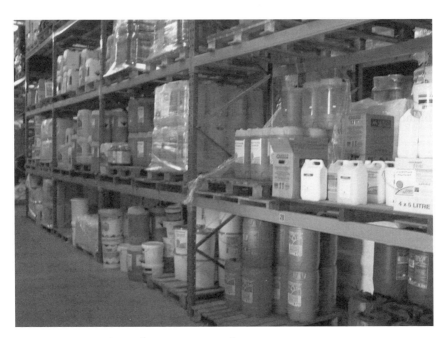

Figure 7.6 Warehouse for veterinary products.

in the light that a single salesperson can command sales of £500 000 or more in this market. It may be possible to double turnover in a short time at the expense of profit. The financial implications of that must be considered. Strategic issues give you standards for controlling the plans.

Now go through the following process:

1. Assess or estimate sales growth, months 1–12, years 1–5.
2. Set target gross margin on product areas to be promoted over the same period as in 1.
3. Assess overheads for the same period. These include costs associated with administration, running the establishment and finance.
4. Prepare a cash flow to establish how much capital is required. As mentioned at the beginning of this chapter selling into the agricultural market requires the funding of debtors. Although it is possible to conduct some depot sales for cash, inevitably most of the business done with farmers will be on monthly credit terms. Don't underestimate this! The higher your sales are the more money you require to fund debtors.

Consider the purchase of £1000 of stock for a single customer. Assume that payment for this stock is made to your supplier on the last day of the month following the month of purchase. Assume also that your customer does not pay you for a further month after that. Obviously the business needs £1000 in cash to fund this customer, this debtor, for 30 days.

In practice, £1000 of purchases will likely divide partly into stock, partly into credit sales and perhaps partly, also, into cash sales. The way to estimate, on an ongoing basis, the cash requirement on the business of a series of purchases and a series of sales (a more realistic way to represent normal trading conditions) is to consider it in terms of debtor days, creditor days and stock level.

A simple formula to use for the debtor and creditor days at any month end is as follows:

$$\text{Debtor days} = \frac{\text{Total outstanding debtors}}{\text{Average daily sales for that month}}$$

$$\text{Creditor days} = \frac{\text{Total outstanding creditors}}{\text{Average daily purchases for that month}}$$

Consider two possible scenarios as shown in Table 7.2.

A calculation needs to be done for the end of each month up to the end of the projected period for which the cash flow is required within the business plan. Creditor days and debtor days need to be estimated for each month. You then have a picture of how much working capital, if any, is required to fund the debtors' ledger. It is important that the subsequent credit control procedures employed by the business are

Table 7.2 Estimation of required capital based on creditor and debtor days

	Debtor days	Creditor days	Capital needed (released)
Scenario 1	45	30	Value of 15 days' purchases
Scenario 2	35	40	Value of 5 days' sales

effective so that the debtors' ledger does not grow beyond the budgeted level. You will see from scenario 2 that suppressing your creditors (paying them later) delivers a positive benefit to your cash flow and can be useful. However, continuity of supply in any business is important. Damaging the goodwill of your suppliers is to be avoided.

It is important to realise that stock control also plays a significant part in stable cash flow. The cost value of any increase in stock hits the cash flow directly. So you will see that increase in debtor days and increase in stock create an immediate need for cash in the business. This is perfectly normal in the course of business but must be anticipated so that the proper provision can be made. Selling medicines into the large-animal market requires additional cash control measures caused by credit sales but of course, the rewards are commensurate with the effort.

When preparing the business plan, allow for a 'buying in' period to the local market place. You need to build a competitive image in the early stages. The 'added value' then takes over and established advice becomes more important and price is discussed less often. The business plan must reflect these potentially lower margins at the start. It might be appropriate to project 20% as the initial gross margin rising to 25% by the end of the first year. An established large-animal veterinary pharmacy may achieve nearer 30%.

Internet selling

As Internet selling gathers volume this will likely be accompanied by reducing margins. If you intend to present your pharmacy as an Internet seller of either companion or large-animal medicines then the detailed requirements for that are outside the scope of this chapter, which is aimed to address traditional methods of trading. Suffice it to say that the setting-up costs are quite different. The establishment of a competent selling site capable of taking orders will set you back in excess of £10 000 and several times that would not be unusual. Catalogue maintenance and site development become significant cost factors. The overhead structure for Internet selling is different and margins are likely to be tighter so the business plan will have a different shape (see chapter 3 and Box 7.1).

Box 7.1 Internet trading

We are not yet seeing the Internet being used greatly in the animal health market for purchasing products. However, with a search engine such as 'Google' and an appropriate 'key word', world-wide information about products is readily available. The more precise one can be, the easier it is to find product-specific items. 'Pet medicines' as a search term would need to be refined; for example to dog medicines and then down to anthelmintics. Web pages might give you product information and price details through links on the master page.

Some providers then require you to contact them by phone, fax or e-mail to place your orders (if it is an order you wish) and make payment by a secure means. With medicines there are often problems according to legal classifications varying across national borders. Most responsible governments are trying to ensure that goods sold to their countries comply with the their home rules, but this is a difficult matter to police, especially if the source is in the developing world. Sales to individuals for their own use can freely transcend national boundaries, but business sales are subject to usual taxes.

European and American countries are trying to devise systems to ensure legal controls are applied evenly and fairly especially in the area of medicines and illicit substances. The EU medicines legislation both for human and animal medicines at present being addressed in Brussels is attempting to deal with these issues. It is realised that the 'IT' world of the immediate tomorrow will dramatically change the way in which many products are bought and sold. The ease with which information is available on the 'net' means a better-informed public, but one where a little knowledge may be a dangerous thing in purchasing products that are dangerous to use without the knowledgeable understanding of the information so readily available.

Douglas Davidson

The pharmacist's involvement

Characteristics of market

- There is a large veterinary pharmacy market in which pharmacist's existing skills can be used to advantage.
- The commercial animal market requires very careful financial planning but the rewards can be considerable.
- To enter either market from scratch invites us to use the help already there from the RPSGB, NPA and other pharmacists.
- The pet market is one that the community pharmacist can enter into very readily and profitably. Throughout this book the legal categories have been given to demonstrate the potential portfolio of products available for distribution pharmacies.

- A *new* product range using our *existing* pharmacy skills is very attractive if we introduce companion animal medicines to the pharmacy at a time when our emphasis shifts more into healthcare. And good animal health contributes to good human health.
- Adding value: professional advice is available in the pharmacy 6 days per week and the pharmacist is always on site. It makes sense to capitalise on that; there is no professional available in the pet shop or the supermarket and the vet is often absent from his surgery. Pharmacy only products are invariably of proven efficacy. This is not always the case with some pet shops where unlicensed products still pervade the service.

The opportunities to promote veterinary pharmacy should not be missed. One pharmacy in Derbyshire has secured temporary registration for pharmacy stands at Crufts for several years, and provides facilities for obtaining advice and selling pet vaccines under the personal supervision of a pharmacist (Figure 7.7).

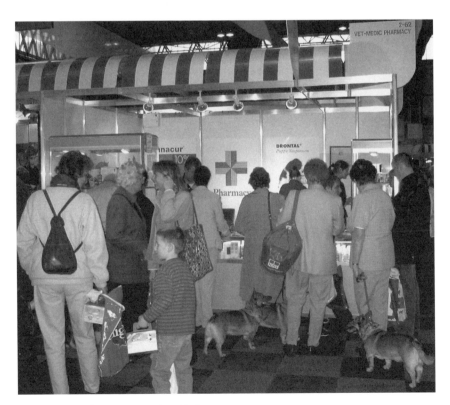

Figure 7.7 Pharmacy stand at Crufts.

Further reading

Banahan B F (1998). *Marketing for Pharmacists*. New York: Haworth Press.

Kayne SB ed. (in press). *Pharmacy Business Management*. London: Pharmaceutical Press.

Kolassa E M (1997). *Elements of Pharmaceutical Pricing*. New York: Haworth Press.

Smith M C, Kolassa E M, Perkins G, Siecker B (2002). *Pharmaceutical Marketing: Principles, Environment and Practice*. New York: Haworth Press.

Part 3

Commercial animals

8

Comparative anatomy and physiology

Colin Chapman

It is necessary to understand human anatomy and physiology to be able to undertake the practice of pharmacy, and so it is also necessary to have a reasonable knowledge of veterinary anatomy and physiology to be able to practise veterinary pharmacy. The many different species of animals and birds could make it appear, at first glance at least, that the acquisition of this knowledge will be very difficult. However, animals and birds have structures and functions not all that different from humans, but there are some significant and important differences. The approach taken in this chapter is to deal with anatomy and physiology by focusing on the differences, most of which can be conveniently sub-divided into those involving skeletal structures, digestive system, respi-ratory tract, reproductive system, tegument and cardiovascular system.

Skeletal structures

All animals have essentially the same skeletal structure, right down to the same number of vertebrae in the neck and similar numbers in the thoracic and lumbar regions (Figure 8.1).

It may seem odd that there are the same number of cervical vertebrae in the necks of giraffes and pigs, seven, but that is precisely the case. However, because most animals have tails there are many more vertebrae overall due to these coccygeal vertebrae, some of which are controversially removed in certain breeds of dog such as Jack Russell terriers and boxers. Additionally there are some very important differences in the bones of the limbs.

The situation in birds is somewhat different: the skull is more like that of reptiles, especially the ability to open the beak ('kinesis'); there are variable numbers of cervical vertebrae; the thoracic vertebrae have ribs attached, and there is fusion of some of these vertebrae ('notarium'); a synsacrum is formed by the fusion of many vertebrae from the tho-racic, lumbar, sacral and caudal regions; several vertebrae support the

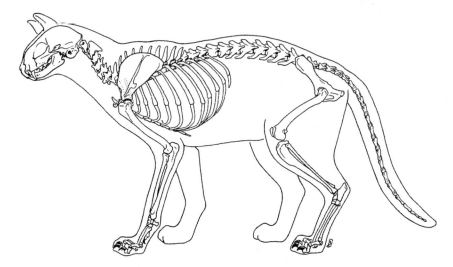

Figure 8.1 Skeleton of a cat. (Adapted from Dyce *et al.*, *Textbook of Veterinary Anatomy*, W B Saunders, 2002.)

tail, including a fused structure ('pygostyle'); the sternum has a large ventral keel in flying birds; and there are some significant differences in the structure of the limbs (Figure 8.2).

The limbs of birds contain the majority of bones found in the limbs of animals but the clavicles are often united to form the furcula ('wishbone'), there are fusions of bones in the metacarpal and metatarsal regions to form the carpometacarpus, tibiotarsus and tarsometatarsus, and the number of digits is reduced to three in the forelimb and four in the hind limb. Most bones have within them components of the air sacs, which occur extensively in the body of birds.

In addition to the bones of the skeleton there can be heterotopic bones that develop by endochondrial or intramembranous ossification such as in the interventricular septum of the heart of cattle, the penis of dogs, and the sesamoid and navicular bones in the feet of horses.

The variations in the structure of the limbs are due in large part to the functions of the limbs and types of locomotion. For example, cats still have remnants of a collar bone ('clavicle') and a clearly distinct radius and ulna in each forelimb because they grasp objects, whereas there is no clavicle and virtually no ulna or fibula in the legs of a horse because the limbs only move forwards and backwards.

The limbs of the horse are unusual for another reason: there is a single digit on each limb (Figure 8.3). In effect, the horse is walking on

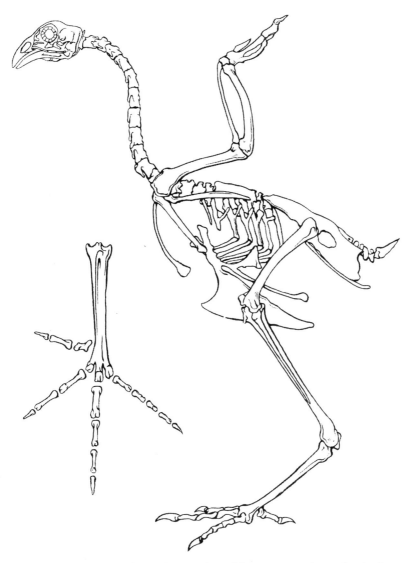

Figure 8.2   Skeleton of a chicken. (Adapted from Dyce *et al.*, *Textbook of Veterinary Anatomy*, W B Saunders, 2002.)

its third fingernail. This means that all but one digit has been lost during the evolutionary process, although tiny remnants of the second and fourth metacarpal bones may remain as 'splint bones' on either side of the third metacarpal bone. The same anatomical structures are also in the hind limbs, except that there is seldom any remnant of the second metatarsal bone. It is hardly surprising that the limbs of horses are such

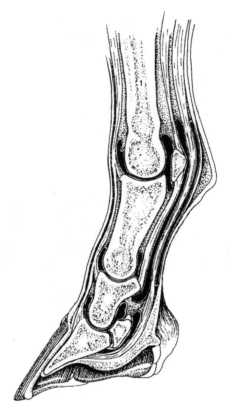

Figure 8.3 Lower limb of a horse. (Adapted from Dyce *et al.*, *Textbook of Veterinary Anatomy*, W B Saunders, 2002.)

a major site of traumatic damage because there is just one digit on each limb carrying an animal that can weigh more than a tonne.

In between humans and horses there is a range of limb modifications, such that dogs usually only have four digits (although, the vestigial fifth digit ('dew claw') may be present on the inner side of both front and hind legs; Figure 8.4), pigs have four digits but only two carry weight ('the trotters'); and ruminant animals, such as sheep, cattle, alpacas and giraffes, have two digits.

Within the skulls of all animals there are sinuses. In sheep and goats the frontal sinuses extend into the horns when these are present. The frontal and other extensive sinuses in the head serve to dissipate the force of impact that occurs when some species of animal head butt each other at considerable speed.

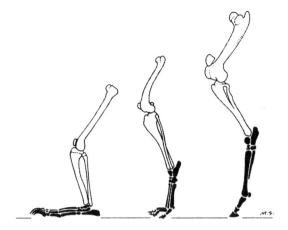

Figure 8.4   Hind limbs of bear, dog and horse. (Adapted from Dyce *et al.*, *Textbook of Veterinary Anatomy*, W B Saunders, 2002.)

Digestive system (see also chapter 9)

The anatomy and physiology of the digestive system in animals and birds is broadly similar to the one in humans. Where differences do occur they reflect changes in structure and function necessary to allow for specialised diets such as a complete reliance on plants by cattle, sheep and goats, or a predatory lifestyle which occurs, to some extent, with dogs and cats.

It is in ruminants that there is the greatest difference, beginning with the absence of some teeth, the presence of a substantial amount of striated muscle in the oesophagus, the production of large amounts of saliva, and the division of the stomach into four compartments (Figure 8.5).

Only one of the compartments of the ruminant stomach, the abomasum, is analogous to the stomach in humans. The other three (rumen, reticulum and omasum) all precede the abomasum, and all have evolved to allow ruminants to be entirely herbivorous. The rumen is effectively a large fermentation vat containing a large number of microorganisms which digest cellulose to produce volatile fatty acids. It undergoes regular contractions which serve to mix the contents and to force food into the reticulum and omasum. The volatile fatty acids produced are absorbed across the stratified squamous epithelium of the rumen to provide a source of energy. The reticulum is a much smaller, muscular, organ which has a central role in the formation of boluses ('cuds') which are regurgitated to be chewed and swallowed ('chewing of the cud').

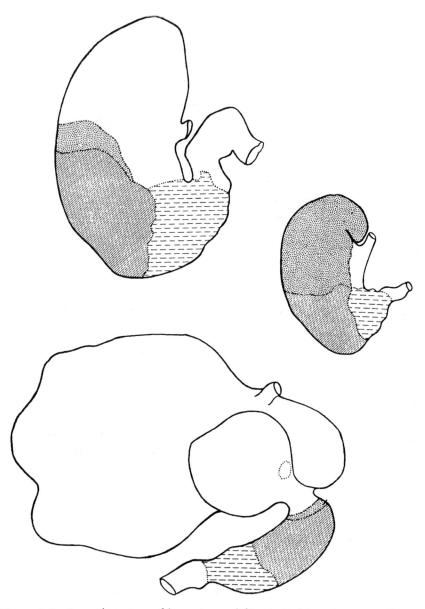

Figure 8.5   Stomach regions of horse (upper left), pig (right) and ruminant (lower left) (clear area is oesophageal region, dark areas are the cardiac and fundic gland regions, and the area with horizontal stripes is the pyloric gland region). (Reproduced from Frandson R D, *Anatomy and Physiology of Farm Animals*, Lea and Febiger, 1970.)

Striated muscle in the oesophagus assists the process. The omasum lies between the reticulum and the abomasum as it is made up of many internal folds, or leaves, which make it well suited for squeezing fluid out of the food passing through it, grinding solid components of the food to some extent, and moving food into the abomasum.

An anatomical structure called the reticular (oesophageal) groove exists in the wall of the reticulum which allows ingested food to pass directly into the omasum, rather than the rumen. This structure permits young ruminants to drink milk without it going into the rumen.

Another major modification of the digestive tract in ruminants occurs with the tooth structure; ruminants do not have upper incisor teeth. These are replaced by a hard pad which allows animals to grasp vegetable matter and to break it off with an upward jerk of the head. The molar teeth are also different in that the dentine and enamel are arranged in a way that facilitates abrasive wear, resulting in sharp edges ideally suited to breaking up plant material.

Horses, rabbits and kangaroos are also herbivores but do not have four compartments to the stomach. Instead the caecum and colon are enlarged and it is in these that fermentation occurs to convert cellulose to absorbable carbohydrates. In horses the caecum can have a capacity of more than 30 L. There is a simple stomach in these animals, and because it is the distal end of the gastrointestinal tract which is modified, rather than the anterior end, there is no regurgitation of food as part of the digestive process.

The animal with a gastrointestinal tract which most closely resembles the one in humans is the pig, and the pig is also an omnivore in that it can eat and digest a range of food types. Further along the spectrum are dogs and cats which are carnivores. The modifications that have been made are to have teeth that can pierce skin and tear meat off bones, and an oesophagus that contains a significant amount of striated muscle that allows food which has been swallowed in a hurry to be regurgitated. The canine teeth in both dogs and cats are spear-like and the molars, particularly the carnassial teeth, structured to produce a shearing or tearing effect.

At the terminal end of the gastrointestinal tract dogs and cats have anal sacs that contain smelly sebaceous material which is extruded in the later stages of defecation. This serves to mark out territory. There are also anal glands in dogs. Both the anal sacs and glands can become impacted or infected in dogs, leading to constipation and other more intractable problems.

The stomach of birds is divided into two parts: the proventriculus and the gizzard, with the gizzard being a 'grinding mill' for seeds and

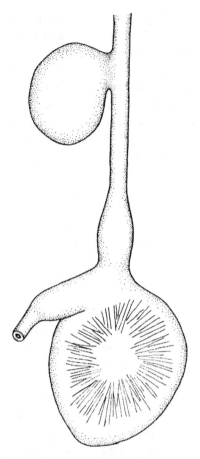

Figure 8.6 Crop (top), oesophagus and gizzard (stomach) of a grain-eating bird. (Adapted from Kent G C, *Comparative Anatomy of the Vertebrates*, W C Brown Communications, 1987.)

other solid material ingested (Figure 8.6). There is also a diverticulum of the oesophagus ('crop') in some birds, particularly the grain eaters, which serves as a storage site that releases food over a period of time for processing in the gizzard. At the end of the digestive tract birds have a chamber ('cloaca') into which the digestive, urinary and reproductive tracts empty.

Respiratory tract

The respiratory tract of animals is very similar to that in humans, except in the horse where there are several unusual anatomical features. One of these makes breathing through the mouth impossible because the soft palate and the epiglottis combine to occlude the opening into the mouth from the larynx. The position of the epiglottis also means that a tube to be passed into the stomach for the purpose of administering medicines must be inserted through the nasal cavity. Another unusual feature is the presence of guttural pouches, each of which can have a volume of up to 500 mL. They are located on either side of the pharynx and are distensions of the eustachian tubes which run from either side of the pharynx to the middle ear. It is reasonably common for the guttural pouches to become infected, leading to chronic respiratory problems and epistaxis. In the larynx there are arytenoid cartilages which serve to close the glottis, the opening to the larynx. If the muscles which are attached to the cartilage become paralysed a condition called 'roaring' can occur in horses.

The purring of cats is believed to be due to the rapid narrowing and widening of the glottis causing air being breathed in and out to vibrate. The ability of many birds to produce elaborate sounds is due mainly to the syrinx, an elaborate structure at the junction of the trachea and bronchi.

Reproductive tract

The anatomy of the female and male reproductive systems in animals is not significantly different from those in humans. Essentially the same structures are present but there are a few differences such as the occurrence of a bone in the penis of dogs, a urethral process extending beyond the tip of the penis in sheep and goats, and a 'fibroelastic' type of structure in the penis of the boar, bull and ram. In the cat the penis points downwards and backwards, and in birds there is no penis but a phallus which in most birds never protrudes. Mating of birds is by a 'cloacal kiss' in which the cloaca of the male is pressed against the cloaca of the female.

There are, however, some significant differences in reproductive physiology, particularly a change from a regular oestrous cycle, as occurs in humans, to oestrous cycles heavily influenced by seasons of the year. Thus, many breeds of sheep are seasonally anoestrus during the colder months of the year, or during periods of short day length; a similar situation occurs in horses. Dogs and cats usually only have oestrous cycles in spring and autumn. To add to the differences, cats only ovulate after mating, and the length of the gestation period varies amongst animals (Table 8.1).

Table 8.1 Duration of pregnancy

Species	Pregnancy (number of days)
Horses	330–345
Cattle	278–290
Sheep	147–155
Goats	145–155
Pigs	112–116
Dogs	62–64
Cats	58–64

Both the visible and the microscopic structures associated with the placenta vary amongst animals to the extent that immunoglobulins are unable to pass from the maternal to the fetal circulation *in utero* in horses, cattle, sheep and goats. This blockage does not occur in dogs, cats or humans. The consequences of the inability of maternal antibodies to cross the placenta means that foals, calves, lambs and kids must obtain protective antibodies in the first milk ('colostrum') within the first 12 to 24 hours of birth.

Two other significant differences occur. The first is that menstruation only occurs in primates, although dogs and cats may bleed in the hours before coming into oestrus or ('heat'), a phase of the cycle known as pro-oestrus. The second is that, apart from elephants, it is only primates that have mammary glands located on the thorax, although dogs, cats and pigs have mammary glands all along the thorax and abdomen.

Integument

There are some very obvious differences in the structure of the skin particularly the type of hair, the specialised thickenings of the skin, and the number and nature of skin glands. There are also a variety of modifications to the nails on the digits, and there are horns and antlers which have no equivalents in humans, other than in mythology.

Hair is a keratinised skin appendage which is shed and usually replaced. It consists of dense keratin and dermal pigments, giving hair a variety of colours. White or grey hair occurs because of reduction in the amount of pigment and an increase in the number of air vacuoles in the hair fibre. Hair can be of three broad types: guard, wool and tactile. The guard hairs form the 'top coat' and generally lie against the skin to give a smooth appearance, but there are variations. For example, the bristle of pigs and the coarse hair in the mane and tail of horses are also guard hairs which have a thick medulla and thin cortex, whereas the hair of the coat of dogs and cats has a thin medulla and thick cortex. In humans the guard hairs are shed continuously but in animals the shedding is intermittent, usually seasonal. Wool hairs are well developed in sheep and have no medulla. Goats and some rabbits have hairs with structures somewhere between guard and wool hairs. Tactile hairs are thicker and longer than guard hairs, with the best example being whiskers on a cat.

Feathers are not a form of hair but modified scales, which are themselves repetitious thickenings of the stratum corneum. There are no scales in mammals except for the legs and tails of rodents. Feathers receive brown, yellow and red pigments but not blue. Any blue colouration is due to reflected light, just like a blue sky.

Footpads are cushions on which animals walk. They are made up of dense cornified epidermis and thick subcutaneous tissue. In dogs and cats there are digital and metacarpal pads, along with carpal pads which have no obvious function. Footpads are incorporated into the hoof of ruminants and pigs ('bulbs') and horses ('frog' and 'bulbs of the heel'). In horses there are also rudimentary metacarpal and metatarsal pads ('ergots') and vestigial carpal and tarsal pads ('chestnuts'). In dogs, pigs and horses the footpads contain sweat glands which serve to mark out 'territories' for these animals.

In addition to the sweat glands in footpads there are also a number of different types of sebaceous and sweat glands in other parts of the body of animals. These include 'conventional' sebaceous glands which produce sebum in all animals, including sheep where it is known as wool fat, and musk deer where it gives rise to perfumes. Pheromones are also present in the sebum of animals particularly dogs and cats. Other sebaceous glands include tail and anal glands in dogs, horn glands in goats, circumoral glands in cats, and glands around the eyes and feet of sheep. Sweat glands are also found in animals but dogs and pigs have few of them. Since one of the ways body temperature is controlled is by sweating, dogs have to pant to make up for an inability to sweat. Horses on the other hand can sweat profusely.

Claws, hoofs and nails are all modifications of the stratum corneum at the ends of the digits, and all have the same basic structure: a hard dorsal plate and a softer ventral plate ('nail bed'). Mention has already been made of the horse's foot being a highly evolved version of the fingernail of humans. The hoofs of ruminants and pigs are similar to those of the horse, whereas the claws of dogs and cats are more like the finger- and toenails of humans.

Horns and antlers are composed of keratin, either as the true horns in cattle, sheep and goats, or hair horns composed of aggregated keratinised hair-like epidermal fibres on the nose of rhinoceros. Antlers and giraffe horns are branched dermal bone, not cornified structures, which are covered with skin ('velvet'). Antlers are usually shed from season to season.

Sensory organs

The sensory organs in animals and birds generally have the same structure and function as those in humans. When there are differences these are more qualitative than quantitative. For example, hearing and smell are acute in dogs, night vision is better in most animals compared with humans, and the ears of animals are 'mobile' to allow the auricles ('pinnae') to be turned towards noise. Within the auricle is cartilage, reasonably stiff in most animals but soft in dogs, and in dogs the external acoustic meatus is 'L' shaped, making it susceptible to infection and difficult to examine clinically (Figure 8.7).

The sense of smell is highly developed in most animals, being aided in this by both the voluminous nature of the nasal cavities in many instances and the highly developed nature of the olfactory epithelium, although this is poorly developed in birds. The vomeronasal organ

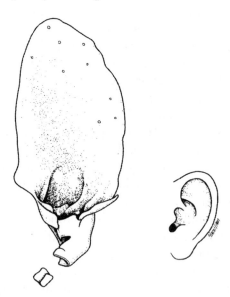

Figure 8.7   Left ear of dog and human. (Adapted from Dyce *et al.*, *Textbook of Veterinary Anatomy*, W B Saunders, 2002.)

(Jacobson's organ) is believed responsible for the lip-curl (flehman) reaction seen when male animals smell urine or vaginal secretions. It is present in many animals but absent in humans.

In the eye the number of rods and cones, the neurosensory cells in the retina, vary in number and distribution among animals, birds and humans. Rods, which only detect images in black and white, and which are most effective in relatively low light intensities, are more common in animals with good night vision. Cones on the other hand are of three types, each detecting one part of the visible spectrum: blue, green or red. Not all animals have colour vision and those that do have the greatest concentration of cones in the centre (fovea) of the eye, with rods more in the periphery. In humans the cones are well developed.

Cardiovascular system

The one notable difference in the cardiovascular system is the composition of blood in birds where there is retention of a nucleus in red blood cells. The lymphatics also differ because there is a bursa of Fabricius in birds but not animals, and there are lymph nodes in animals but not in most birds. The resting pulse rate varies among the animal species (Table 8.2).

Veterinary medicines (see also chapter 3)

Peculiarities of anatomy and physiology of animals and birds has resulted in the development of specialised dose forms, the administration of drugs by unusual routes, and some important differences in pharmacodynamics and pharmacokinetics.

Table 8.2 Resting pulse, respiratory rates and body temperature

Species	Pulse rate[a]	Respiratory rate[b]	Temperature[c]
Horses	30–40[d]	10–15	38
Cattle	60–80[e]	30–50	38.5
Sheep	70–90	15–35	39
Goats	70–90	30–60	39
Pigs	70–120	30–60	39
Dogs	70–120	20–35	39
Cats	120–140	15–40	38.5
Hamsters	300–600	–	–

[a]Beats per minute; [b]breaths per minute; [c]rectal (degrees Celsius); [d]colts 70–80; [e]calves 100–120

The majority of unusual dose forms have been developed for ruminants, particularly devices that can be placed in the rumen to deliver drug or mineral over a long period of time. These devices are usually 'boluses' with enough weight to be trapped in the rumen, or have 'wings' to prevent them being regurgitated.

An unusual route of administration used in cattle is based on the fact that the upper part of the rumen is located just below the skin in the left paralumbar fossa, a distinct indentation high on the flank just behind the ribs. It has proven possible to inject drugs, usually anthelmintics, directly through the skin in the fossa and into the rumen, the so-called intraruminal injection.

However, a more common way of administering anthelmintics is by way of 'drenching guns' which are devices that permit the repeated oral dosing of many animals in succession by way of a syringe which is put into a repeat action gun-like device with a long nozzle. Drugs and minerals can also be administered indirectly by applying medication to feed or putting it in water, by placing medicated licks in easily accessible places, and by painting medication on the flank of cattle so that it is licked off.

In order to treat the ectoparasites that commonly infest sheep, cattle and goats a number of 'pour-on' formulations have been developed, largely superseding the older plunge and spray dips which were used to fully wet animals with insecticides. The older forms of treatment were quite difficult to manage because the repeated use of the plunge dips and the recycling of water in spray dips resulted in the insecticides being 'stripped' and having to be replaced or topped up at regular intervals.

The oral dosing of horses can be by 'stomach tube', with the tube having to be passed through the nose. It requires considerable expertise to do this, so oral paste formulations were developed and these have greatly simplified the oral administration of drugs to horses. Pastes are now used for other species of animal as well.

There are a few drugs that behave differently in animals, largely because of differences in physiology. This is particularly the case with aspirin, paracetamol (acetaminophen), monensin and the avermectins. The metabolism of aspirin is slow in cats because of reduced glucuronyl transferase activity. The half-life is four to five times longer than in dogs or humans, which means that aspirin should only be administered once daily to cats.

The situation with paracetamol in cats is much more serious due to the toxicity that arises as a result of defective conjugation of the drug in the liver. Normally, paracetamol is metabolised by phase 2 mechanisms, such as conjugation with glucuronide or sulfate, to form non-toxic metabolites. In the cat these pathways are grossly ineffective so phase 1 mechanisms are utilised, resulting in highly toxic metabolites. To add to the problem, the metabolites would normally be dealt with by intracellular glutathione, but this is also a defective system in the cat. The net result is that paracetamol kills cats, due to methaemoglobinuria and liver necrosis, at doses as low as a single 500 mg tablet.

Monensin and avermectin are reported to be toxic in some circumstances. Monensin and several other carboxylic ionophores are used to control coccidiosis in poultry and to promote growth in cattle. Should they be given inadvertently to horses there can be myocardial and skeletal muscle necrosis, resulting in death due to congestive heart failure. Giving leftover feed for cattle to horses is a common cause of poisoning. Avermectins are used extensively to kill both internal and external parasites in animals but toxicity has been reported when this drug is used in rough-haired collies, and when abamectin is used in Murray grey cattle. In both cases the toxicity manifests as tremors and coma.

In addition to the differences in the anatomy and physiology of animals and birds, there are behavioural characteristics that make animals different in many respects to humans. However, the variations in behaviour are quantitative rather than qualitative, such that the fight and flight reflex is exaggerated in horses and subservient behaviour is exaggerated in some dogs. To further complicate matters, there are animal husbandry and environmental factors that can have a big influence on the health and welfare of animals. The net result is that diseases of animals will be unlike those in humans in many cases or will occur far more frequently in animals. However, there are also many diseases in common. It is against this diverse background that veterinary pharmacy has to be considered.

Further reading

Dyce K M, Sack W O, Wensing C J G (2002). *Textbook of Veterinary Anatomy*, 3rd edn. Philadelphia: W B Saunders Company.

Frandson R D (1992). *Anatomy and Physiology of Farm Animals*, 5th edn. Philadelphia: Lea and Febiger.

Kent G C (1987). *Comparative Anatomy of the Vertebrates*, 7th edn. Oxford: W C Brown Communications.

9

Animal nutrition

Graham Crawley

This chapter will briefly discuss the significant variations from human systems that occur in farmed mammals, with the emphasis on ruminants. It will also consider some of the specific diseases or syndromes that arise when there is an inadequate provision of food. The feed problem can be in quantity, quality or composition, or any combination of these. General malnutrition occurs, but will not be discussed as the effects and results are similar in all species including humans. Most of the few cases which occur in the UK arise from neglect nowadays and are rarely due to ignorance.

Background

Animals are traditionally described as being carnivores, omnivores or herbivores depending on what they eat. However, we now know that this is an oversimplification. Most species are omnivorous (mixed feeders), some having a preference or tendency to ingest a high proportion of animal tissue (the carnivores), and rather more species having a preference or tendency to ingest mainly plant material (the herbivores). Feral sheep on some of the Shetland islands have been seen to catch and partially eat young seabirds, as have deer on the island of Rhum.

The animals at the herbivorous end of this spectrum have problems. Herbage is a less concentrated source of nutrients than animal tissues, necessitating a greater intake of food and hence a significantly larger proportion of the body volume being dedicated to digestion. In addition, the release for absorption of the carbohydrates, proteins and other nutrients that are present is hindered by the rigid cellulose structure of plant cell walls. This is particularly important for ingested herbage as distinct from grains and other concentrate rations.

This means that successful herbivores have had to develop systems that enable them to obtain these nutrients by breaking down the cell walls. Many mammals are not good at making cellulase enzymes. They have to rely on the bacteria and protozoa that are resident as commensals in the gastrointestinal tract to rupture the cell walls. This has involved changes in both the anatomy and the physiology of the gastrointestinal tract (see chapter 8), all the way from the mouth to the large intestine. Humans achieve this objective by cooking their food, which also tends to degrade the nutrients.

It should also be remembered that herbivores are prey species. This controls their feeding patterns and hence influences how they should be fed and managed when they are being reared and maintained in a farm environment – the more their management can allow their normal behaviour patterns the better. For instance, ruminants such as cattle and sheep tend to eat a large quantity quickly with a minimum of mastication, and set about chewing and digesting it later on. Equines, which have, proportionally, a much smaller stomach, prefer to eat little and often, and they chew the food well before swallowing.

It is interesting to remember that it was only in the mid-nineteenth century that Claude Bernard first proposed the theory of the stable chemical composition of the *milieu interieur*, thereby starting the study of biochemistry and metabolism. Since then we have learned a considerable amount about the biochemical techniques and mechanisms which evolved to maintain this internal stability, while providing the biochemical requirements for reproduction, growth, milk production, immune responses, energy for movement, etc. We now know that, at least from a metabolic standpoint, pigs are very similar to humans, so there will be little mention of them here, whereas ruminants (and the other herbivores) do have major differences from humans. Hence this chapter will address mainly ruminant nutrition and metabolism. Not only do the ruminants have major variations from monogastric animals, but they are by far the most important of the domesticated herbivores in UK agriculture.

Considering the variations in the architecture of the gastrointestinal tract and in the sources of the major nutrients, to a quite surprising degree the fundamental metabolic pathways are similar in all the main species. To illustrate the most extreme divergence in structure and diet, compare the felines as carnivores with the ruminants, which are herbivores (see Table 9.1). Not only is there a major difference in the proportions of the gastrointestinal tract, there is also a much greater gastrointestinal tract volume relative to body size in herbivores.

Cats, the most carnivorous of domesticated animals, have a small stomach and a relatively short intestinal tract but, as predators, are able to ingest large quantities relative to their body weight. However, they

Table 9.1   Gastrointestinal tract proportions

	Stomach(s)	*Intestines*
Ruminant	70%	30%
Feline (monogastric)	30%	70%

will then not need to feed for several days (some predators can survive for months without feeding or needing to feed). On the other hand, ruminants have a very large 'stomach' (250 L plus in adult cattle), which is divided into well-defined areas. In relation to body size, the intestines are much longer, and are more convoluted and of greater diameter, although they make up a smaller proportion of the total gastrointestinal tract volume. Like all herbivores, they must eat large quantities every day. It only takes 12 hours for food to pass right through the gastrointestinal tract of a cat, but it takes 4 days in a cow!

Ruminant specialisation

'Ruminant' is the name given to those species of mammals that swallow food as soon as it is ingested with little if any preliminary mastication, and later bring the food back up to the mouth in boluses for thorough chewing. This retrieval of food for further chewing is called rumination. The species that do this include cattle, sheep, goats, deer, camels and other camelids, and even giraffes. So, despite the rather ponderous nature of the system, it must be efficient to have survived the rigour of evolutionary selection in a wide variety of species.

As Table 9.2 shows, ruminants are born with a gastrointestinal tract in which the 'stomach' area is very different from that in adults. This is because, as with all mammals, the newborn ruminant lives on a milk diet. Hence, their 'stomach' must be able to clot and then digest milk efficiently and there is no requirement for rumination. The only 'stomach' of the four that meets these requirements is the abomasum. As the animal grows older it starts to eat grass or hay, and some concentrate rations, the proportions of the stomach alter (see Table 9.2) with a dramatic increase in the size of the rumen and reticulum (reticulo-rumen), and rumination will start.

When food is swallowed it enters the reticulo-rumen, where it stays for 2–3 days. From there it moves into the omasum and then the abomasum, before entering the small intestine. Most of what is usually called the 'stomach' in ruminants bears little resemblance to that organ in simple-stomached or monogastric species. In ruminants the whole

Table 9.2 Bovine stomachs

| | Ratio of sizes with age expressed as % | | |
	Rumen and reticulum	Omasum	Abomasum
Birth	38	13	49
8 weeks	60	13	27
36 weeks	65	25	11
72 weeks	85	7	8

organ is divided into different sections (usually four). The first sections are, in essence, a vast dilation of the oesophagus, which can more properly be compared to the crop in birds – except that the crop is mainly a storage organ. The first sections in ruminants play a major role in digestion (i.e. the breakdown of food) and, to a much lesser extent, absorption. Only the final section has any real similarity to the single stomach in non-ruminant species, but it is still not the same as a monogastric stomach. The various sections or areas can be easily differentiated by both the structure of the internal surface and the thickness of the 'stomach' wall (see Table 9.3). The anatomy of the stomachs in an adult bovine is shown in Figure 9.1.

The ruminant animal will graze for a period of time (or eat silage, hay or concentrate ration), swallowing what it ingests without chewing the food. It will then usually lie down and start rumination. Careful observation will reveal that roughly every 30 seconds the animal will

Table 9.3 Bovine stomachs: the function of the stomachs in ruminants

Name	Function
Rumen	>70% of the total volume. In this area the fermentation of ingested food occurs by microbial activity
Reticulum	This, although being structurally distinct, is functionally an extension of the rumen; but it will also act as dustbin for non-plant materials (stones, soil, pieces of metal etc.) inadvertently swallowed when the animal is grazing
Omasum	This, although small, has an extensive surface area created by the presence of many very large folds in the internal surface (hence in abattoir slang – 'The Bible'). The functions are not fully understood, but are probably involved in the scavenging of monovalent ions
Abomasum	Functionally this is the part most similar to a monogastric stomach, but the contents are much less acidic

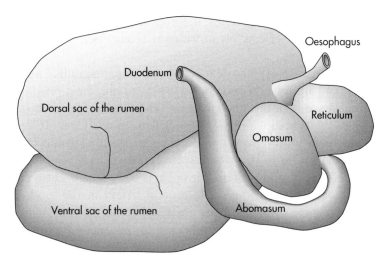

Figure 9.1 Diagram of the anatomy of the stomachs in an adult bovine.

have a small eructation and then start chewing. The chewing starts as a bolus of food comes into the mouth along with the voided gas. After being chewed, the bolus will be swallowed again and the process is repeated. Rumination will only occur in animals that are restful and relaxed. It will not occur if they are walking, apprehensive or otherwise distracted or disturbed.

The eructation is critically important. The fermentation in the reticulo-rumen produces several hundred litres of gas (mainly methane and carbon dioxide) each day. If the animal cannot void the gas it will become bloated, with a grossly distended rumen and abdomen, and will die very soon afterwards if the condition is not treated. Thomas Hardy described the effects very well in *Far From The Madding Crowd*.

The reticulo-rumen contains, in addition to food, a liquid suspension of bacteria and protozoa, numbered in many millions per millilitre. These organisms are responsible for the fermentation of feed that is the function of these stomachs. Chewing during rumination and the subsequent fermentation help to break down the cellulose-based cell walls, giving access to the starch and other nutrients that are contained in the cells. As with all the gastrointestinal tract, the muscles in the walls of these stomachs have an inherent motility. In the reticulo-rumen this ensures that there is thorough mixing of the ingested food with the fermentative organisms, and it also creates feed boluses, which are pushed up into the end of the oesophagus. This movement into the lower end of the oesophagus stimulates reverse peristalsis, which moves the food up to the mouth. The presence of the reticulo-rumen or fermentation chamber has major effects on nutritional requirements and digestive function.

Firstly, because of microbial activity, ruminants, unlike any other mammals, can utilise non-protein nitrogen for the creation of amino acids, and hence peptides and proteins. These molecules then become available to the animal when the microorganisms die. Up to 10% of the animal's protein requirement can be created from inorganic nitrogen. While this may seem to be rather esoteric, it does have major implications for costs, as non-protein nitrogen is very much cheaper than protein nitrogen. Rumen digestible protein (RDP) in the food can be broken down in the rumen and absorbed by microorganisms, which will in time die and release the protein back into the rumen liquor. Here it will either be recycled through more bacteria or pass into the intestine for absorption by the animal. Other proteins (i.e. undigestible protein, UDP) are not digested in the rumen and pass straight through into the intestine. Achieving the correct balance of these three protein sources is an important but difficult art.

The balance is important as it is one of the requirements needed to optimise the function of the rumen by maintaining the correct microbial population; and the better the rumen functions the more efficient is the animal in growth, milk production, etc. For the same reason, it is also necessary that the diet contains an adequate supply of the correct type of fibre to optimise rumen function. Sometimes this is difficult to achieve. For instance, in very high-producing dairy cows at peak lactation the demands for all nutrients are very high, and it is not easy to formulate a diet which meets all these requirements and at the same time contains sufficient fibre, whilst being fed to the animal within its appetite. In particular, if there is a negative energy balance then serious problems can occur; this will be discussed later. The dry matter content of the food, rather than the total volume of the food, mainly controls the quantity that an animal will eat in a day.

As a consequence of the microbial activity in the rumen–reticulum complex, deficiencies of the water-soluble vitamins are very unusual in ruminants. Two such deficiencies occasionally occur and these will be discussed later in the chapter.

The early stages of energy metabolism in ruminants are radically different from those in monogastric species, even though they all use the tricarboxylic acid (TCA) cycle for the final release of energy through ATP and ADP. Energy is absorbed from the food mainly as free fatty acids (FFAs), which are propionic, butyric and acetic acids. Of these, in typical circumstances, over 80% is propionic acid. A small proportion of energy is absorbed as glucose. This is only used for central nervous system functions and the production of milk sugars. If there is insufficient glucose absorption to meet this demand, gluconeogenesis will occur from propionic acid, pyruvate or even proteins. The FFAs are absorbed mainly in the rumen, and to a lesser extent in the small intestine. When the FFAs have been absorbed they will be converted to pyruvate and then move on to enter the TCA cycle as a source of energy (see Figure 9.2).

If it is not required for immediate use, the energy will be converted into lipid as a concentrated energy store, used for gluconeogenesis, or converted to glycogen and stored. The biochemical mechanisms for the production of energy by the TCA cycle are identical to those that occur in monogastrics, i.e. the ATP–ADP system.

Equines are interesting because they have combined both systems for energy absorption and production. The stomach and small intestine function as in other monogastric species, and the enlarged large intestine acts as a fermentation system for FFA production. This function of the

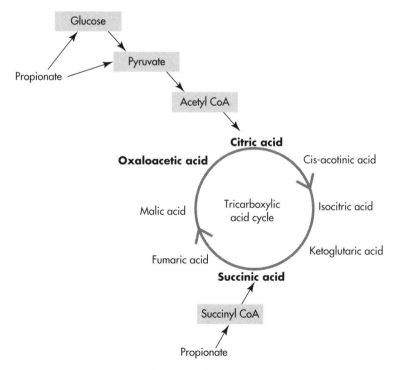

Figure 9.2   The tricarboxylic acid cycle.

Table 9.4 Problems that can arise when there is either incorrect feeding or metabolic demands are greater than the animal can manage

Major nutrients	Major minerals	Trace compounds	Physical problems
(1) Energy	(2) Calcium	(5) Thiamin	(12) Bloat
	(3) Phosphorus	(6) Vitamin B_{12}/cobalt	
	(4) Magnesium	(7) Vitamin E/selenium	
		(8) Copper	
		(9) Iron	
		(10) Iodine	
		(11) Vitamin D	

large intestine has been adopted by a variety of other species, and they are usually referred to collectively as 'hind gut fermenters'.

To return to the ruminants, we will now look at problems that can and do arise when there is either incorrect feeding or metabolic demands that are greater than the animal can manage, and sometimes a combination of both.

These problems will be considered in three groups (see Table 9.4): those related to the major nutrients; the problems related to the major minerals, such as calcium; and those related to nutrients that are required in very small amounts – vitamins and trace elements.

Energy balance problems

Whilst the biochemical problem is very similar in cattle and sheep metabolically, the times of the usual problem in cows and the problem in sheep are very different, as are the clinical symptoms. In cattle, it occurs in dairy cows as they reach peak lactation. In sheep, it occurs in ewes in late pregnancy when they are carrying more than one fetus. Recently, a syndrome in cattle has been described that is much more similar to the sheep syndrome with regard to symptoms, timing and refractoriness to treatment.

Cattle

There are two syndromes related to energy problems in cattle.

The main energy-related disease has a variety of names, including ketosis, slow fever and acetonaemia. This abundance of names confirms that this syndrome has been recognised for many years and can cause significant problems. The incidence has decreased since the introduction of loose housing and the feeding of silage. It usually occurs 6–8 weeks after calving in dairy cows that calve during the period when they are housed. The problem arises when cows, as they move towards peak lactation, cannot ingest sufficient food to provide all the energy needed to meet the enormous demands that this entails, and an energy deficit arises. As descibed above, there is a limit to the quantity of food that they can eat, and there has to be sufficient roughage in the total food intake to maintain efficient rumen function. Hence, it is not possible to feed just concentrates in order to avoid the energy deficit. The cow will start to metabolise body fat stores in significant quantities. This causes the production of clinically significant amounts of the ketone bodies, which are β-hydroxybutyric acid and aceto-acetic acid together with their decarboxylation products isopropanol and acetone. These then produce a metabolic acidosis. This causes the cow to become lethargic, reduce milk production, become constipated and stop eating concentrate rations, which makes matters even worse. If left untreated the animal will usually recover very slowly, after a dramatic loss of body weight and an almost complete cessation of milk production.

Some people can detect the presence of ketone bodies in milk, breath and urine by smell but there is a reliable biochemical test that can be used to confirm the diagnosis.

Treatment with a single dose of corticosteroid and a high-energy feed will virtually always produce a rapid and reliable response, but usually the cow will not produce as much milk in that lactation as she should. In ruminants it has been shown that ethylene glycol (antifreeze) is a very good high-energy drench, and pharmaceutical-grade preparations are available. Oral glucose is not effective and is not used. It would be absorbed by the rumen microorganisms and never arrive in the small intestine, where it could be absorbed. A small dose given intravenously can be beneficial to support the main therapy.

The other fairly recently described form of energy deficiency in cattle is called 'fat cow syndrome'. It occurs 7–10 days after calving in dairy cows and just before calving in beef cows, usually those that are carrying twins (compare with sheep; see next section). There is total anorexia and recumbency, with a normal temperature, pulse and respiration. It is difficult to treat and death may occur within14 days. It is usually caused by overfeeding the cow with energy when she is not lactating. This causes liver damage, which reduces the cow's ability to metabolise many things, but importantly, in this case, energy. This leads to metabolic acidosis, as described below. This syndrome was first described in the 1980s.

Sheep

The clinical problem in sheep is called 'twin lamb disease'. It occurs duing the last 3–4 weeks of pregnancy, almost exclusively in ewes carrying more than one lamb. Hence the name of the syndrome. In sheep the problem arises because the ewe is in a fairly delicate balance in late pregnancy. As the fetuses grow they put more demands on the ewe's metabolism. Unfortunately, at the same time they occupy an increasing amount of the abdominal volume. This reduces the quantity of food that the ewe can ingest in a day, hence reducing the available metabolic energy and other nutrients. It is when this situation tilts towards an energy deficit that twin lamb disease starts, again due to a metabolic acidosis.

Clinically affected ewes will initially be seen to be dull and not move with the rest of the flock. They will not eat their concentrates, hence they have even less metabolic energy and a vicious spiral develops as they metabolise more body fat and hence become more ketotic. As the disease develops, the ewes become blind and even less active. If left, they will rapidly lose body condition and die.

Treatment of twin lamb disease is not easy and there is no standard therapeutic regime. As the ewe is in late pregnancy, corticosteroids cannot be given as the fetuses could be damaged. Various treatment strategies have been tried, including repeated intravenous glucose injections and very high parenteral doses of multivitamins. The only reasonably effective trcatment regime is of use only when the ewe is detected early in the course of the disease. Repeated treatments with high doses of ethylene glycol, twice daily initially, have been proved to be beneficial.

Calcium deficiency

The calcium balance in animals is controlled by many factors, which are essentially the same as in humans (see Figure 9.3). However, the variations in blood calcium level are larger than in humans, and disease will result when the level drops too low. It is also possible for cows or ewes to have blood calcium levels that are well below the supposedly critical level without any clinical symptoms. As with energy problems, the timing of calcium problems and the clinical manifestations are different in cattle and sheep, as are the greatest demands on the calcium pool, which are milk production in cattle and multiple fetuses in ewes. The equivalent disease in humans is true eclampsia, which occurs well into lactation. Among the domesticated species, only cats and dogs produce a clinical syndrome similar to true eclampsia in humans.

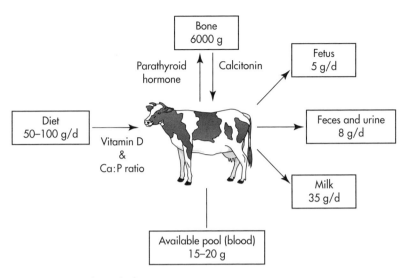

Figure 9.3 Calcium balance.

Probably the single most important point to understand is that true calcium deficiency is very rare. The usual problem is hypocalcaemia or reduced blood calcium level, even though there is sufficient calcium in the body to correct the situation. Figure 9.3 highlights how close the demand for calcium is to the daily intake, and how low the calcium reserves are in the body. The drop in blood calcium occurs rapidly and there is no reserve which the body can activate rapidly. This is because most of the calcium in the body is tightly bound in hard tissues, such as bones and teeth. It takes a long time for the body to release useful amounts of calcium from these tissues. So when there is a rapid decline in blood calcium level, the body is not able to respond fast enough to rectify the problem. Paradoxically, in some animals this will lead to the onset of clinical disease, whereas other animals, with very similar or even identical blood chemistry, will be clinically normal.

Cattle

Hypocalcaemia is a problem in dairy cattle. The incidence of this disease increases with age, or probably more correctly with the number of pregnancies, and some breeds of cattle are more prone to the problem even within the dairy breeds. For instance, the Channel Island breeds are much more likely to develop hypocalcaemia than Friesians. The syndrome will most frequently happen from 3–4 days before calving to 2–3 days after calving and is usually called 'milk fever' or, more correctly, 'parturient paresis'. The latter term is more correct because a raised temperature is not one of the symptoms that occurs in this disease, but there is paresis. The symptoms vary depending on whether the problem starts before, during or after calving. Let us ignore the calf for a moment; the symptoms that develop are directly related to the effects of calcium on the function of nerve cells or neurones.

Initially, there will be slight drowsiness with a mild degree of unsteadiness. This quite rapidly develops into a marked unsteadiness with stiff straight legs due to spastic paralysis. The animal will transfer its weight from one hind leg to the other in a very characteristic paddling movement. At the same time gastrointestinal tract motility slows down and no dung or urine will be voided. The animal then progresses to loss of balance and will fall over to lie in lateral recumbency. It will stop eructating so the rumen will swell which can lead to death if there is no treatment.

If the problem starts during calving, in addition to the above parturition stops until treatment is given. This can lead to the death of the calf. If the problem occurs soon after calving then it will stop the expulsion of the placenta (afterbirth), which can lead to metritis and subsequently to reduced fertility. This can be a serious problem, as cows must calve regularly to maintain their annual milk production. If confirmation of the diagnosis is required, serum calcium levels are measured easily and are very reliable (c.f. hypomagnesaemia).

Treatment is by injecting calcium borogluconate, which is a non-irritant solution of calcium formulated as 20 and 40% solutions in 400 mL bottles. In mild or early cases it can be given subcutaneously, but in more advanced cases the calcium must be given intravenously. Either solution can be used subcutaneously but only the 20% can be used intravenously. If the 40% is given by this route there is a severe risk of causing cardiac arrest. When treating a clinical case intravenously it is good practice to give a subcutaneous injection to act as a depot for continued treatment. When giving large-volume subcutaneous treatments, the fluid must be at body temperature when it is injected. If it is cold all the blood vessels around the injection site constrict and the fluid will not be absorbed. If it is given cold it is often possible to feel the fluid still present where it was injected 12 hours later.

When a cow that is already recumbent and showing all the symptoms is treated intravenously, there is a rapid and dramatic response. She will very quickly become more alert, lose the spastic paralysis and move into sternal recumbency. This enables her to eructate, which will reduce the rumen distension and make her much more comfortable. She will then quickly progress to standing and passing urine and feces, and may even be eating again within a short time.

The above description is true for uncomplicated hypocalcaemia. However, often there are complications in the form of reduced levels of other chemical components of the blood, such as phosphorus, magnesium and energy. These do not alter the clinical picture but can complicate treatment. A selection of calcium borogluconate solution formulations with some or all of these components has been developed. They are often used for pre-emptive subcutaneous treatment but can also be given therapeutically, either intravenously or subcutaneously.

Sheep

In sheep the equivalent syndrome is called lambing sickness. This nearly always starts soon after lambing but produces a similar clinical picture to that already described. Unfortunately, during late pregnancy and early lactation the ewe is living on a metabolic knife-edge for energy, calcium and magnesium. So any interruption in food intake will disturb blood calcium, blood magnesium and energy levels, so that the clinical and biochemical findings tend to be similar whatever the original problem was. So treatment is usually for all three conditions and does not depend on making a clear, specific diagnosis, which is difficult. The main need is to differentiate the metabolic syndromes from other causes of malaise in peripartum ewes.

Phosphorus deficiency

While this occurs in some countries, it is very rare in the UK. True phosphorus deficiency will cause pica or depraved appetite. Cows and sheep will chew on old bones and/or lick soil, both of which are abnormal behaviour patterns but are not exclusive to phosphorus deficiency. These behaviours are important because they may expose the animals to organisms such as *Clostridium botulinum* (see chapter 10).

A long-held belief holds that phosphorus deficiency will cause infertility, but there is a considerable debate on this topic. However, there will be reduced fertility when the cattle have become so thin that they are unable to ovulate or sustain an implanted embryo. This is similar to the amenorrhoea which develops in human females with advanced anorexia nervosa. In these situations the effects on reproduction are secondary to the loss of condition; they will occur whatever causes the loss of condition and are not directly due to the specific problem.

The other symptom that has been associated with phosphorus problems in the UK is 'dog-sitting'. This is when cows sit up on their hindquarters just like an alert dog. This is a very unusual behaviour as cattle normally stand up hind end first.

Much more common is an incorrect calcium : phosphorus ratio, the effects of which vary depending on which way the ratio has changed. Ideally the ratio should be between 2 : 1 and 1 : 1. When the ratio rises, i.e. there is too much calcium, then bone fractures occur. When the ratio changes in the other direction, i.e. there is too much phosphorus, then rickets, osteomalacia and arthropathy will occur.

The only way that this ratio can be determined is by analysing bone samples from a dead animal. Traditionally, the analysis is done on rib bone. Although the result is not useful for the dead animal, these are herd problems, so the result indicates whether there should be dietary adjustment for the rest of the animals in the group.

Magnesium deficiency

As with calcium absorption, a variety of factors influence the bioavailability of magnesium. However, in this case the factors are external and include the concentrations of various ions in the feed, particularly the sodium : potassium ratio. Magnesium absorption increases with a rising ratio until it reaches a plateau at a ratio of 5. The type of protein in the herbage changes during the growing season, and the protein in early grass reduces magnesium availability. Also important is the time that food dwells in the intestine; the longer the better, so again early grass, which speeds up the transport of food, is a problem.

Figure 9.4 shows that balance is even finer than the calcium situation. It is extremely difficult for the animal to release any magnesium from the hard tissues to try to correct any drop in the blood magnesium level. A further complication arises because the turnover rate of the magnesium pool is very fast, so a change in availability has a rapid effect on the blood magnesium level. As with calcium, the clinical disease is due to hypomagnesaemia, which may or may not be accompanied by whole-body magnesium deficiency. Animals can survive for days or weeks with blood magnesium levels well below the critical level, and only develop the typical clinical symptoms after a sudden surprise or stress. When an animal develops the disease it is important to realise that many of the other animals within the group will also have a low blood magnesium level, and will be at risk.

In both cattle and sheep the disease is called 'staggers' or 'grass staggers'.

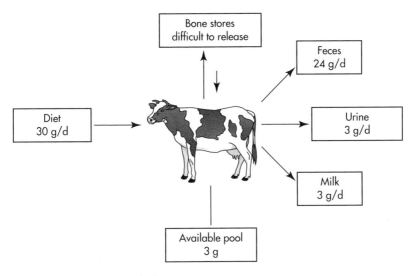

Figure 9.4 Magnesium balance.

Cattle

The problem typically occurs within 2–3 months of the animals being turned out from winter housing onto spring grass. Whereas milk fever will develop over several hours, staggers is much more rapid and animals can go from apparent normality to death within less than 2 hours. Again the effects are on the function of the nervous system. The first symptom is hyperaesthesia, an exaggerated response to external stimuli. Incoordination, paralysis, recumbency and death quickly follow if no treatment is given. Diagnosis on clinical symptoms is not always easy and laboratory techniques can be misleading. Although the problem is hypomagnesaemia, immediately before death there is a sudden release of magnesium into the blood. Hence ante-mortem and postmortem serum magnesium levels are not useful. The most reliable postmortem sample for magnesium analysis is the aqueous humour from the anterior chamber of the eye.

Treatment is by the subcutaneous injection of magnesium sulfate solution, but the act of putting an injection needle through the skin may cause a fatal seizure.

Intravenous treatment is very hazardous and should only be done by a veterinary surgeon because of the risk of cardiac arrest.

Obviously, with such a dramatic and dangerous disease, prevention is very important. Unfortunately, most magnesium salts are unpalatable, so it is difficult to give magnesium by mouth, and due to its rapid turnover the magnesium has to be given every day. Magnesium lactate is reasonably palatable and is also water-soluble, so it can be added to drinking water as long as there is no other source of water available. If there is, the stock will preferentially drink from that.

Another approach is to take advantage of the fact that objects with high specific gravity are retained in the reticulo-rumen. A 'bullet' has been developed which stays there and dissolves away over a 10-week period, releasing magnesium at a steady rate. If these bullets are administered immediately after the cattle are turned out, they protect the animal during the high-risk period.

Sheep

In sheep, staggers usually occurs just before lambing, and is the third part of the periparturient metabolic complex. The symptoms are similar to those in cattle but are difficult to differentiate from the other deficiencies that occur at this time. If differentiation is needed ante-mortem, then the rate of onset and development of the syndrome may be helpful. Twin lamb disease takes days, hypocalcaemia takes several hours and hypomagnesaemia takes 1–2 hours.

Treatment in sheep is by subcutaneous injection of a calcium borogluconate combination solution and/or magnesium sulfate solution.

Trace compounds

These are required in milligram amounts per day by cows, and include some vitamins and some of the essential trace elements. The essential trace elements are a group of elements – usually metals or semi-metals – that have been proved in some very careful feeding trials to be essential in very small amounts for normal metabolism. The reason that they are essential, but at very low levels, is that their only function is as constituents of enzymes. Hence very little is required, but if there is insufficient to maintain enzyme production there will be dramatic metabolic effects. The other point of importance is that, for most of them, if an excess is given they will be toxic, so treatment regimes have to be considered carefully.

There are 24 essential trace elements in all. Deficiencies of 15 of them have only been seen in experimental conditions. Of the remaining nine, three have not been recorded in the UK, and of the final six, zinc deficiency has been seen fewer than ten times in animals other than pigs. Even in pigs zinc deficiency is very rare now, so we will concentrate on the five trace elements listed in Table 9.4 (above).

As has been mentioned already, deficiencies of water-soluble vitamins are rare in ruminants because of bacterial and protozoal activity and the presence of water-soluble vitamins in some raw cereals, but there are two problems that can occur.

Thiamine (vitamin B_1)

Occasionally, insufficient thiamine is absorbed to meet the animal's needs. What actually happens is that the normal amount of the vitamin is produced but it is broken down before it can be absorbed. So there is a conditioned or induced deficiency. This only occurs in ruminants, so it is reasonable to assume that the degradation is in the reticulo-rumen part of the gastrointestinal tract. It is not known what causes the presence of thiaminase, which is responsible for the breakdown.

The effects are dramatic. The animal has increased cerebrospinal fluid pressure, which leads to severe headaches, blindness, marked depression and finally coma and death. There is also marked necrosis of the cerebral cortex, hence the technical name of cerebrocortical necrosis. Farmers and stockmen sometimes call this disease 'brain rot'.

Treatment is by the repeated injection of large doses of thiamine, either alone or if it is not available alone, as a multivitamin preparation.

Vitamin B_{12} and cobalt

These two will be discussed as one topic because cobalt is an essential part of vitamin B_{12}. If there is a deficiency of cobalt there will be a shortage of vitamin B_{12}. In farm animals, deficiencies of this vitamin do not occur for any other reason.

Vitamin B_{12} has very different functions in monogastric species than in ruminants. In monogastric animals the main activity is as an enzyme for haemoglobin production. So a vitamin B_{12} deficiency causes pernicious anaemia.

Whilst vitamin B_{12} does have this activity in ruminants, of far greater importance is the critical role it has in the absorption and metabolism of FFAs for energy production.

There are two functions of this vitamin in energy metabolism. The first is that it is involved in the absorption of FFAs across the rumen wall. It acts as a carrier that helps to transfer the FFAs into the circulation, thus providing the animal with its major source of energy.

It is also involved in the insertion of propionate into the TCA. Vitamin B_{12} is the enzyme that converts L-methyl malonyl-coenzyme A into succinyl-coenzyme A. This is the last step in the pathway which enables propionate to enter the TCA cycle (see Figure 9.5). If there is insufficient vitamin B_{12} the animal will experience an energy deficiency. There will also be an accumulation of methyl malonic acid, which will be excreted in the urine.

Sheep

Cobalt deficiency is most commonly seen in sheep. It is usually called 'pine', but other names, such as 'moss ill', are occasionally used. It occurs in growing lambs after they have weaned themselves. The lambs grow slowly, or not at all. Their fleece is dry and has a harsh appearance, tears stain the hair below the eyes; the animals appear depressed and are susceptible to infections, particularly with gastrointestinal worms.

Diagnosis of pine can be by measuring the serum vitamin B_{12} concentration or by the concentration of methyl malonic acid in the urine. In either case, at least six animals should be sampled in any group to give a representative picture.

In general practice the response to treatment is fast; there is an obvious improvement in the alertness of the lambs within 24–36 hours, which confirms the diagnosis before the laboratory results are available.

Treatment can be with vitamin B_{12} injections, but more usual and economic is oral treatment with cobalt. The response to treatment is almost as rapid after oral administration as it is after injection of vitamin B_{12}. Parenteral treatment with cobalt is totally ineffective as the animal cannot excrete the cobalt into the rumen, where it is needed so that the microorganisms can incorporate it in order to manufacture vitamin B_{12}. Oral treatment with cobalt can be in a drench, either as a trace element

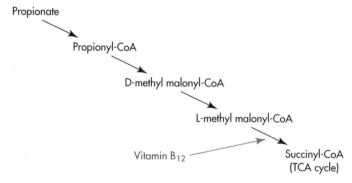

Figure 9.5 The metabolism of propionate into the TCA.

formulation, or as a supplement in anthelmintic drenches. When the condition has been recognised on a farm the pasture can be treated with cobalt sulfate or cobalt chloride. As cobalt is a relatively safe trace element it is possible to put sufficient cobalt on the pasture to last 3 years. This will stop the disease occurring, which is obviously better that having to treat animals when production losses have already occurred.

Cattle

Cobalt deficiency is not seen in cattle very often, but is recognised as a cause of reduced milk yield in dairy cows.

Treatment will be by mouth or by pasture supplementation. Also, the cobalt salt can be watered onto silage three times weekly if the condition is diagnosed after the grass has been harvested. Again there is a rapid response to treatment.

Vitamin E and selenium

These will be discussed together because, although they have different actions, some of these actions are very closely related. It has been shown that selenium, as glutathione peroxidase (GSHPx), can offset a vitamin E deficiency and vice versa. They cannot replace each other totally, but will do so up to about 80% of the daily requirement.

Vitamin E acts by reducing the production of lipid peroxidases and selenium is a constituent of the enzyme glutathione peroxidase, which breaks down the lipid peroxides (see Figure 9.6). These are very

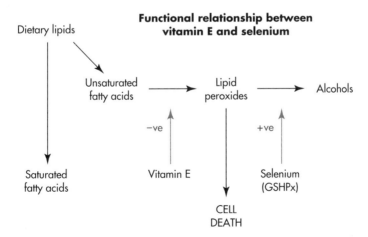

Figure 9.6 Vitamin E and selenium.

important functions as the lipid peroxides are very dangerous molecules that will cause cell-wall damage, leading to the death of the cells. As lipid peroxides will be formed in many types of cell, there is a wide variety of clinical manifestations of vitamin E and/or selenium deficiency. Selenium is also a constituent of the enzyme iodothionine iodinase. This converts the thyroid hormone precursor T_3 to the active hormone T_4. Thyroid hormone has many functions, among which is the activation of the polymorphonucleocytes. These are responsible for the innate non-specific immunity, which is the first line of defence against invading microorganisms. Thyroid hormone is also involved in cell-mediated immunity and the utilisation of brown fat. These important functions of the second seleno-enzyme are unrelated to vitamin E, and widen the spectrum of symptoms found in selenium deficiency.

The clinical symptoms of vitamin E and/or selenium deficiency can be grouped into four categories according to their effects on reproduction, muscles, production and resistance to infection.

Effects on reproduction

Most of the effects occur in females. There can be adverse effects on all stages of the reproductive cycle in cows and ewes. These will include:

- Failure to conceive.
- Embryonic death.
- Abortion, vitamin E and/or selenium deficiency.
- Stillbirth.
- The birth of weak calves.
- Retention of the fetal membranes after birth, which can lead to metritis and reduced fertility.

As most or all of the profit from cows and ewes comes from the production of live healthy offspring and full milk production, these are very serious problems. These effects alone can dramatically reduce the profitability of a herd or flock without any of the other prblems associated with a vitamin E and/or selenium deficiency.

In males there is evidence that the quality of the semen is reduced, which may not matter too much for natural service but can be important in the diluted and frozen semen used in artificial insemination.

Effects on muscles

Vitamin E and/or selenium deficiency will cause degeneration of striated muscle cells in calves and lambs. This is called white muscle disease because the affected muscles are pale and watery, and as the condition develops the damaged muscle cells are replaced with white fibrous tissue. The onset is usually sudden, happening particularly when the stock are grazing young fresh grass, which often has a high unsaturated fatty acid content that puts great demands on the lipid peroxide control systems. Often the lesions are bilaterally symmetrical. The symptoms depend on which muscles are involved. The main syndromes are as follows:

- When the muscles used for locomotion are affected the animal will either be very reluctant to move or will lie down and refuse to move at all.
- When the muscles used for chewing and swallowing are affected the animal will be reluctant to eat or drink.
- When the respiratory muscles are affected the animal will show difficulty and pain when it breathes. Visually, this can look very similar to pneumonia, but by definition pneumonia is an infection of the lungs.
- If the cardiac muscles are involved, there will be sudden death, which is usually not observed. The attack occurs when the animal is excited; it will make a sudden grunt, fall over and die within less than a minute.

Effects on production

The effects on production include reduced growth rate in growing animals, reduced milk yield in lactating dairy cows and reduced wool growth in sheep.

Effects on resistance to disease

Vitamin E and/or selenium deficiency will cause a reduced response to disease in several ways. Firstly, as described above, polymorphonucleocytes will be able to phagocytose (surround and ingest) invading microorganisms but are not able to kill them. There is a reduced immune response, both humoral and cellular, to pathogens. These changes mean that the animals will be much more susceptible to infections. This will be seen as an increased level of disease in general rather than of particular diseases. A case study in humans showed that people with lower selenium status were more likely to develop cancer, and there are numerous reports in the literature showing that, in split-herd trials, selenium and/or vitamin E supplementation in deficient herds reduces diseases ranging from pneumonia to mastitis.

As there is no tissue in the body that acts as a selenium store and because selenium has a very low safety margin, effective treatment must use a continuous low-level technique.

Effective long term treatment may be with:

- A persistent slow-release injection of selenium.
- Oral treatment by feed supplementation.
- Administration of soluble selenium-containing boluses that are retained in the reticulo-rumen, where they will release selenium over many months.

There is no persistent vitamin E injection, and oral supplementation with vitamin E is expensive and not very long-lasting. There are short-term injections of vitamin E and a soluble selenium salt. However, they appear to have little or no advantage over the long-term treatments unless there is a total deficiency of vitamin E.

Copper deficiency

Copper was one of the earliest elements to be proven to be an essential trace element. It is a component of at least 15 enzymes that have a wide variety of functions (see Table 9.5).

The copper absorption and deficiency story is complex because there are two types of deficiency. Primary deficiency occurs when there is not enough copper in the rations to meet the animal's needs. Secondary deficiency occurs when there is sufficient copper but other ions or molecules in the rations make the copper unavailable to the animal. The two most important ions in this category are molybdenum and iron. The difference between primary and secondary deficiency is important when treating copper deficiency.

The symptoms of copper deficiency are different in cattle and sheep.

Cattle

In cattle the clinical symptoms are mainly associated with ill-thrift and poor production. There will be scouring (diarrhoea) caused by the copper deficiency, which therefore will not respond to treatments such as antibiotics or anthelmintics. There is a reduced growth rate, together with poor hair colour and appearance. This change in the coat has been used as a diagnostic tool in the past, but a variety of other conditions will produce exactly the same changes in the coat. There will be an increased tendency for bones to fracture. Because of abnormal cartilage development at the growth plates in the long bones there will be arthritis, which occurs particularly in the pedal joints.

For many years there was lively discussion as to whether copper deficiency causes infertility, with eminent scientists on both sides of the

Table 9.5 Some of the more important cupro-enzymes

Enzyme	Symptoms of deficiency
Ferroxidase	Anaemia, growth retardation
Cytochrome oxidase	Amyelination Anaemia Scouring Growth retardation, increased susceptibility to infection
Desaturase	Growth retardation Amyelination
Lysyl oxidase	Bone fractures, growth retardation, increased susceptibility to infection
β-Hydroxylase	Scouring
Superoxide dismutase	Increased susceptibility to infection, growth retardation
Tyrosinase	Achromotrichia (reduced hair colour)

argument. Copper depletion studies finally resolved the difference of opinion. It was shown by very elegant work that, in addition to causing copper deficiency, excess molybdenum independently causes infertility. It was also shown that infertility does not occur in primary copper deficiency. The debate was interesting because both sides were correct and what mattered was the type of copper deficiency.

The diagnosis of copper deficiency in cattle is not easy. It cannot be done on clinical grounds as there are no symptoms that are exclusive to copper deficiency. The measurement of copper in blood samples is only useful as confirmation when the deficiency is well advanced. The blood level drops late as the symptoms develop, so it cannot be used to assist pre-emptive treatment. For this purpose the most reliable test would be liver copper concentration, but liver biopsy is not a practicable proposition in general practice. If an animal dies or is sent for slaughter, a portion of the liver can be retained for analysis. Liver is the tissue of choice because it acts as a store or reservoir of copper. Hence, the concentration of copper in the liver is a very good indicator of overall copper status.

Treatment has to be long-term as the animals need to maintain correct copper status all the time to maximise their efficiency. It can be with copper oxide needles, which stay in the rumen and slowly dissolve, releasing copper over several months. Treatment can also be with copper injections. These have to be very carefully formulated and developed as copper is very irritant in cattle. Preparations have to be carefully chelated to reduce this side-effect.

Sheep

Under British farming systems, by far the most important effect of copper deficiency in sheep is swayback. This condition does not occur in cattle. When copper-deficient ewes are pregnant, the developing fetus(es) are unable to produce sufficient myelin to completely myelinate the central nervous system. One of the functions of myelin is to act as electrical insulation around nerve cells and fibres. Poor myelination will cause electrical impulses travelling along a nerve cell axon to jump to another, parallel cell. This means that the brain cannot be certain of the origin of the nervous impulses it receives. This can lead to anything from mild incoordination when a lamb is walking to total flaccid paralysis, depending on the degree of demyelination. The condition cannot be treated, so slaughter on welfare grounds is the only option in all but the most mild cases.

The effects on growth are rarely of sufficient severity to be a serious problem. As the wool from British sheep is relatively coarse and is not valuable, the effects on wool quality are not important. However, in countries like Australia, where the wool produced is of very high quality and lambs are worth very little, the adverse effect on wool quality is by far the most important effect of copper deficiency in sheep.

The diagnosis of copper deficiency in sheep is usually done by confirming the presence of swayback, as there is no other cause of this condition. The prevention of swayback is relatively easy because myelination occurs between days 100 and 120 of pregnancy. As long as the ewe has a good copper status for that period, then swayback will not develop.

This can be achieved by long-duration copper injection or by the use of copper oxide needles. In sheep it is essential to only treat ewes that are copper-deficient and to give the authorised dose. This is because sheep are susceptible to copper poisoning, some breeds being much more sensitive than others.

Iron deficiency

Iron deficiency will cause anaemia. The only situation where iron deficiency is a significant problem in farmed stock is in piglets that are born and reared on concrete. If they are reared outside, there is enough iron on the sow's udder and teats for the piglets to absorb all that they need. Trials have confirmed that parenteral treatment with 200 mg iron in the first 3 days of life will correct the problem and the piglets will be much healthier and grow much faster. To reduce irritancy, the iron is formulated as a complex of iron and dextran. It is not possible for the sow to transfer more iron across the placenta so there is no advantage to giving her more iron during pregnancy (see chapter 11).

Iodine deficiency

In all species iodine is an integral part of thyroid hormone.

In ruminants a lack of thyroid hormone due to iodine deficiency does not cause hypothyroidism as it is seen in humans with goitre, reduced basal metabolic rate (BMR), cretinism, etc. The only consistent finding is that if heifers or cows that are in calf become iodine-deficient they will often abort. The aborted fetus will have an enlarged thyroid gland, which confirms the diagnosis.

Treatment is either by supplementing the concentrate ration or making iodised mineral licks available.

Vitamin D deficiency

The treatment of young sheep before their first winter with vitamin D has, in a few instances, been shown to result in larger and fitter sheep at the end of the winter, but these were not fully controlled trials.

Bloat (see also chapter 10)

There are two types of bloat. The more common one, called 'frothy bloat', is where the fluid in the rumen forms a foam with the gas that should be expelled, due to changes in surface tension. This usually occurs as a result of the ingestion of an excess of some plant types, such as some species of clover. The foam stops the gas being eructated, but treatment with silicone preparations to break down the foam is often successful.

The other type of bloat occurs when an obstruction in the oesophagus stops eructation. Initially, this type of bloat has to be treated by making a hole through the abdominal wall into the rumen. Care must be taken to let the pressure down slowly to minimise the risk of shock to the animal. When the immediate crisis is over, the identification and treatment of the obstruction can proceed.

Always remember one of the sayings of Confucius:

'We have not succeeded in answering all our questions. Indeed, we sometimes feel that we have not completely answered any of them. The answers we have found only serve to raise a whole new set of questions. In some ways we feel as confused as ever. But we now feel that we are confused on a higher level and about more important things!'

Further reading

David D (1998). *Equine Nutrition*. Oxford: Blackwell Science.

Davis C L, Drackley J K (1998). *Development, Nutrition and Management of the Young Calf*. Ames, Ia: Iowa State University Press.

Greenhalgh J F, Morgan C, Edwards R (2002). *Animal Nutrition*. London: Prentice Hall.

Underwood E J, Suttle N (1999). *The Mineral Nutrition of Livestock*. Cambridge, Ma: Cabi Publishing.

10

Diseases of cattle, sheep and goats

Colin Chapman

When dealing with the diseases of cattle, sheep and goats it is important to keep in mind that the susceptibility of these animals to disease is heavily influenced by the ways in which they are managed by farmers, by the nature of the environment where they graze or are housed, and by the unique structure of their digestive tract. This is analogous to the situation with diseases of humans, where factors such as lifestyle, occupation and longevity heavily influence the occurrence of many common health problems. Thus, animals kept on pastures badly contaminated with feces are likely to be exposed to large numbers of parasite eggs and larvae, those allowed access to toxic plants are at risk of poisoning, and those which commit dietary indiscretions are liable to develop bloat or suffer the consequences of hardware disease (discussed below). A further consideration is that these animals usually live in groups, such as herds, flocks and mobs, so for most diseases there will be measurable morbidity and mortality rates and there will be common predisposing factors, such as recent transport or handling, the same sources of feed and drinking water, and high stocking rates.

For several diseases, the first hint of trouble is the sudden death of a few animals in a group, sometimes accompanied by signs of ill-health in the others. For many other diseases the most common presenting signs will be less severe, and these include the following: clearly evident weight loss; diarrhoea, bloat and other manifestations of abdominal discomfort; lameness associated with diseases and disorders of the feet and limbs; nervous system disorders, ranging from excitement to depression and somnolence; respiratory symptoms, including dyspnoea, coughing and nasal discharge; disorders of the skin and other visible parts of the body; and disorders of reproduction, including infertility, abortion, mastitis and urinary tract disorders. It is possible to categorise and discuss the diseases according to these broad presenting signs, as will be done in this chapter, but in doing so it must be stressed that some diseases cross the boundaries, so that pregnant cows affected by salmonellosis, for example, can manifest both diarrhoea and then abortions.

There are several striking features of the diseases of cattle, sheep and goats, most of which are quite unlike those that most pharmacists will have ever encountered before; there are very many plants that may cause problems.

Some diseases of ruminants can be contracted by humans, particularly those causing abortions; this is something that must be taken into account when people seek health advice from pharmacists in rural settings. Another feature is the different approach that has to be taken with the use of pharmaceutical products, particularly the challenge of keeping drug residues out of milk and meat, the need to consider operator safety because of the drugs and chemicals used or the methods of administration, and the need to avoid carcass damage when injections are used (see chapter 3).

Sudden death

Sudden death of cattle, sheep and goats is not necessarily associated with diseases that have very short time-frames: the frequency of observation must be taken into account. In fact, 'sudden death' may have occurred over several days but have only just been discovered. Nevertheless, there are diseases that can kill animals quickly, such as anthrax, some diseases caused by *Clostridia* spp., acute liver fluke infections, poisonings with cyanogenic plants and those containing nitrates, and blue-green algal poisoning. These diseases are very different from those causing sudden death in humans, where the major causes are cardiovascular accidents, such as stroke, massive gastrointestinal bleeding and sudden cardiac death, and drug overdoses.

Clostridial diseases (see also chapter 2)

Clostridial diseases are usually acute and are not contagious. Thus, outbreaks are due to common predisposing causes. The bacteria responsible are commonly present in soils with a high organic content and in the intestinal tracts of healthy animals. There are several important clostridial diseases: blackleg (*Clostridium chauvoei*); bacillary haemoglobinuria (*C. haemolyticum*); tetanus (*C. tetani*); malignant oedema (*C. chauvoei, C. novyi* type A, *C. septicum, C. sordellii* or *C. perfringens* type A); braxy (*C. septicum*); black disease (*C. novyi* type D, also called *C. oedematiens*); pulpy kidney (*C. perfringens* type D); lamb dysentery

(*C. perfringens* type B); big head (*C. novyi* type A); struck (*C. perfringens* type C); abomasitis (*C. sordellii*); and botulism (*C. botulinum*). In each case, the pathogenesis is associated with one or more exotoxins.

Tetanus

Tetanus is caused by a potent, heat-labile neurotoxin produced by *C. tetani*. This bacterium, like all *Clostridium* species, grows in an anaerobic environment. In the case of tetanus, this is usually the deep cuts that may accompany the castration and removal of tails from lambs, and dog bites. The symptoms of tetanus are generalised stiffness, spasms and prolapse of the third eyelid. Tetanus spores are extremely common on farms, especially in yards. Interestingly, susceptibility to tetanus differs among animal species, horses being highly susceptible, sheep moderately so, and cattle the least susceptible.

Enterotoxaemia

Enterotoxaemia caused by *C. perfringens* type D (pulpy kidney) is associated with a protoxin that leads to the sudden death of calves, lambs and kids, usually after a heavy intake of food or a change of food. The condition is precipitated by gut stasis, allowing the proliferation of *C. perfringens* type D in the upper small intestine. Often it is the biggest and best animals that are found dead, without any previous hint of trouble. A closely related condition has been reported in adult sheep in the UK, but it is associated with *C. perfringens* type C rather than type D.

Another form of enterotoxaemia, lamb dysentery, occurs most commonly in cold and wet regions where ewes are confined to small yards or to sheds. The causative organism, *C. perfringens* type B, proliferates in the intestine of susceptible lambs, resulting in damage to the gastrointestinal tract and causing obvious abdominal discomfort, fetid diarrhoea and the sudden death of very young lambs.

Both haemorrhagic enteritis and braxy (bradshot), two other clostridial diseases of lambs, are similar to lamb dysentery except that haemorrhagic enteritis is confined to only a few places in the UK and braxy is caused by a different microorganism, *C. septicum*. Braxy follows trauma to the abomasum (the fourth stomach) by frosted grass or gastrointestinal parasites.

Infectious necrotic hepatitis (blackleg) is more common in cattle than sheep. The causative organism, *C. chauvoei*, is ingested by animals and, by unknown means, gets into muscles and other tissues, where no

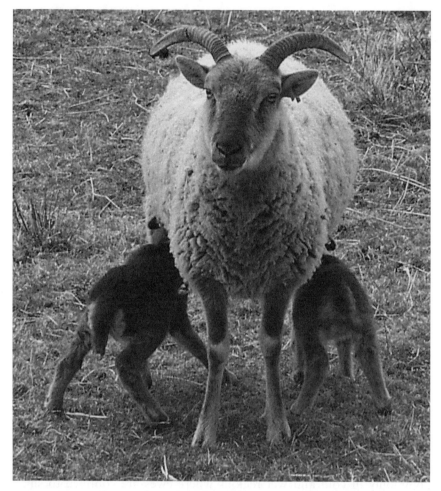

Figure 10.1 Rare Soay ewe with lambs (northern Scotland, 2003).

immediate harm is caused. However, bruising or wounding may produce anaerobic conditions which favour activation of the spores in the tissues, resulting in the release of toxins and rapid death. Animals seen alive with blackleg show symptoms associated with toxaemia, such as rapid breathing and profound depression, along with some evidence of localised swelling and lameness. 'False blackleg' can be caused by *C. septicum*, *C. novyi* or *C. perfringens*, and is better classified as a form of malignant oedema.

Malignant oedema (gas gangrene) is an acute wound infection caused by one or more different species of *Clostridium*. It is usually associated with the contamination of wounds with soil. Once in the wound, the various *Clostridium* species produce toxins that result in gangrene of the skin and oedema in the subcutaneous tissue. There may be frothy exudation associated with the wound. A high fever is always present and affected animals die within 24–48 hours as a result of toxins being absorbed into the bloodstream.

The pathogenesis of black disease is similar to that of blackleg, but the causative organism and precipitating factors are different. It is a disease that is more common in sheep than cattle. The causative organism, *C. novyi*, is trapped in the liver, where it causes no harm until activated by events which cause liver damage, such as migrating liver fluke. Toxins are then released and death soon follows. A condition of rams called 'big head' is a different version of black disease in which *C. novyi* is activated in the tissues of the head after fighting among rams.

Bacillary haemoglobinuria (redwater) is more common in cattle than in sheep and, like both blackleg and black disease, is associated with spores lodging in the tissues. In redwater, *C. haemolyticum* spores are trapped in the liver and perhaps the muscles, and are activated by migrating liver fluke or other causes of tissue necrosis. The toxins produced lead to the destruction of red blood cells, resulting in haemoglobinuria, jaundice, fever and death. In Australia, acute leptospirosis is a more likely cause of haemoglobinuria in cattle. In sheep it is often caused by chronic copper poisoning.

Outbreaks of botulism are more common in birds than either sheep or cattle. The disease is caused by a toxin released by *C. botulinum*, an organism that proliferates in decomposing animal matter and sometimes in plant material. A major problem with botulism arose in feedlot cattle in Queensland, Australia, a number of years ago, when chicken manure and decomposing chicken carcasses were incorporated into the feed for the cattle. The toxins of *C. botulinum* produce paralysis without the development of histological lesions.

There is no effective treatment for animals acutely affected with any of the clostridial diseases, but prevention is easily achieved by the use of multivalent vaccines, provided they are used properly. It should be kept in mind that calves, lambs and kids born to vaccinated dams are protected by maternally derived colostral antibodies for up to 16 weeks. Antisera are available for the short-term protection for animals at risk.

Anthrax

The causative organism of anthrax, *Bacillus anthracis*, forms spores that persist in soil for many years and, when climatic conditions are favourable, can be ingested by ruminants. Fortunately, this is not common because the spores contaminate only limited areas of the countries where the disease occurs, and climatic conditions seldom favour outbreaks. When ingested, and sometimes when they are inhaled, the spores are activated and the bacteria are able to invade, leading to profound toxaemia and shock. Acutely affected animals will often be found dead with blood discharging from all external orifices, while other animals may appear profoundly depressed and 'toxic', and will develop profuse diarrhoea. Treatment of affected and at-risk animals must be instituted quickly with daily intramuscular injections of procaine penicillin (25 mg/kg) or oxytetracycline (5 mg/kg). Animals that die must be disposed of properly and quarantine measures introduced. Decontamination is difficult, but formaldehyde solutions are reasonably effective. Vaccination of all animals in an endemic area is usually required to control an outbreak and prevent further problems.

Liver fluke disease

Fasciola hepatica, the common liver fluke of sheep and cattle in temperate regions, and *F. gigantica* (in warmer climates) are parasites with world-wide distribution. The life cycles of both involve specific semi-aquatic snails as intermediate hosts, so liver fluke infection may occur when animals graze on irrigated pastures or near swamps and streams in endemic areas. Snails are infected by miracidia which hatch from eggs passed in the feces of infected animals; after a period of development, the parasite larvae leave the snails to form cysts on plants at the water's edge. It is from these plants that sheep and cattle are infected. Liver damage is caused by the juvenile parasites migrating from the intestines into the liver and then to the bile ducts. The number of parasites migrating through the liver determines the extent of damage. Sheep are more susceptible to sudden death because a relatively small number of parasites can cause considerable damage. Cattle, on the other hand, are more likely to develop chronic fascioliasis, seen clinically as emaciation and chronic ill-health. Treatment of acute fascioliasis with oral triclabendazole (10 mg/kg for sheep and 12 mg/kg for cattle) may be effective because the anthelmintic kills migrating parasites. Treatment every 6 weeks will be necessary in endemic areas. Several drugs can be used to treat chronic fascioliasis: closantel (10 mg/kg orally); clorsulon (20 mg/kg by subcutaneous injection); albendazole (7.5 mg/kg for sheep and 10 mg/kg for cattle, both orally); nitroxinil (10 mg/kg by subcutaneous injection); and oxyclozanide (15 mg/kg for sheep and

10 mg/kg for cattle, both orally). The killing of snails with copper sulfate was popular once but this approach is dangerous because copper is toxic to ruminants. The avoidance of heavily infested areas, the draining of swamps and the strategic drenching of animals at risk are more effective ways to control this disease.

Toxic plants

A common cause of sudden death is the ingestion of toxic plants, of which there are many.

Cyanide poisoning

Plants such as sorghum, quince and honeysuckle contain cyanogenic glycosides which can be converted to hydrocyanic acid in the rumen and absorbed into the body, where they prevent aerobic respiration in the cells. Acutely affected animals quickly develop respiratory distress, restlessness and tremors, and then become recumbent, suffer convulsions and die. Characteristically, the gums of the poisoned animals are bright red. By contrast, animals that ingest small amounts of the toxic plants over long periods are affected differently: sheep develop goitre; cattle, sheep and goats develop ataxia and cystitis; and animals give birth to deformed offspring. Treatment of acute cyanide poisoning is with repeated intravenous injections of sodium nitrite and sodium thiosulfate solution (5 g sodium nitrite and 15 g sodium thiosulfate in 200 mL of water, then give 50 mL to sheep and goats, and 200 mL to cattle). There is no specific treatment for chronic cyanide poisoning.

Nitrate poisoning

Plants containing high concentrations of nitrate can also cause sudden death in ruminants due to conversion of nitrates to nitrites by microorganisms in the rumen. The nitrites result in methaemoglobinaemia and consequent anoxia, cyanosis and death. The clinical signs are very similar to those seen with cyanide poisoning, except that the gums are brown and the blood a dark colour.

The toxicity of the many plants that can cause nitrate poisoning, such as rape, turnips and cereal crops, can be exacerbated by the excessive use of nitrogenous fertilisers. Water containing high concentrations of nitrate can also be toxic. Cattle are more susceptible than sheep, and hungry animals are more susceptible than well-fed ones, because of the more rapid ingestion of toxic plants. Monensin can be dangerous to use when nitrate toxicity is possible because it facilitates the conversion of nitrates to nitrites in the rumen. Nitrate poisoning usually results in outbreaks that are characterised by the sudden onset of respiratory distress and a high mortality rate. Treatment with at least two doses of methylene blue (2 mg/kg by slow intravenous injection) given 6 hours apart may be successful in converting the methaemoglobin back to haemoglobin. A dose of 20 mg/kg can be given, but is likely to be toxic.

Water bloom

Blue-green algae of several different species cause a bloom on dams, lakes and waterholes when conditions favour overgrowth of the organisms, such as hot weather, shallow water, and high concentrations of nitrogen and phosphorus. The algae contain neurotoxins and hepatotoxins, which are released when these cyanophytes die or are damaged, causing acute neurological signs, dyspnoea and the sudden death of many animals, and varying degrees of anorexia, jaundice and photosensitisation in others. Outbreaks occur when animals drink directly from contaminated water, particularly if winds push the water bloom to the edges, and particularly in flocks of sheep, which, unlike cattle, are not inclined to wade into the water to drink. There is no effective treatment, so prevention and control are the only effective approaches when water bloom is abundant. Measures that can be used are pumping water from the contaminated supply to troughs; the use of floating booms to keep the blue-green algae away from the edges; adding gypsum to the water to flocculate/precipitate the algae and some nutrients; and preventing the contamination of water supplies with animal feces.

Bracken fern poisoning

Bracken fern (*Pteridium aquilinum*) poisoning can have three major consequences, depending on the amount ingested and the species of animal: acute bracken poisoning (haemorrhagic fever); bovine enzootic haematuria; and bright blindness in sheep. Acute poisoning can cause sudden death, preceded by diarrhoea with melena, and bleeding from the mouth, nose, rectum and vagina. It looks like anthrax. Cases of acute poisoning occur mostly in cattle grazing large amounts of young bracken fern, the cause being a toxic glycoside that results in serious bone marrow depression and thrombocytopenia. Bovine enzootic haematuria follows the long-term ingestion of small amounts of bracken fern. The predominant clinical sign is blood in the urine due to bladder wall lesions caused by the toxic glycoside, and a gradual loss of body weight. Bright blindness is also due to the glycoside, but sheep are the only species affected by this disease and the lesions are in the retina. Sheep with this condition are bright and alert but are blind. There are no specific treatments possible for any of these conditions, and control has to be aimed at limiting access to the plants. Thiamine is not a treatment, even though it is used for this purpose in horses: the diseases in horses and ruminants after the ingestion of bracken fern are different.

Other causes

Snakebite is a rare clinical disease of ruminants, yet it is often blamed for sudden death, particularly in Australia, where snakes are more commonly encountered. The low number of deaths probably reflects the low venom load that occurs if animals of large body weight are bitten. When sudden death of livestock occurs, or when there are neurological signs suggestive of snakebite, other more likely causes should be sought. A positive diagnosis of snakebite can only be made if there is the identification of venom in the tissues, blood or urine. Should snakebite be confirmed, then specific antivenin is the only treatment.

Other, more likely, causes of sudden or unexplained death of a single animal are: trauma associated with fighting, cardiac rupture after penetration by a foreign body in hardware disease, aspiration pneumonia, and acute bloat. When several animals die suddenly, the likely causes, in addition to those already mentioned, are acute phalaris poisoning, grass tetany, acute interstitial pneumonia, lightning strike, the ingestion of toxic plants (such as hemlock and oleander) or ionophore poisoning associated with the accidental ingestion of toxic amounts of monensin, lasalocid or salinomycin.

Neurological disorders

Neurological disorders are usually evident as behavioural changes, ataxia, seizures, depression, blindness, paresis or varying degrees of paralysis. Some are age-related, such as enzootic ataxia (swayback) of lambs, due to copper deficiency in pregnancy (see chapter 9), whereas others are associated with exposure of animals to a common source of infection or to pastures containing toxic plants. In addition to the diseases that have already been discussed, in which neurological signs precede the rapid death of affected animals, such as occurs in botulism, tetanus and after the ingestion of cyanogenic glycosides or nitrates, there are several important diseases of ruminants in which neurological signs are the most prominent manifestations. These include diseases caused by infections (listeriosis, scrapie, louping ill, rabies and bovine spongiform encephalopathy), metabolic abnormalities (pregnancy toxaemia and ketosis), acute mineral deficiencies (hypocalcaemia and hypomagnesaemia), hypoglycaemia secondary to liver disease, poisonings (lupinosis and lupin poisoning, and phalaris and ryegrass staggers) and traumatic injuries to the brain or spinal cord. Neoplastic and degenerative diseases of the nervous system of ruminants are extremely rare.

Hepatic encephalopathy

Neurological symptoms can be associated with liver and biliary disease because of the consequent fall in blood glucose. When this fall is acute, hyperexcitability and convulsions result but when the fall is much slower there is drowsiness and lethargy. Liver failure also means that the normal detoxification mechanisms are compromised, resulting in neurological symptoms. The accumulation of ammonia in the blood is yet another reason for nervous signs. A great number of largely unpalatable plants contain pyrrolidizine alkaloids, including ironweed (*Amsinckia* spp.), wild lucerne and rattlepods (*Crotalaria* spp.), Patterson's curse, Salvation Jane and vipers bugloss (*Echium* spp.), heliotrope (*Heliotropium* spp.) and ragworts and fireweeds (*Senecio* spp.). Pyrrolidizine alkaloids are metabolised in the liver to toxic metabolites that lead to progressive hepatic dysfunction, so the clinical signs take some time to become evident but then have a sudden onset. Two problems arise: hepatic encephalopathy, which leads to neurological symptoms, and toxaemic jaundice, the latter being much more common in sheep. Toxaemic jaundice is associated with an accumulation of copper that can be suddenly released to cause a haemolytic crisis characterised by a sudden onset of depression, weakness and jaundice, followed by death. Copper accumulation can also occur in sheep grazing pastures dominated by subterranean clover (*Trifolium subterraneum*), which does not cause liver damage but still facilitates the retention of copper. This so-called phytogenous copper poisoning can be controlled by the regular administration of molybdenum in combination with sodium sulfate in feed or licks, or by molybdenum applied to the pasture.

Toxic plants

Incoordination due to plant-derived chemicals and toxins acting directly on the central nervous system is reasonably common. For example, phalaris staggers can follow the ingestion of canary grasses (*Phalaris* spp.) due to the actions of dimethyltryptamine, an analogue of serotonin. Affected animals become excitable and uncoordinated when disturbed. Some may walk on their knees, others hop, and a few may lie on their sides and paddle with their legs. It is not uncommon for some animals to die suddenly at the beginning of an outbreak, but for those that survive there can be complete recovery. No specific treatment is available but the oral administration of cobalt (at least 28 mg each week) will greatly reduce the occurrence of the problem.

Ryegrass staggers is a bit different in that this condition is caused by a mycotoxin and it is a transient problem. The mycotoxin is produced by a fungus, *Neotyphodium lolii*, growing on ryegrass when climatic conditions are favourable. The disease is only evident when animals are disturbed, causing them to fall easily and to thrash around when trying to get up. Left alone, all will recover so no treatment is required, other than to move the animals off the contaminated pasture. Annual ryegrass toxicity is a different disease caused by the seed heads of annual or Wimmera ryegrass, and several other grasses, becoming infested by nematode larvae carrying *Corynebacterium rathayi*. Galls form on the seed heads, inside which a corynetoxin is produced. Affected animals fall when disturbed and begin convulsing. Many die. There is no treatment other than intramuscular chlordiazepoxide (20 mg/kg), which is too expensive unless the animal is particularly valuable.

The popularity of lupins as food for cattle and sheep in some parts of the world has resulted in an increased occurrence of lupinosis, due to fungal contamination of lupin seeds and stubble, particularly after summer rains, and lupin poisoning, due to neurogenic alkaloids in the seeds and pods. Similar alkaloids can be found in other plants, such as laburnum and broom. The occurrence of lupin poisoning has decreased over time due to selective breeding programmes that have resulted in virtually non-toxic 'sweet' lupins. When poisoning does occur, it is an acute neurological disorder which has a high mortality rate. Lupinosis is a form of hepatic encephalopathy due to the mycotoxin phomopsin, produced by a saprophytic fungus, *Diaporthe toxica*. Affected sheep become depressed and will not eat, and most develop jaundice and photosensitisation. Withdrawal of sheep from toxic lupin stubble and symptomatic treatment is all that can be done.

Metabolic disorders

Pregnancy toxaemia

Pregnancy toxaemia (twin lamb disease) can occur in ewes during the later stages of pregnancy if food intake is insufficient to meet the metabolic requirements of the ewes. As explained in chapter 9, ketosis develops due to the breakdown of body fat and proteins to generate energy. The ketone bodies produced lead to neurological signs, but in the early stages of twin lamb disease the clinical signs are vague and non-specific, often resulting the condition being detected only when it has progressed to the stage where affected animals wander aimlessly, grind their teeth and stop feeding. It is not just a disease of ewes carrying twin lambs: pregnant ewes carrying one lamb, particularly those that are very fat or those in which feed intake is reduced by inclement weather, intercurrent disease, stressful situations or very wet pastures, can succumb to this metabolic disease. Diagnosis is based to a large extent on the circumstances surrounding the occurrence of the disease, along with its insidious onset and progressive nature. In the more advanced stages of the disease there is a smell of acetone on the breath. Treatment is difficult and often unsuccessful. If the ewe is still eating, the quality and quantity of feed should be improved. If individual ewes are to be saved, caesarean section may be necessary or lambing induced by giving intramuscular dexamethasone (20 mg). Oral propylene glycol (500 mL twice a day for 3 or 4 days) may prove effective if the disease is detected early in its course.

Acetonaemia

Acetonaemia (ketosis) in cattle has the same underlying pathogenesis as pregnancy toxaemia in sheep: a negative energy balance resulting in the mobilisation of body fat, except that in cattle it usually develops in the first few weeks after calving due to the failure of gluconeogenesis to keep up with the loss of glucose in milk. It can also be due to diseases that decrease food intake, such as abomasal displacement, hardware disease, severe mastitis and starvation. There are two forms of acetonaemia – wasting and nervous – although these forms are really the two ends of a spectrum. In the wasting form there is a rapid loss of weight, a large drop in milk production and moderate depression. In the nervous form there are episodes of delirium, such as aimless walking, head pressing, depraved appetite and exaggerated chewing. Treatment is with intramuscular dexamethasone (50 μg every second day) or betamethasone (50 mg/kg every second day), along with intravenous dextrose solution 50% (500 mL) or oral propylene glycol (250 mL twice daily for 2 days then 150 mL daily for a further 2 days). Glycerin can be used instead of propylene glycol, at the same dose.

Polioencephalomalacia

Polioencephalomalacia is a neurological disorder that has an ill-defined metabolic origin. It occurs most commonly in feedlots and seems to be associated with a high intake of grain or molasses. Affected animals exhibit severe neurological symptoms that include depression, ataxia, blindness and convulsions, and most will deteriorate to the point where they sit down and give the impression of staring into the sky ('stargazing'). Recovery of severely affected animals is unlikely. The clinical signs and circumstances are reasonably distinctive but consideration must be given to other causes, such as hypomagnesaemia and listeriosis. Treatment with intravenous thiamine (15 mg/kg) every few hours may be effective early in the course of the disease. Frusemide (furosemide) (1 mg/kg), mannitol (up to 70 g intravenously) and dexamethasone (2 mg/kg) may reduce the cerebral oedema that accompanies polioencephalomalacia.

Acute mineral deficiencies (see chapter 9 for detailed coverage)

Both hypomagnesaemia and hypocalcaemia can cause neurological disorders. Low blood magnesium concentrations are the underlying cause of grass tetany, and periparturient paresis (milk fever) is associated with low blood calcium concentrations. There are situations in which both occur at the same time. The acute and subacute forms of the disease are more common in cattle than in sheep and goats. The acute form is seen as a sudden onset of neurological signs, such as repeated episodes of frantic running and convulsions, leading to death of the animal. Sometimes the animals are simply found dead, depending on how frequently they are observed. In subacute cases the neurological signs are less dramatic and may include a staggering or stiff gait and increased sensitivity to noise. There is a fine balance between the intake and excretion of magnesium in ruminants, and little possibility of reserves being mobilised quickly in adult animals. As a consequence, loss of magnesium during lactation and the ingestion of lush spring pasture containing low sodium : potassium ratios, a situation that inhibits magnesium absorption in the rumen, can trigger hypomagnesaemia. In cattle, hypomagnesaemia is common when lactating cows are turned onto lush pastures (lactation tetany), when beef cattle graze grass-dominant pastures in spring, and when young cereal crops are grazed (wheat poisoning). The occurrence of hypomagnesaemia in sheep is usually associated with lactating ewes grazing young spring pastures. Treatment is with a combined solution of calcium and magnesium: cattle should be given a 500 mL intravenous infusion containing 25 mg/mL calcium borogluconate and 5 mg/mL magnesium hypophosphite, and sheep should be given 50 mL. Subcutaneous injections of magnesium sulfate (25 mg/mL) should follow, cattle getting 200–400 mL and sheep 50–100 mL. It is usually necessary to remove affected animals from the lush spring pastures and give them hay treated with magnesium mixed with molasses and water. Prevention can be achieved by giving susceptible animals additional hay and magnesium supplements, including the administration of intraruminal devices containing magnesium.

Milk fever is primarily a disease of dairy cattle caused by the sudden reduction of serum calcium concentration during lactation, usually in the first 2–3 days after calving. It is characterised by hypersensitivity and excitability in the early stages followed by depression, anorexia and sternal recumbency. Without treatment the condition progresses to coma and death. Diagnosis is reasonably straightforward, based on the circumstances and clinical signs, but alternatives must be considered, such as toxic conditions and traumatic injuries associated with calving. Treatment is aimed at restoring serum calcium concentrations; this is done by carefully administering 400–800 mL of calcium borogluconate solution (25 mg/mL), giving a portion intravenously to begin with and the balance by subcutaneous injection. Response to therapy should be reasonably rapid, and is seen usually as cows standing and regaining normal bodily functions within 2 hours.

There are situations in which cows are unable to stand after treatment for milk fever. Such animals are called 'downer cows'. The most common cause is severe damage to muscles during prolonged recumbency. If nursing and nourishment can be provided full recovery is likely, particularly if soft bedding is used or the affected animals are moved to softer ground. Rolling affected animals from side to side several times each day may help, but lifting devices are dangerous because they can inflict injuries. They are certainly not worth persevering with if the affected animal makes no attempt to stand when helped to do so. Despite intensive nursing, there are downer cows that fail to improve, probably because of traumatic injuries sustained at calving, such as obstetric paralysis, dislocated joints and acute bacterial infections of the udder or peritoneal cavity.

Microbial infections

Ovine encephalomyelitis (louping ill) is a viral disease of sheep that is endemic in parts of the UK. Similar diseases of sheep may also occur in other parts of Europe.

The causative flavivirus is transmitted by a tick, *Ixodes ricinus*, and can cause Lyme disease in humans (see chapter 13).

The clinical signs in affected sheep vary from virtually nothing to mild tremors and a bounding gait (hence the common name for the disease) to severe ataxia and death. Hand-feeding of affected sheep and sedation may be successful, using intramuscular xylazine (0.05–0.2 mg/kg), midazolam (4 mg/kg) or acetylpromazine (0.05–0.1 mg/kg). Some animals will recover and be resistant to reinfection, although residual neurological signs may persist. A vaccine that provides protection for up to 2 years is available. Because lambs are protected for about 3 months after birth by colostral antibodies, vaccination at about this age is necessary in endemic areas. Tick control can be achieved using pour-on insecticidal formulations.

Circling disease

Another form of meningoencephalitis is circling disease, caused by *Listeria monocytogenes*, in sheep and other ruminants in temperate climates. This neurological disease is usually acquired by the ingestion or inhalation of the organism from the animal's environment. In addition to the neurological symptoms, there may be other manifestation of the disease, such as abortions and various forms of septicaemia. When *L. monocytogenes* localises in the brain the distribution is usually not symmetrical, so that the neurological signs can be unilateral, such as walking in circles and lopsided facial paralysis. Listeriosis has symptoms that resemble pregnancy toxaemia, polioencephalomalacia, and even rabies. Treatment can be attempted with antibiotics, such as intramuscular procaine penicillin (25 mg/kg daily for 10 days).

Humans can be infected with *L. monocytogenes* by handling tissue from infected animals, such as placenta, by consuming contaminated milk or milk products, and from the environment, leading to meningitis and septicaemia.

Scrapie (see also chapter 2)

This is a neurological disease of sheep that has some unusual aspects. The first is that the infectious organism has never been fully characterised or understood, yet it is known to exist and to be transmitted from ewes to lambs. The second is that it seems to have given rise to the organism that causes bovine spongiform encephalopathy. The onset of scrapie is slow and barely noticeable, so that the first signs may occur when the disease is well advanced. These signs include tremors and a lack of coordination of the limbs, accompanied by intense itching ('scrapie') and gradual emaciation. It is a progressive disease for which there is no treatment and no vaccine. It occurs predominantly in the UK, and is not found in New Zealand and Australia.

Bovine spongiform encephalopathy (see also chapter 2)

Bovine spongiform encephalopathy (BSE), also called mad cow disease, may have arisen as a result of feeding cattle with meat and bone-meal derived from sheep affected by scrapie.

    The BSE epidemic began in Great Britain in 1986, and the disease then spread to other countries. A case of BSE was reported in the USA in December 2003. It seems to be a zoonotic disease, because variant Creutzfeldt–Jakob disease, a progressive neurological disease, has arisen when people have eaten contaminated beef products.

    The onset of BSE is slow and insidious, beginning with slight ataxia, evidence of apprehensive behaviour and disorientation, and heightened sensitivity to light and sound. Some cattle become aggressive when handled. The disease is slowly progressive, most affected animals displaying strange behaviour and becoming emaciated. There is no effective treatment. The incidence of BSE has declined since the introduction in Great Britain of a ban on the feeding of meat and bone-meals of ruminant origin to cattle.

Border disease

Border disease of newborn lambs is a congenital disorder caused by a virus closely related to both the classical swine fever virus and the bovine viral diarrhoea and mucosal disease virus. The affected lambs are undersized, with hairy fleeces, and have involuntary tremors ('hairy shakers'). Those that survive recover gradually to remain a source of infection for other sheep. The fertility of flocks in which the virus is endemic is well below expected levels. There is no specific treatment.

Bizarre neurological signs, such as aggression and belligerent behaviour accompanied by incoordination and several other symptoms of nervous system dysfunction, are suggestive of rabies, a disease that occurs in most countries but not New Zealand, Australia, the UK and Scandinavia (see chapter 8). It is caused by a lyssavirus that is usually transmitted to cattle, sheep and goats through bites by rabid dogs and foxes. The incubation period can range from weeks to months, and treatment with antisera and vaccination is seldom attempted. Control is achieved through strict quarantine and by vaccination strategies, including the vaccination of wildlife.

Other causes

There are a number of diseases in which neurological disorders are not the main feature, such as caprine arthritis encephalitis, grain overload and toxoplasmosis (all of which are discussed below) and a number of diseases that tend to occur in only one animal in a herd, flock or mob, such as spinal cord or brain abscesses and a range of congenital abnormalities. There are four parasitic diseases that can cause neurological symptoms: coenurosis, sarcocystosis, neurofilariasis and cerebrospinal nematodiasis. Coenurosis is caused by larvae of a dog tapeworm, *Taenia multiceps*, migrating to the brain of sheep and forming space-occupying lesions. This results in asymmetrical neurological signs indistinguishable from those associated with a brain abscess or tumour, such as compulsive circling, ataxia, postural abnormalities and head-pressing. In regions where *T. multiceps* is endemic the regular treatment of farm dogs with praziquantel (5 mg/kg orally) will minimise contamination of the pastures where sheep graze. Affected sheep are seldom treated.

Sarcocystosis is a disease also caused by an intestinal parasite of dogs, this time by a group of protozoan parasites that can also infect cats. Cattle, sheep and goats can be intermediate hosts for these parasites, being infected from contaminated pastures and developing visible clinical symptoms if large numbers of parasites are ingested. The vast majority of infections cause no symptoms but sheep have been reported to develop ataxia, trembling and ataxia. Chronic infections may cause weight loss, and abortions associated with sarcocystosis are known to occur. Amprolium (100 mg/kg orally each day for several weeks) or salinomycin (4 mg/kg orally for 30 days) may treat affected sheep successfully. Cooking all meat fed to dogs and cats on farms in endemic areas should minimise problems with these parasites.

Both neurofilariasis and cerebrospinal nematodiasis have restricted geographical distribution, even though the parasites that cause these conditions are reasonably widespread, and there are other diseases, such as cowdriosis (heartwater) and cerebral babesiosis, which are also caused by parasites and occur only rarely.

Respiratory disorders

Respiratory disorders can lead to a range of clinical signs, the most prominent of which are coughing, nasal discharge and abnormal breathing, particularly dyspnoea. In addition there may be abnormal respiratory sounds, cyanosis due to poor oxygen exchange, evidence of thoracic pain, and bleeding from the nose. The most common cause of respiratory disorders in cattle, sheep and goats is infection with pathogenic microorganisms. Interestingly, ruminants seldom get the respiratory diseases that are widespread in the human population, such as asthma, chronic obstructive pulmonary disease complex, and cancers of the lung. In cattle, respiratory diseases are often due to the interaction of pathogens with animal husbandry practices, such as methods of weaning calves, the quality of housing and the various stresses associated with transport. Components of the so-called bovine respiratory disease complex include enzootic pneumonia of calves, shipping fever, a number of specific viral and bacterial infections, fog fever and hypersensitivity pneumonitis. In sheep, the respiratory diseases include two distinctive nasal conditions (nasal bot larval infestation and enzootic nasal tumour), along with viral, bacterial and parasitic infections of the lungs.

Goats can contract the same respiratory diseases as sheep, and have one distinctive additional disease: contagious caprine pleuropneumonia, an acute respiratory disease caused by *Mycoplasma capricolum* ssp. *capripneumoniae*. This disease, which seems to be confined to Africa and Asia, can be treated with long-acting tetracycline (20 mg/kg intramuscularly) or tylosin (10 mg/kg intramuscularly) daily for several days. Vaccines are available.

Bovine respiratory disease complex

Enzootic pneumonia

Enzootic pneumonia of calves is typical of bovine respiratory disease complex in that various pathogens combine with environmental and husbandry factors to cause outbreaks of mild to severe respiratory problems, particularly at the time that immunity obtained through colostrum begins to wane. The primary pathogens are *Mycoplasma* spp., assisted by a parainfluenza-3 virus, bovine respiratory syncytial virus, *Chlamydia* spp. and *Pasteurella* spp. Calves housed in humid and cramped conditions are particularly susceptible. Transmission of the pathogens is by aerosol and direct contact. Affected animals develop a harsh, hacking cough and varying degrees of fever. Most will recover but secondary bacterial infections will exacerbate the condition. Treatment with long-acting oxytetracycline (20 mg/kg intramuscularly) is given to prevent this complication. Overall control of enzootic pneumonia has to address the multifactorial nature of the disease, meaning that better housing, less crowding and better weaning practices are necessary.

Pneumonic pasteurellosis

Pneumonic pasteurellosis (shipping fever) is similar in many respects to enzootic pneumonia but occurs in older calves and under different circumstances. The typical situation is that calves are brought into feedlots and are subjected to multiple stress factors in the process. The outbreak of pneumonia occurs 1–2 weeks later and lasts for several weeks. Affected animals become depressed and develop fever and a cough, and there is usually a mucopurulent nasal discharge. Most calves will recover. Treatment is again aimed at limiting the possibility of secondary bacterial infections making the situation worse. Antibiotics can be given individually or as mass medication in feed and water. A range of antibacterial drugs is used, including sulfamethazine (100 mg/kg) and oxytetracycline (5 mg/kg) in water for 7 days, or long-acting oxytetracycline intramuscularly (20 mg/kg), or tilmicosin (10 mg/kg) subcutaneously. Control can be achieved by management strategies, such as preconditioning and conditioning to minimise the stress on calves moving into feedlots, and the use of vaccines and prophylactic antimicrobial drugs.

Bovine respiratory syncytial virus

Bovine respiratory syncytial virus infections predominate in young calves, causing an interstitial pneumonia that predisposes to secondary bacterial infections. The causative parainfluenza-3 virus is less pathogenic than other respiratory pathogens, so it usually results in subclinical or mild respiratory conditions; however, it can predispose animals to secondary bacterial infections. Bovine herpesvirus-1 is more complex because it is associated with several diseases in cattle: infectious bovine rhinotracheitis (IBR); infectious pustular vulvovaginitis; balanoposthitis; conjunctivitis; abortion; encephalomyelitis; and mastitis. Cattle with IBR develop fever and respiratory signs characterised by a mild cough, a stringy nasal discharge and inflammation on the inside of the nasal cavity ('red nose'). The clinical course of IBR is from 4 to 7 days but will be longer and more severe if secondary bacterial infections complicate the picture. Pregnant cows may abort days to weeks after recovering from IBR. The bovine viral diarrhoea virus may also cause respiratory problems but usually only in conjunction with other pathogens. The treatment of all viral pneumonias is by way of antimicrobial drugs to prevent or control secondary infections, and the use of anti-inflammatory drugs, such as ketoprofen, to reduce fever and so limit any loss of production.

Acute bovine pulmonary emphysema

Acute bovine pulmonary emphysema (fog fever) is due to hypersensitivity to moulds. It occurs in cattle moved from dry to lush pastures on some occasions and seems to be associated with the ingestion of large amounts of tryptophan. This is converted by microorganisms in the rumen to 3-methylindole, which is toxic to lung tissue, causing interstitial pneumonia. Fog fever affects several animals at once, 3–4 days after the change of pasture. It has a sudden onset and a high mortality due to the extensive involvement of the lungs. Treatment is barely worthwhile, so the best course of action is prevention by careful husbandry and by the oral administration to animals at risk of monensin (200 mg/head/day) or lasolacid, both of which inhibit the microorganisms that convert tryptophan to 3-methylindole.

Acute respiratory disease in sheep

Acute respiratory disease in sheep is usually caused by *Pasteurella haemolytica*, sometimes aided by parainfluenza viruses and adenoviruses. Pneumonic pasteurellosis in sheep is an acute disease that may cause the sudden death of some animals and severe respiratory distress in many others in a flock. There are two other possible clinical manifestations of pasteurellosis: septicaemia and mastitis. Treatment is with long-acting oxytetracycline (20 mg/kg). Vaccines are used to prevent outbreaks.

Aspiration pneumonia

Aspiration pneumonia is a common respiratory disorder in all three species, and is due to clumsy attempts to administer liquids by means of stomach tube or drenching gun, and can also occur when animals suffering from milk fever inhale regurgitated material because the swallowing reflex is diminished. Large quantities of liquid can quickly kill the animal, and a small volume containing solid matter, particularly microorganisms, will probably result in pneumonia. Small volumes of clear solutions may be absorbed rapidly and cause little trouble. Antibiotics, such as long-acting oxytetracycline (20 mg/kg intramuscularly) should be given for several days in all cases in an attempt to prevent pneumonia.

Parasitic infections

Nasal bot

The nasal bot (*Oestrus ovis*) causes nasal discharge in sheep because the maggots migrate into the nasal cavity and to the frontal sinuses, where they cause catarrhal inflammation. These maggots can remain in the nasal cavity for several weeks before being expelled by sneezing. Nasal bot flies are abundant in the warmer months, particularly in areas of high rainfall, and females can profoundly irritate sheep by flying around their faces and darting into the nostrils to deposit the larvae. Sheep can often be seen on hot days standing in groups with their heads together in an attempt to keep these flies away from their faces. This can result in a loss of productivity. Once the larvae are expelled they burrow into the ground, where they pupate before emerging as adult flies. Treatment with ivermectin (0.2 mg/kg orally) or closantel (7.5 mg/kg orally) as single doses in late summer to prevent the build-up of heavy infestations and then again in winter to remove larvae, is necessary to control this troublesome fly.

Parasitic bronchitis (husk or hoose)

Parasitic bronchitis occurs in cattle and is due to the bovine lungworm, *Dictyocaulus viviparus*; in sheep and goats it is due to *D. filaria*, *Muellerius capillaris* and *Protostrongylus rufescens*. Bovine lungworm is widespread in cold and temperate climates, where larvae on pastures can survive for long periods. Adult parasites live in the trachea and bronchi, and the eggs produced are coughed up and swallowed. Larvae hatch from the eggs and pass in the feces to contaminate the pasture, from where they can be ingested by calves and older cattle. The ingested larvae migrate across the intestinal wall, enter the bloodstream and get trapped in the lungs, where they migrate to the bronchi and trachea to cause inflammation. Good resistance to infection and to reinfection occurs, so respiratory disease is usually brief and occurs only in calves. A large number of parasites can cause acute respiratory distress, whereas the much more common subacute form of the disease leads to laboured breathing and coughing. Treatment with any one of several anthelmintics is usually successful: intramuscular ivermectin (0.05 mg/kg); oral moxidectin (0.02 mg/kg); moxidectin as a pour-on (0.05 mg/kg); or oral benzimidazoles, such as albendazole (7.5 mg/kg), febantel (7.5 mg/kg), fenbendazole (5 mg/kg), netobimin (7.5 mg/kg) and oxibendazole (4.5 mg/kg). Intraruminal devices containing anthelmintics are also available. Control can be achieved by minimising the exposure of calves to contaminated pastures and by vaccinating calves with irradiated larvae. Strategic drenching of calves at risk is worthy of consideration. Parasitic bronchitis in sheep and goats is uncommon and relatively unimportant. Infected sheep are treated with the same anthelmintics as those used to treat bovine lungworm.

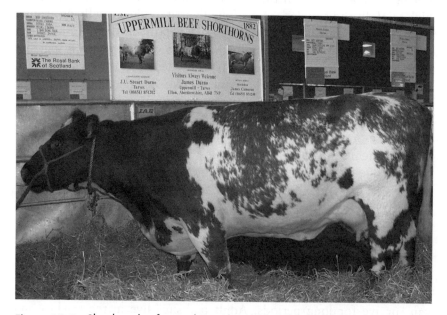

Figure 10.2 Shorthorn beef animal (Royal Highland Show, Edinburgh, 2003).

Respiratory tract tumours

Sheep and goats can develop tumours of the respiratory tract, principally pulmonary adenomatosis (jaagsiekte) and enzootic nasal tumour. Both are endemic in many countries (but not Australia and New Zealand), and enzootic nasal tumour has not been reported in the UK. Both are believed to be caused by retroviruses. Enzootic nasal tumour is a contagious condition in which adult sheep and goats develop low-grade cancerous changes in the nasal cavities, leading to persistent nasal discharge, coughing and dyspnoea. There are no effective treatments for either of these infections, only control by culling affected animals and the imposition of strict quarantine measures. Sheep pulmonary adenomatosis is a different sort of tumour that usually causes affected sheep, and sometimes goats, to lose body weight and to develop respiratory distress. A characteristic clinical sign is the passing of copious amounts of fluid from the nostrils when the head is lowered. Death from pneumonia is the usual outcome.

A progressive pneumonia called maedi-visna, which was first reported in Iceland, now affects sheep in many countries (but not Australia and New Zealand). A retrovirus that is related to the human acquired immune deficiency syndrome (AIDS) virus, to equine infectious anaemia virus and to the caprine arthritis encephalitis virus is responsible. The symptoms are like those of sheep pulmonary adenomatosis but there is no tumour. Instead there is pneumonia that gets worse over time, resulting in laboured breathing and emaciation. Culling and quarantine are used to control this endemic disease.

Other causes

Nitrate poisoning, poisoning due to hydrocyanic acid, and blue-green algal poisoning can all cause acute respiratory symptoms in the period leading to the death of affected animals, and have already been discussed. Another acute respiratory disease is bovine malignant catarrhal fever, a complex viral disease that is transmitted to cattle from sheep or wildebeest and causes mucosal lesions, profuse oculonasal discharge and dyspnoea. Fortunately, it is a rare disease, as is rinderpest, a viral disease very similar in appearance to malignant catarrhal fever, and peste des petits ruminants (goat plague or kata), a contagious disease of goats and sheep, both of which are confined to parts of Africa, Asia and the Middle East.

Abdominal problems

There are many diseases that can cause abdominal discomfort in ruminants, many of which are not associated with the gastrointestinal tract: other organs and structures may be involved, particularly the kidneys and urinary tract. Damage to the reproductive tract in cows, ewes and does, such as may occur if there is torsion or rupture of the uterus, can also cause abdominal discomfort. Often peritonitis will accompany this damage, in which case there will be fever and toxaemia in addition to the abdominal pain. Peritonitis can also be associated with perforation of the gastrointestinal tract in hardware disease, following the perforation of abomasal ulcers and as a consequence of rumenitis after acute carbohydrate indigestion.

In this section, the causes of abdominal discomfort that are not associated with diarrhoea will be discussed; the causes of diarrhoea will be considered in the next section. The signs of abdominal discomfort can vary. There may be an upward arching of the back with the limbs tucked underneath the body, or the back may be arched downwards and the legs placed widely apart (the 'saw horse' posture), or the affected animal may adopt a 'dog-sitting' position. Some animals will lie down and bellow, and there may be persistent straining with or without diarrhoea. An important approach in all cases of abdominal discomfort is the relief of severe pain associated with distension of the wall of the organ or structure in the abdominal cavity. For cattle, sheep and goats, a number of non-steroidal anti-inflammatory drugs can be used: carprofen (1.4 mg/kg subcutaneously or intravenously each day); phenylbutazone (10–20 mg/kg intravenously daily); flunixin (2.2 mg/kg intravenously daily); sodium salicylate (100 mg/kg orally twice daily); ketoprofen (3.0 mg/kg intramuscularly or intravenously daily); and meloxicam (0.2 mg/kg subcutaneously each day).

Hardware disease

Hardware disease (traumatic reticuloperitonitis) is a common cause of abdominal discomfort in cattle. It can be a localised or diffuse condition and is caused by the penetration by sharp objects, such as nails and wire, from the reticulum into the surrounding tissues and organs. Therefore, the vagus nerve, diaphragm, heart, lungs, liver and spleen can be involved, leading to a complex range of clinical signs. Some of these are given specific names, such as vagus indigestion, diaphragmatic hernia and traumatic pericarditis. In all cases there is peritonitis that causes abdominal pain, fever, ruminal atony and a sharp fall in milk production. Diagnosis is difficult and the prognosis is guarded. Treatment with antibiotics, usually penicillin, long-acting tetracyclines or trimethoprim-potentiated sulfonamides, may be effective in some cases. Magnets are sometimes administered orally in an attempt to prevent recurrence. Often surgery is needed but may not be effective.

Grain overload

Rumenitis, or inflammation of the rumen, has several causes, including grain poisoning, ulceration and fungal infections. Ingestion of large amounts of grain, particularly by animals not accustomed to doing so, can lead to acute carbohydrate engorgement (rumen overload), which is characterised by anorexia, depression, weakness and diarrhoea. Some walk in a drunken manner and abdominal pain is often not evident. The ruminal fluid becomes highly acidic, so treatment is aimed at correcting the ruminal and systemic acidosis using intravenous 5% sodium bicarbonate solution (5 L to cattle over a period of 30 minutes) along with oral dosing with magnesium oxide or magnesium hydroxide (up to 500 g for cattle and up to 50 g for sheep). However, the best course of action is usually a rumenotomy, which involves surgically opening the rumen, removing its contents, and then placing rumen fluid from another animal ('cud transfer') in the rumen along with a small amount of hay.

A less severe dietary problem is simple indigestion, which also occurs if a lot of grain is eaten or if animals consume indigestible roughage, such as straw and bedding. It is essentially a mild form of grain overload which has much less severe clinical signs and often resolves spontaneously. It was once common to give affected animals gastric stimulants ('rumenatorics'), such as nux vomica (strychnine), ginger and tartar emetic, and to administer magnesium oxide to counteract the expected acidosis in the rumen. However, there is no evidence that rumenatorics serve any useful purpose, and magnesium oxide can lead to metabolic alkalosis and electrolyte disturbances more often than not. Cud transfer, using a stomach tube rather than rumenotomy, is usually a far more effective approach.

Ulceration

There are several causes of ulceration of the various parts of the gastrointestinal tract of ruminants. Viruses, especially the bluetongue virus and the virus that causes peste des petit ruminants, both of which have limited geographical distribution, cause ulceration of the buccal mucosae in addition to the range of other symptoms they cause. Ulceration also occurs due to mechanical and chemical insults and mycotoxins from mouldy hay. Ulcers commonly occur in the abomasum in high-producing dairy cows, in cattle in feedlots, and in cattle that have left-sided abomasal displacement. Affected animals suddenly develop abdominal discomfort. Treatment is with antacids such as magnesium oxide (2 mg/kg), magnesium trisilicate (up to 16 g for cattle) and aluminium hydroxide (15–30 g for cattle and 2 g for sheep, three times a day) but not sodium bicarbonate, because it may generate too much carbon dioxide in the rumen and lead to bloat. Kaolin and pectin can also be used. Proton pump inhibitors, such as omeprazole, or the H_2-receptor inhibitors, such as cimetidine, can be used, but the cost will be very high.

Abomasal displacement

In addition to ulceration are several other conditions of this 'normal' stomach that are important, particularly left-side displacement of the abomasum.

Left-side displacement of the abomasum

Left-side displacement of the abomasum (LDA) occurs mostly in large dairy cows in the weeks after calving. Cows on high-grain diets are the most susceptible, possibly because these diets can lead to distension and atony of the abomasum, making it easier for it to be twisted under the rumen and to lodge on the left side of the peritoneal cavity. Affected animals exhibit clinical signs that are very similar to simple indigestion, milk fever and reticuloperitonitis. Treatment by rolling the cow may be effective but surgery is usually necessary. Prevention can be achieved to a large extent by careful management of the diet of pregnant and lactating dairy cows, and by the administration of intraruminal capsules containing monensin.

Right-side distension and displacement of the abomasum

Right-side distension and displacement of the abomasum (RDA) is another problem that occurs. It also occurs most commonly in dairy cows fed on high-grain diets in the weeks after calving. The condition also occurs in calves. When there is only RDA, the clinical signs are very similar to LDA, but when there is volvulus the discomfort is far more severe and the prognosis much worse. Treatment with calcium borogluconate (500 mL of a 25% solution given subcutaneously or, carefully, intravenously) may assist by increasing abomasal motility. Fluids and electrolytes given orally have been shown to be beneficial. Surgery may be required.

Obstruction

Obstruction of the omasum, abomasum or intestines can lead to abdominal discomfort of varying intensity. Impaction after the ingestion of tough and fibrous plants, especially in extremely cold weather, is often the cause, and sometimes it occurs under drought feeding conditions due to the ingestion of sand and soil. However, the most common causes of obstructions are intestinal accidents in the form of volvulus, intussusception, strangulation, compression and torsion, including a specific form of caecal torsion ('red gut') encountered in sheep in some parts of the world. Functional obstruction due to paralytic ileus can also occur. The clinical signs of obstruction will vary from mild to severe abdominal discomfort, making it difficult to differentiate from other causes of 'acute' abdomen, such as renal colic and urethral obstruction. Surgery will often be required.

Bloat (see also chapter 9)

A distinctive form of abdominal discomfort is bloat, or distension of the ruminant forestomach with gas. This is more of a problem in cattle than in sheep and goats. The condition can be subdivided into primary and secondary bloat, both of which are associated with the trapping of either free gas or foam in the rumen. It occurs in ruminants because of their unusual stomach structure and because of the fermentation process that occurs in the rumen where the contents are constantly being processed with the assistance of microbes, which produce cellulase. This and other enzymes convert plant materials into volatile fatty acids, methane, carbon dioxide and ammonia, assisted by copious quantities of saliva, which keeps the rumen contents buffered and in a fluid state. An important component of the process is regurgitation (eructation), by which the contents of the rumen are forced back to the mouth, where the food is re-masticated, mixed with saliva and re-swallowed. This is called chewing the cud. When more gas is produced in the rumen than is eliminated by eructation or belching, such as when there is blockage of the oesophagus, or if stable foams are formed in the rumen, bloat occurs. In cases of primary bloat the animals should be removed from the causative pasture and treated according to the severity of the condition. The options range from an emergency rumenotomy made through the mid-point of the left paralumbar fossa, release of the gas with a large-bore trocar and cannula, promotion of salivation by using a stick tied in the mouth, and the passage of a stomach tube. Antifoaming agents, such as poloxalene solutions (aim for a dose of 25–50 g) or dimeticone (50–100 mL) should be used when possible, and re-administered if necessary. The treatment of secondary bloat requires resolution of the actual cause. To prevent primary bloat there are several strategies: careful management of the access of cattle to lush young pastures or to grain in feedlots; strategic administration of antifoaming agents by a variety of means; and the use of intraruminal devices containing monensin. Abomasal bloat is a different condition; it is reasonably common in young calves, lambs and kids overfed on milk replacer, particularly if it is warm. Affected animals can be grossly distended soon after being fed and may die from asphyxia in severe cases. It has been found that adding formalin (formaldehyde solution 37%) to the milk replacer (1 mL to each litre) minimises the problem.

Other causes

Acute abdominal pain caused by urinary tract disease is very uncommon in ruminants. One possible cause is pyelonephritis and another is urethral obstruction (urolithiasis), which is discussed below. Liver disorders can also cause abdominal discomfort but more usually lead to jaundice and nervous signs. Contagious bovine pyelonephritis can lead to intermittent obstruction of the ureters with pus and tissue debris, leading to episodes of colic. It is more common in adult cows than in bulls or steers and is caused by infection of the urinary tract with *Corynebacterium renale*. This microorganism can be transmitted between animals by contact, including mating, and by catheters used by veterinary surgeons. Affected animals, in addition to exhibiting signs of abdominal pain, frequently try to urinate and may pass bloodstained urine. Most will lose weight and productivity. Treatment with intramuscular procaine penicillin (25 mg/kg daily for 3 weeks) is effective early in the disease but much less effective later.

Diarrhoea ('scouring')

Abdominal discomfort may accompany conditions in which diarrhoea is a major feature, but for many diseases the discomfort is minimal or absent. For example, in parasitic gastroenteritis and Johne's disease there is chronic diarrhoea, often semisolid rather then liquid, and no evidence of abdominal pain. In the diseases that cause diarrhoea, the consistency of feces can range from soft to liquid, the colour from pale to dark, and the odour from mild to putrid; the feces may contain anything from a small amount of fibrous material, mucous or foreign material to a lot of each of these components. Each of these characteristics can provide clues about the cause of the diarrhoea. As a guide to what constitutes diarrhoea, the normal output of feces in cattle is 25–45 kg each day, and for sheep and goats it is 0.5–1 kg daily.

The causes of diarrhoea include inflammation, malabsorption, local stricture and overload of the gastrointestinal tract, particularly in young animals. In addition, a number of bacteria release toxins capable of causing 'secretory' diarrhoea, due to intestinal hypersecretion, and the rapid passage of intestinal contents in stressful or excitable situations can cause 'neurogenic' diarrhoea. A sudden change of diet commonly causes diarrhoea, probably because of intestinal hypermotility.

Parasitic gastroenteritis

Diarrhoea, with or without a dramatic loss of body weight, due to intestinal parasites is frequently encountered in cattle, sheep and goats, but not all parasites cause diarrhoea; *Haemonchus contortus* and *H. placei* (barber's pole worms) are more likely to cause constipation. However, most roundworms do so, the main parasites being *Teladorsagia (Ostertagia)* spp., *Trichostrongylus* spp., *Cooperia* spp. and *Nematodirus* spp. These parasites are often grouped together and called 'trichostrongylids'. There are also a number of protozoa that can cause diarrhoea; for example, *Eimeria* spp. cause coccidiosis, an acute diarrhoea common in animals kept in highly contaminated and muddy conditions.

The trichostrongylids have a direct life cycle, passing via the feces to contaminate the pastures where ruminants graze. Generally, the milder the environmental conditions the longer the parasites' eggs and larvae survive, with the exception of *H. contortus* larvae, which are more common in summer rainfall regions. Animals of all ages ingest the larvae, and the more that are ingested the greater the problem that will occur. The ingested larvae are able to penetrate the mucosae of the abomasum and spend time in the tissues surrounding the stomach and small intestine. Days or weeks later, the larvae mature and return to the lumen of the intestines, causing damage to the intestinal wall in the process, leading to parasitic gastroenteritis (PGE). The migrating larvae of *Teladorsagia* spp. are particularly pathogenic because they undergo arrested development in the intestinal wall at times of the year when environmental conditions are harsh, and are released en masse in time for the eggs to pass onto the pasture in spring or autumn. The specific form of PGE caused by this parasite is called ostertagiosis.

Two types of PGE occur: type I arises in situations where the parasites complete their life cycle without being retarded in the wall of the abomasum; type 2 occurs when there is the mass emergence of larvae from the wall of the abomasum. Any immunity to trichostrongylids that develops wanes at about the time that ruminants, particularly sheep, give birth to their offspring, resulting in a large number of worm eggs passing onto the pasture, a phenomenon known as the periparturient egg rise. *Nematodirus* spp. are a little different from the other trichostrongylids in that the larvae develop within the eggs, rather than hatching out and being subjected to the environmental conditions, and ruminants develop good resistance to reinfection, so that it is mainly a parasite of young animals, particularly lambs and kids.

Animals infested with trichostrongylids become unthrifty, many develop diarrhoea, and some may die. Lambs infested with *Nematodirus* spp. are more dramatically affected, most of them developing profuse watery diarrhoea. Fecal egg output can be very high, plasma pepsinogen concentrations are raised, and moderate anaemia develops. Treatment with broad-spectrum anthelmintics is necessary, ideally in a strategic way to maximise efficacy and to minimise resistance. Ivermectin (0.2 mg/kg orally or intramuscularly, or 0.5 mg/kg as a pour-on for cattle) is commonly used, and the newer avermectins and moxidectins are also popular and effective. The other large group of anthelmintics is the benzimidazoles (albendazole, febantel, fenbendazole, oxfendazole (all 5 mg/kg) and mebendazole (15 mg/kg), all given orally). Levamisole (7.5 mg/kg orally or 10 mg/kg as a pour-on for cattle) can also be used but can be toxic in goats. Goats may require higher doses of all anthelmintics because of more efficient drug metabolism. Anthelmintics should be used in such a way as to minimise the development of resistance: the correct dose should be used. Regularly change from the avermectins to the benzimidazoles; turn treated animals onto clean pastures; and use fecal egg counts to guide treatment. The available drugs are summarised in Table 10.1.

Coccidiosis

Coccidiosis is a disease of calves, lambs and kids raised under crowded conditions, and usually begins with the sudden onset of profuse, foul-smelling diarrhoea in housed animals and those in feedlots or muddy paddocks where the protozoa that cause the disease are able to contaminate feed and water. The parasites causing coccidiosis are host-specific *Eimeria* spp., although cross-infection between goats and sheep is possible. The life cycle of the parasites is direct. Oocysts are passed in the feces of infected animals into the environment and, in cool and moist conditions, these sporulate and can survive for several years unless conditions get hot and dry. The ingestion of a large number of sporulated oocysts leads to disease. However, it is a self-limiting disease because infected animals quickly develop resistance to reinfection. Treatment centres on the provision of rehydration therapy. The prevention and control of outbreaks requires attention to the precipitating factors, such as overcrowding and stress, and the use of coccidiostats over a period of 1–4 weeks. Those most commonly used are amprolium (25 mg/kg orally or 35 mg/kg in feed), monensin (2 mg/kg orally or 20 mg/kg in feed), lasalocid (25–100 mg/kg in feed), sulfadimidine (140 mg/kg orally or 35 mg/kg in feed) and decoquinate (1 mg/kg orally or 50–100 g/tonne of feed).

Colibacillosis

A common cause of diarrhoea in newborn ruminants is one or more pathogenic strains of *Escherichia coli*, giving rise to the term 'colibacillosis' to describe the condition. However, other pathogens are also involved, particularly rotaviruses, coronaviruses and *Cryptosporidium parvum*. Often pathogenic microorganisms combine with other factors, such as overcrowding, poor hygiene and reduced immunity in artificially reared calves, lambs and kids deprived of colostrum, to trigger outbreaks of 'white scours'.

Coliform septicaemia can also occur in which there is sudden death, particularly in animals that have been deprived of colostrum, and it is usually impossible to distinguish coliform septicaemia from the other possible causes of septicaemia in new-born ruminants, such as *Salmonella* spp., *Listeria monocytogenes* and *Pasteurella* spp. Acute

Table 10.1 Endoparasiticidal products for cattle, sheep and pigs

Drug name	Parasite target	Species	Product name (UK)
Abamectin	Roundworms and lungworms	Cattle	Enzec (Merial)
Doramectin	Roundworms Type II ostertagiosis Nasal bots	Ruminants, pigs Cattle Sheep	Dectomax (Pfizer)
Eprinomectin	Roundworms and lungworms Type II ostertagiosis	Cattle	Eprinex (Merial)
Ivermectin	Roundworms and lungworms Type II ostertagiosis Nasal bots	Ruminants, pigs Ruminants Sheep	Ivomec, Oramec, Panomec (Merial), Noromectin (Norbrook), Rycomec (Young's), Virbamec (Virbac)
Moxidectin	Roundworms Type II ostertagiosis Nasal bots	Ruminants Cattle Sheep	Cydectin (Fort Dodge)
Albendazole	Roundworms, lungworms, Tapeworms, adult liver fluke	Cattle and sheep	Albenil (Virbac), Albex (Chanelle), Allverm (Young's), Endospec (Bimeda), Rycoben (Young's), Valbazen (Pfizer),
Febantel	Roundworms Lungworms Tapeworms	Ruminants, pigs Ruminants Sheep	Bayverm (Bayer)
Fenbendazole	Roundworms Type II ostertagiosis Lungworms	Ruminants Ruminants, pigs	Fenzol (Norbrook), Flexadin (Vetaquinol), Panacur (Pfizer) Zerofen (Chanelle)

Flubendazole	Roundworms and lungworms	Pigs	Flubenol (Janssen)
Mebendazole	Roundworms and lungworms Tapeworms	Sheep	Chanazole (Chanelle) Ovitelmin (Janssen)
Netobimin	Roundworms and lungworms Tapeworms, adult flukes Type II ostertagiosis	Ruminants	Hapadex (Schering-Plough)
Oxfendazole	Roundworms and lungworms Tapeworms Type II ostertagiosis	Ruminants	Autoworm; Systamex (Schering-Plough), Bovex (Chanelle), Parafend (Norbrook), Performex (Novartis)
Thiophanate	Roundworms Type II ostertagiosis	Ruminants, pigs	Nemafax (Merial)
Levamisole	Roundworms and lungworms	Ruminants	Anthelpor (Young's), Armadose (Bayer), Chanaverm (Chanelle), Decazole (Bimeda), Levacide (Norbrook), Levacur (Intervet), Niratil (Virbac), Nilverm (Schering-Plough), Ripercol (Janssen), Sure LD (Young's), Vermisole (Bimeda)
Morantel	Roundworms	Ruminants	Exhelm (Pfizer), Paratect (Pfizer)
Closantel	Immature and adult flukes Nasal bots, haemonchus	Sheep	Flukiver (Janssen), Flukol (Janssen)
Nitroxynil	Immature and adult flukes Some roundworms	Ruminants	Trodax (Merial)
Triclabendazole	Immature and adult flukes	Ruminants	Fasinex (Novartis)

Products listed above are classified as pharmacy merchant supplies 'PML'. It is important to check product authorisation information to confirm species and application details.

neonatal diarrhoea can quickly lead to dehydration, so the mainstay of treatment is rehydration therapy using commercially available preparations. The use of antimicrobial drugs and the reduction of risk factors are also steps that should be taken.

Salmonellosis

Acute diarrhoea in older ruminants is often caused by *Salmonella* spp., the most common pathogens being *S. typhimurium*, *S. dublin*, *S. newport*, *S. anatum* and *S. montevideo*. In addition to causing acute diarrhoea, this group of bacteria is responsible for septicaemia in very young animals, chronic enteritis, abortions in cattle and sheep, and human infections associated with contaminated food (see chapter 2). There can also be 'silent' infections and carrier states. In some countries salmonellosis is a significant disease of dairy cattle and sheep kept at high stocking rates, particularly if there is some sort of stress, including transport and intensive grazing. In calves, acute enteritis associated with salmonellosis is clinically similar to the symptoms of coccidiosis, viral diarrhoea and cryptosporidiosis. In adult cattle the condition resembles mucosal disease, acute intestinal obstruction, winter dysentery and bracken fern poisoning. In sheep there are similarities with coccidiosis and internal parasitic infections. Perhaps the most distinctive features of acute enteritis caused by *Salmonella* spp. are the fever and putrid diarrhoea that follow it, then the acute dehydration that results. Early treatment of affected animals with trimethoprim-sulfonamide preparations is effective but may induce carrier states in recovered animals. Fluid and electrolyte therapy is necessary when there is severe dehydration. Vaccines are available and have reasonable efficacy, and should be used in conjunction with good hygiene and quarantine measures (see also chapter 2).

Bovine virus diarrhoea

A disease complex called 'bovine virus diarrhoea, mucosal disease' occurs in most countries but, despite the high prevalence of infection, there is a low rate of occurrence of any of the specific entities: acute mucosal disease; acute diarrhoea; abortion and stillbirth; haemorrhagic disease; and congenital abnormalities. Most cattle are subclinically affected by the bovine mucosal disease virus (BVDV) and remain a possible source of infection to others in the herd. When acute diarrhoea occurs it is rapidly fatal, particularly in younger animals. The mucosal disease entity is a bit different in that affected animals suddenly become depressed and salivate profusely before the onset of tenesmus and watery diarrhoea. Many animals that develop mucosal disease die. Infection of cows with BVDV during pregnancy can cause abortions, stillbirths and fetal abnormalities. However, this reproductive entity of the disease complex may often only be evident as poor fertility in a herd of cows. The haemorrhagic entity is characterised by a tendency to bleeding in affected animals, showing up as bloody diarrhoea, epistaxis, and haemorrhages in the buccal mucosae. There is no specific treatment for any of the disease entities. Instead, control measures are necessary, such as quarantine, test and slaughter, and the use of vaccines.

Other causes (see also chapter 2)

Viral diarrhoea of newborn ruminants resembles colibacillosis, cryptosporidiosis and coccidiosis in that there is the sudden onset of profuse diarrhoea, mostly in calves. Several viruses are responsible, including rotaviruses and coronaviruses, and therefore no specific treatment is possible. Oral and parenteral fluid therapy is the best approach to treatment, accompanied by control measures such as ensuring that the calves receive adequate colostrum and that the cows are vaccinated during pregnancy.

Cryptosporidiosis, caused by *Cryptosporidium parvum*, is a milder form of diarrhoea, in large part because this protozoan parasite induces malabsorption rather than secretory diarrhoea. Fluid therapy is the best treatment, along with halofuginone (100 µg/kg orally each day for 7 days) or paromomycin (100 mg/kg orally each day for 11 days) if specific therapy is necessary.

Winter dysentery is a highly infectious disease of cattle and is probably caused by a coronavirus. The disease usually occurs as an outbreak of explosive diarrhoea lasting only a few days, sometimes accompanied by severe dehydration. Johne's disease, another cause of diarrhoea in cattle, also causes a loss of body weight; it is discussed in more detail in the next section of this chapter. The ingestion of a number of plants can result in diarrhoea. Acute bracken fern poisoning has already been described as a possible cause of sudden death in cattle, and it can also cause acute diarrhoea; other possible causes are common box bush (*Buxus sempervirens*), chicory (*Cichorium intybus*) and privet (*Ligustrum vulgare*). Arsenic poisoning was once a common cause of acute diarrhoea but there are few cases now that this toxic compound is seldom used on farms.

In sheep, diarrhoea can also be associated with infection by *Campylobacter jejuni* (weaner scours or weaner colitis) and *Yersinia enterocolitica* (yersiniosis), both of which are uncommon, and both of which usually cause ill-thrift rather than more serious consequences.

Weight loss

There are diseases of cattle, sheep and goats in which the predominant clinical problem is a loss of body weight (ill-thrift). Sometimes the cause is obvious, such as starvation, chronic diarrhoea, lameness, external parasites and chronic respiratory diseases. Starvation can occur because of reduced availability of adequate food but can also occur in the midst of plenty because of poor feeding practices, particularly when hobby farmers are involved. It must be kept in mind that when it is necessary to hand-feed animals there is a strong likelihood that there will be shy feeders among a group, that there will be too little trough space for all animals to feed freely, that the feed provided will not be nutritionally balanced, and that too little feed will be provided from time to time.

Johne's disease

A common cause of weight loss in cattle and sheep when there is adequate feed is Johne's disease. The causative organism, *Mycobacterium avium paratuberculosis*, was thought for a time to have an association with Crohn's disease in humans but this has never been proven.

It is the ability of this bacterium to survive for long periods in the environment and to resist host defences in cattle and sheep that makes it a formidable pathogen that is very difficult to treat or control. In ruminants the pathological mechanisms associated with Johne's disease are essentially the same, but in cattle the disease manifests with chronic intractable diarrhoea and progressive weight loss, whereas in sheep diarrhoea is not a feature. Infection is acquired by the ingestion of contaminated pasture and water. Calves may also pick up infections from the udders of cows that have been soiled with feces. After ingestion, the bacteria pass to the intestines, where they can enter Peyer's patches to infect macrophages in the mucosa and submucosa. Some bacteria also pass to the regional lymph nodes. In most cases, a cell-mediated immune response will eliminate the infection, a situation which is most likely to occur in adult animals. In a reasonably small proportion of animals the infection will persist and lead to a chronic enteritis, characterised by thickening of the mucosa and consequent malabsorption. It can take many years before affected animals lose the ability to absorb nutrients from food, and although their appetite and general health appear good, these animals progressively lose weight and will eventually become emaciated and die. Even prior to the occurrence of clinical signs the bacteria are shed in the feces in large numbers, thus contaminating the pasture and water supplies. The disease in cattle can be divided into four stages: silent infection; subclinical disease; clinical disease; and advanced clinical disease. In the final stage, infected animals suffer extreme weight loss and develop watery diarrhoea. Prior to that, the feces remain reasonably solid, diarrhoea may only be intermittent and weight loss only slight. Even when Johne's disease is endemic in a herd of cattle the incidence of clinical disease rarely exceeds 5% of adult animals, and the mortality rate will be less than 1% per year. Because there is no fully effective treatment for the disease, the way the condition is handled is by trying to control it, usually by identifying and eliminating clinically affected and serologically positive animals, accompanied by improved management and hygiene to minimise the spread of infection. In some countries vaccination is used to prevent clinical disease, but vaccines do not prevent infection.

Parasitic infections

Eperythrozoonosis, a disease of sheep characterised by weight loss and jaundice following a period of stress, occurs in many parts of the world. The causative organism is a rickettsia, *Eperythrozoon ovis*, which parasitises and destroys red blood cells, leading to anaemia and jaundice. The organism is transmitted between sheep by biting insects. Eperythrozoonosis can be treated by a single intramuscular injection of long-acting oxytetracycline (20 mg/kg). Cattle are commonly infected with *E. wenyonii* but seldom develop clinical disease.

Weaner ill-thrift in sheep, a condition characterised by a loss of weight at weaning and failure to thrive after that, may also be caused by *E. ovis*, but other causes are possible: intestinal parasitism; trace element or vitamin deficiency; poor pasture palatability; and overcrowding.

Parasitic gastroenteritis, particularly haemonchosis in sheep and ostertagiosis in cattle, and chronic liver fluke disease are parasitic infections that commonly cause weight loss. Haemonchosis is caused by an atypical gastrointestinal trichostrongylid, *Haemonchus contortus*, which occurs more commonly in warmer regions and feeds on blood, resulting in anaemia and weight loss rather than diarrhoea. A large infestation can cause death. Treatment is with the same broad-spectrum anthelmintics as those used for other trichostrongylids, except that resistance to these drugs is common and other anthelmintics may have to used, such as those used in liver fluke disease.

Mineral deficiencies (see also chapter 9)

Copper deficiency

Copper deficiency is a world-wide problem which can be primary, due to soil deficiencies, or secondary, due to the excessive ingestion of molybdenum or sulfate. In cattle, copper deficiency causes unthriftiness that is characterised by a rough coat, reduced milk production, and poor growth of calves. There may be persistent diarrhoea (peat scours) and the alarming 'falling disease', in which cows literally drop dead. In sheep the principle manifestations are fleece abnormalities, including loss of pigment in black wool, scouring and unthriftiness. Lambs may be born with swayback or develop enzootic ataxia. Treatment is with copper. Oral drenching with copper sulfate (1 g for sheep, 4 g for calves and 8 g for adult cattle) each week for four weeks is effective. It is also possible to inject long-acting copper formulations, such as copper grey cinate (60 mg for calves and 120 mg for adult cattle every two weeks for 3 months). The alternatives are controlled-release glass copper oxide needles or copper oxide powder in rumen boluses.

Cobalt

Cobalt is required by cattle, sheep and goats for the synthesis of vitamin B_{12}, and there are many parts of the world where soils are deficient in cobalt. A reduction in vitamin B_{12} causes inappetance, leading to loss of body weight and reduced wool and milk production. The condition has to be differentiated from copper deficiency, Johne's disease, high intestinal worm burdens and starvation. Oral dosing with cobalt sulfate (1 mg/kg/day) or intramuscular injections of vitamin B_{12} (100–300 μg each week) is suitable for sheep. Cobalt oxide pellets are available for oral administration.

Selenium deficiency

In ruminants a deficiency of selenium can lead to ill-thrift and inefficient reproduction, and to enzootic muscular dystrophy (white muscle disease and stiff lamb disease) in calves, lambs and kids born to mothers that had low intakes of selenium during pregnancy. Acute enzootic muscular dystrophy can cause sudden death of young ruminants, whereas stiffness and lameness are the main features of the chronic form of the disease.

Other causes

Disorders of the mouth, jaw and throat can obviously result in a loss of weight if the problem is persistent, as can occur if there is a loss of teeth, actinobacillosis ('wooden tongue') or even rickets. Wooden tongue is caused by *Actinobacillus lignieresii*, a bacterium normally found in the mouth of ruminants, which can enter the underlying tissues in the mouth if there are abrasions and cuts. Once in the tissues, *A. lignieresii* causes inflammation followed by formation of a solid granuloma. Affected cattle may be unable to chew properly because of a swollen or deformed tongue, whereas sheep usually develop lesions around the jaw, face and nose but still may have difficulty eating. Sodium iodide solution given intravenously (10 mg/kg) as a single dose or as three daily doses is effective in many cases. The solution can also be given subcutaneously to sheep, and procaine penicillin (10 mg/kg intramuscularly daily for 5 days) can be used for both sheep and cattle.

There are many plants that can cause unthriftiness, many of which can also cause other clinical signs, depending on the amount ingested by cattle, sheep and goats. For example, the long-term ingestion by sheep of the soluble oxalates from soursob (*Oxalis pescaprae* or *Oxalis cernua*) leads to chronic nephrosis and the consequent loss of body condition. Acute oxalate poisoning, on the other hand, is a quite different condition in which clinical hypocalcaemia is caused by the ingestion of large quantities of any plant containing soluble oxalates, such as halogeton and rhubarb, leading to the precipitation of calcium oxalate in the blood. It is treated in the same way as hypocalcaemia caused by other means, but animals may still die from renal failure.

Progressive weight loss of cattle was once a common result of tuberculosis, caused mostly by *Mycobacterium bovis* and much less commonly by *M. tuberculosis*. It is eradicated from many countries, although wildlife reservoirs, such as brushtail possums in New Zealand and badgers in parts of the UK, have made this virtually impossible. Sheep and goats are largely resistant to the clinical effects of tuberculosis but not to infection. The clinical signs in cattle, apart from emaciation, will depend on where the lesions are located. Many are in the lungs; others may be in the intestines, reproductive tract and udder.

 Infected cattle can be a source of infection to humans so the usual approach taken is test and slaughter. Treatment is seldom attempted.

Other causes of weight loss are discussed elsewhere in this chapter and include the wasting form of acetonaemia and chronic bracken fern poisoning.

Lameness

Lameness in cattle, sheep and goats is often due to injuries, and usually only one or two animals in a group are affected. When many animals are lame there should immediately be suspicion of foot rot, foot scald or foot abscesses in sheep, and even bluetongue or foot-and-mouth disease. Mineral and trace element imbalances can also cause lameness, and young animals are susceptible to a further range of diseases, such as joint-ill, white muscle disease and rickets.

Foot rot and related conditions

Among the common causes of lameness in sheep are foot scald (benign foot rot), foot rot and infectious bulbar necrosis. Other causes include contagious ecthyma and strawberry foot rot, and, in some parts of the world, the bluetongue and foot-and-mouth disease viruses. In foot scald the skin between the digits is damaged by frosty pastures, constant wetting or trauma, so allowing penetration of the subcutaneous tissues by bacteria, particularly *Fusobacterium* spp. and *Actinomyces pyogenes*. These lead to interdigital dermatitis. Unless there is further infection of the wound, the lesion remains localised, although it may get so severe as to result in substantial swelling and suppuration. Most sheep in mob would be lame, often in more than one foot. Treatment with long-acting tetracycline (a single 20 mg/kg intramuscular injection) should be effective.

Foot rot is a more severe condition in which additional bacterial invasion leads to separation of the hoof from the underlying tissue, and a strong, distinctive odour. Foot rot only occurs where there is contamination of the pastures with *Dichelobacter nodosus*, a factor that has led to eradication programmes and the development of vaccines. Treatment with a single dose of long-acting tetracycline or procaine penicillin is usually effective. Spread must be minimised by adopting quarantine measures, restricting movement of sheep and the use of footbaths. Copper sulfate solution (5%), formalin solution (5%) and zinc sulfate solution (10%) are suitable for use in the footbaths. None of the vaccines available is fully effective.

Foot abscesses, particularly in the heel, occur in wet conditions, especially in pregnant ewes. Usually only one foot, and even one digit, is affected. Treatment is by surgical drainage and accompanying antibiotic. Wet and muddy conditions, along with cuts and scratches to the interdigital skin, can lead to foot rot in cattle. This occurs because bacteria from the environment, especially *F. necrophorum*, contaminate the wound to exacerbate the inflammation that follows any trauma, and lead to the foot becoming swollen and sore. The digits are pushed apart by the swelling, there is a foul odour, and the affected animal is acutely lame and lethargic. Treatment with antibiotics, such as penicillin and oxytetracycline given intramuscularly, is usually required. Local treatment using good wound management principles may also be necessary and preventive measures should be taken to reduce further trouble in the herd.

Foot trauma

Lameness in cattle, sheep and goats can also be due to trauma, such as sole trauma and white line disease. Interdigital cracks and hyperplasia (corns) and laminitis also occur. Sole trauma and white line disease are associated with trauma, either because the animals bruise the sole of one or both digits of a foot by standing on a hard and sharp object or because there is separation of the fibrous junction between the sole and wall of the hoof (the white line), allowing dirt and gravel into the underlying tissue. Either way, there is acute lameness due to inflammation and infection. Frequently there is an abscess at the site. It is usual for only one foot to be affected, unlike lameness associated with foot rot, laminitis or foot-and-mouth disease. Diagnosis is aided by the use of hoof testers, which are devices that look like an oversized pair of pliers with claw-like ends. These are used to apply pressure to various parts of the hoof in order to elicit a pain response from the animal, and so localise the site of the lesion. Once the lesion is located, the horny tissue above it is usually cut away with a sharp hoof knife to relieve the pressure and to allow drainage and flushing of the site, and antibiotics and anti-inflammatory drugs are administered if warranted. If only one digit is affected, a cow slip can be applied to the unaffected digit to redistribute the weight and reduce the lameness. The application of a thick bandage to the foot may be necessary in cases of white line disease so as to prevent further dirt and gravel entering the wound.

If the foot is caught in a tight space, such as in a gutter, or the digits are splayed, there can be trauma to other parts of the hoof structure. One of the more common consequences is interdigital cracking with underlying haemorrhage and inflammation. This condition is treated along the same lines as sole trauma and white line disease, with the addition of hoof trimming if the horny tissue is overgrown and contributes to the problem. Sometimes the overgrowth is severe enough to result in deformity of the hoof and corkscrew claw results, a condition that cannot be corrected satisfactorily.

Interdigital hyperplasia occurs more commonly in the heavy beef breeds of cattle, usually in the hind limbs, due to splaying of the digits. It appears as a firm, tumour-like lump in the interdigital space and may cause lameness. The only treatment is surgery followed by tight bandaging to keep the digits together. Laminitis in cattle – and in sheep and goats for that matter – is the same disease as the one that is much more common in horses. It may range in severity from subclinical to acute to chronic, and affects more than one foot and usually more than one animal in a herd. The treatment adopted will depend on the severity of the condition. Only the acute form requires the administration of anti-inflammatory drugs, such as ketoprofen, and perhaps antihistamines.

Foot-and-mouth disease

An outbreak of foot-and-mouth disease (FMD) may be caused by one of several distinct strains or serotypes of a picornavirus. These are highly virulent viruses that can infect sheep, pigs, cattle and wild ruminant animals.

There have been isolated reports of FMD being transmitted to humans.

The number of infected animals increases rapidly at the start of an outbreak, and all animals develop fever and vesicular lesions on the mouth, feet and teats. Young animals can be killed and the older ones lose productivity very quickly. Diagnosis of the disease is based on the characteristics of the outbreak and on sophisticated laboratory tests to determine not only the presence of the virus but also the strain or serotype. A carrier state arises in recovered animals. The disease is endemic in many parts of the world. Outbreaks are known to occur in other parts of the world, but FMD has not been recorded in Australia, New Zealand, Japan or Indonesia for many years. Spread of the virus is by direct contact or by aerosols, the latter being a particularly potent method because infected animals pass large amounts of virus in exhaled air and in secretions. The virus is also transmitted in infected milk and animal products, such as occurred in the FMD outbreak in the UK in 2001 following the illegal importation of meat products from Asia. The usual response to an outbreak of FMD in a country or region normally free of the disease is to slaughter all infected and at-risk animals, and to impose strict quarantine and movement restrictions. There is no specific treatment. Vaccination is not considered feasible as a control measure for outbreaks because the spread can be so rapid; it is an approach that can be used in endemic areas, but confers only brief protection against the specific strain of the virus used to make the vaccine. Eradication of FMD is complicated by the possible reservoirs of infection, including wild deer, and the possible survival of the virus for several months in cool and moist conditions. See Box 10.1 for experience of FMD in practice.

Box 10.1   Resilience through adversity – a pharmacist's view of foot-and-mouth diease

It could never happen to us. North Cumbria is a quiet area of north-west England where the daily routine rarely changes. An area totally dependent upon livestock farming, but with many deep and rich characters that make one really understand where the true value of community pharmacy lies – the people.

Longtown auction mart. is the largest sheep auction in the country, trading up to 20 000 sheep in a single day. Sometime between the 15th and 22nd of February 2001, harvest came early, only this time it was the Grim Reaper. Some infected sheep passed through the auction, mixing with sheep and farmers throughout the area and triggering a disaster. We can still only guess at the extent of the implications for the whole economy of North Cumbria, an area with sparse population and little opportunity to diversify into tourism.

We wake each morning to hear the names of farms confirmed with foot-and-mouth whose owners are friends as well as customers. As the numbers of our customers confirmed grows to exceed £200 000 worth of turnover, and the continuation of the cull threatens to exceed half of our turnover, one turns to some fundamental SWOT analysis and 'out of box' thinking.

During this crisis, my pharmaceutical skills continue to be called on to solve the most varied practical problems. How do you change the pH of 500 000 gallons of slurry outside of the range 6–9, so that it can be safely disposed on the land of an infected farm? More to the point, how do you relay that information to a man who has not only lost his livelihood (and remember the compensation only reimburses him for the value of his livestock), but also participated in the destruction of cows that he's nurtured for years? How do you decrease livestock-handling equipment ready for sterilisation? All this whilst consideration of other fundamental questions. How do you coordinate other businesses in the town to effectively lobby MPs and ministers to attract funding for the local economy? Which of the many important points do you emphasise in a time-limited meeting with Rt Hon. Michael Meacher MP who is heading up the Rural Task Force? But most fundamentally, what is to happen to our staff when there are no livestock left in North Cumbria for them to treat?

(continued)

Box 10.1 (continued)

Well, virtually all the businesses in the town have very little option to realign. The feed company can only sell bulk feed to farmers, how does the auction trade if there are no sheep or cattle? Even the doctor can only treat human patients. But the pharmacist has a broad scientific training and is qualified in many areas. Most specifically he or she has greater knowledge than any other on the 'High Street' in pharmacology and therapeutics, be that for human or animal medicines. In fact, most animal medicines are identical in formulation and use to human medicines. In addition the pharmacist has communication skills and high numbers of pet owners passing through his or her premises.

If this crisis has taught me anything, it is to have as many strings to my bow as possible, otherwise there'll be a bleak future. A fact that my father-in-law realised too late when he was forced to close his butcher's shop when Asda opened up round the corner.

If a community pharmacy is to provide a comprehensive pharmaceutical service, it should be an ethical obligation to provide that service to animals as well as humans. Every community pharmacy in the land can, and should, provide a range of pet medicines, whether that pharmacy be rural or urban. Pharmacists already have the breadth of knowledge to advise and sell these products. With the abolition of Retail Price Maintenance and the relaxation of restriction on the granting of NHS contracts, the more strings the UK pharmacists have, the better.

Phil Jobson

Other viral diseases

Caprine arthritis encephalitis virus

Goats are susceptible to caprine arthritis encephalitis (CAE) virus, which causes lameness in addition to other problems. There has been a rapid spread of CAE since it was first identified about 20 years ago. In kids and young goats the virus infection leads to incoordination and then paralysis, whereas in older goats CAE manifests as chronic, progressive arthritis in several joints, especially the carpal joint (big knee), and as indurative mastitis (hard bag). There is no specific treatment and there is no vaccine, so affected animals have to be treated symptomatically and measures put in place to prevent horizontal and vertical transmission of the virus. Such measures might include the feeding of heat-treated colostrum and pasteurised milk to kids that are segregated from the does at birth, frequent serological testing, and the disinfection of any equipment that may be used between infected and non-infected herds, using benzalkonium chloride, cetrimide or chlorhexidine.

Bluetongue

Bluetongue is an arthropod-borne orbivirus infection which causes a range of symptoms in sheep, one of which is profound lameness due to laminitis and inflammation of the tissues above the hooves. Most blue-tongue infections of cattle and goats are inapparent. Affected animals also develop a very distinctive purple discoloration of the mouth and tongue (bluetongue), mucopurulent nasal discharge, and sometimes wryneck. Recovery takes a long time, loss of production can be significant, and no specific treatment is available. Vaccination is the only effective form of control.

Mineral deficiencies (see also chapter 9)

Lameness is also a feature of the chronic form of enzootic muscular dystrophy (white muscle disease and stiff lamb disease), whereas in acute disease there is usually the sudden death of young calves, lambs and kids due to myocardial damage, a condition that can be confused with enterotoxaemia. Both forms of the disease are caused by selenium deficiency with or without a concurrent vitamin E deficiency. White muscle disease becomes evident in lambs 1–4 months after birth, showing up as generalised weakness and stiffness. There may be respiratory distress in some lambs. Affected animals lose body condition and will probably die without treatment provided by the intramuscular injection of selenium (as sodium or potassium selenite, 0.1 mg/kg) and vitamin E (usually as *dl-α*-tocopherol, 3–5 mg/kg), as a single treatment. Control and prevention can be achieved by providing additional selenium and vitamin E to pregnant animals and to both mothers and their young after birth. Selenium is available for subcutaneous injection (0.1 mg/kg), as a slow-release subcutaneous injection (1 mg/kg every 3 weeks), intra-ruminal pellets (500 mg in each pellet will last up to 2 years), and oral formulations (0.05–0.1 mg/kg). Top-dressing of pastures (10 g selenium/hectare) can provide up to 12 months' protection.

It is necessary to differentiate white muscle disease from enzootic ataxia and swayback, both of which are associated with copper deficiency, border disease (hairy shaker disease) and daft lamb disease. Copper deficiency will affect a group of animals and usually cause unthriftiness, such as faded coat colour in cattle, loss of crimp and gloss of wool, and persistent diarrhoea (peat scours or teart) in all three species of ruminant. These clinical signs are not diagnostic because malnutrition, intestinal parasitism, cobalt deficiency and a number of external parasites can also result in the same signs. Copper deficiency in lambs and kids causes incoordination and ataxia, both of which are associated with defective myelination of the spinal chord due to copper deficiency in pregnancy (swayback) or in the first weeks after birth (enzootic ataxia). Dosing with copper, in the form of injections, intra-ruminal devices, salt licks or pasture sprays, can prevent primary copper deficiency. The reduction of the amounts of interfering substances, particularly molybdenum and sulfate, will also assist. Caution must be exercised when administering copper because it can accumulate in the liver only to be suddenly released to precipitate intravascular haemolysis and death. Early treatment of enzootic ataxia and swayback with copper sulfate can be effective. Treatment later in the course of these related diseases is unlikely to be successful.

Other causes

Infectious arthritis

Infectious arthritis (joint ill) is common in ruminants, particularly newborn animals following the spread of bacteria in the blood from navel infections acquired at birth. In older animals, cases of infectious arthritis are more commonly due to trauma or the spread of bacteria from infected wounds, or infections with *Haemophilus somnus* in cattle or *Mycoplasma* spp. in cattle, sheep and goats. In young animals several joints are commonly involved, whereas in older animals there is usually involvement of only one or two joints. Lameness, pain and fever are seen during the acute stages of infectious arthritis, with swelling of affected joints likely later in the course of the disease. Treatment over several days with antibiotic is necessary; long-acting tetracycline, procaine penicillin and potentiated sulfonamides are the drugs of choice.

Osteodystrophy

Osteodystrophy in ruminants is due primarily to nutritional causes and genetic abnormalities. The usual nutritional cause is deficiency in calcium or a calcium/phosphorus imbalance, such as can occur when animals are fed incorrect rations, resulting in rickets and osteomalacia. In both cases there is lameness, loss of weight or failure to thrive, and probably distortions and fractures of the long bones. The administration of calcium, phosphorus and vitamin D is necessary to treat these conditions.

Ergot alkaloids

Ergot alkaloids produced by fungi growing on tall fescue (*Festuca arundinacea*) can cause lameness in cattle during cold weather (fescue foot) due to gangrene of the extremities. Interestingly, in hot weather ingestion of the same alkaloids from infected tall fescue pastures results in a different syndrome, fescue summer toxicosis (summer slump), in which there is sharp drop in weight gain or productivity in cattle and sheep. These diseases have to be controlled by management strategies that limit exposure to tall fescue contaminated with fungi.

Cerebellar hypoplasia

Cerebellar hypoplasias, due to genetic abnormalities or infections *in utero* with bovine viral diarrhoea virus and bluetongue virus, occurs in calves and lambs. One form is daft lamb disease. These are normally one-off disorders in which the affected animal is severely incoordinated.

Disorders of the tegument

External parasites are responsible for many of the disorders of the skin and wool, hair or fibre of ruminants, particularly sheep, because wool provides both a sanctuary and a target for many of these parasites. Other common skin disorders include photosensitisation, a range microbial infections including scabby mouth, mycotic dermatitis, cheesy gland, ringworm and poxvirus infections, some significant skin cancers, and various types of dermatitis. It is often not appreciated that many of the skin conditions which occur in humans also affect animals, so there are cases of udder impetigo, vitiligo due to freeze-branding, seborrhoea in the form of greasy heel, and defective pigmentation due to copper deficiency.

Ectoparasites

External parasites can be divided into five groups: flies and their maggots, lice, ticks and mites. The range of ectoparasiticides used to treat the various conditions resulting from infestation is summarised in Table 10.2. One of the flies that causes problems in sheep is *Melophagus ovinus* (sheep ked), a flightless insect that lives entirely on the skin where it feeds on blood by puncturing the skin, causing intense pruritus.

Table 10.2 Ectoparasiticidal products for cattle, sheep and pigs

Drug name	Parasite target	Species	Product name (UK)
Amitraz (Amidines)	Lice, mites, ticks Keds, lice, ticks Lice, mites	Cattle Sheep Pigs	Taktic (Intervet) Top line (Intervet) pigs only
Abamectin	Lice, mites, warble-fly larvae	Cattle	Enzec (Merial)
Doramectin	Lice, mites, horn flies, warble-fly larvae Lice, mites Psoroptes ovis (sheep scab)	Cattle Pigs Sheep	Dectomax (Pfizer)
Eprinomectin	Lice, mites, warble-fly larvae	Cattle	Eprinex (Merial)
Ivermectin	Lice, mites, horn flies, warble-fly larvae Lice, mites Psoroptes ovis	Cattle Pigs Sheep	Ivomec, Panomec (Merial) Noromectin (Norbrook) Virbamec (Virbac)
Moxidectin	Lice, mites, horn flies, warble-fly larvae Psoroptes ovis	Cattle Sheep	Cydectin (Fort Dodge)
Dimpylate (diazinon) (O-P compound)	Keds, lice, ticks, blowfly strike, Psoroptes ovis	Sheep	All Seasons Fly & Scab Dip, Coopers' (Schering-Plough) Osmonds Gold Fleece Sheep Dip (Bimeda, Virbac) Paracide Plus (Battle, Hayward & Bower)

Active ingredient	Target parasites	Species	Products
Phosmet (O-P compound)	Lice, mites, warble-fly larvae Lice, mites	Cattle Pigs	Poron 20 (Young's) Porect (Young's)
Cypermethrin	Lice, flies Lice, ticks, headflies, blowfly strike *Psoroptes ovis*	Cattle Sheep	Deosan Dysect Pour-on (Fort Dodge) Auriplak fly & Scab Dip (Virbac), Crovect (Young's), Ecofleece Sheep Dip (Bimeda), Provinec (Novartis), Robust (Young's), Vector (Young's)
Deltamethrin	Lice, flies Keds, lice, ticks, headflies, blowfly strike	Cattle Sheep	Spot on Insecticide, Coopers' (Schering-Plough)
Flumethrin	Keds, lice, ticks, *Psoroptes ovis*	Sheep	Bayticol Scab & Tick Dip (Bayer)
Permethrin	Lice, mites, flies	Cattle	Auriplak (Virbac), Flypor (Young's), Swift (Young's), Ridect Pour-on (Pfizer), Vetrazin (Novartis)
Cyromazine (triazine derivative)	Blowfly strike prevention	Sheep	Vetrazin (Novartis)

Products listed above are classified as pharmacy and merchant supplies (PML). It is important to check product authorisation information to confirm species and application details.

Affected sheep scratch, bite and rub, leading to self-inflicted damage to the wool and skin (cockle). Shearing followed by dipping or jetting or the application of pour-on insecticides is usually effective, provided that all sheep are treated.

Blowflies

In some parts of the world blowflies are much more troublesome than the sheep ked. Several blowflies are capable of producing myiasis, a condition in which the maggots burrow into the subcutaneous tissue after being deposited on wounds or soiled wool and skin by adult female flies. Primary blowflies are the ones that are the first to deposit maggots. These include *Lucilia* spp. and *Calliphora stygia*, the maggots of which cause tissue damage and serous exudation, which attracts secondary blowflies, of other species, to deposit larvae on the site. Blowfly strikes can spread rapidly and contain thousands of maggots. Severe strikes can kill sheep. Animals that have been severely struck usually stop eating and kick or bite the infested site. There is often a distinctive pungent odour. Most strikes are at sites where there is soiling, such as around the anus and tail, or where there are wounds, such as after shearing or dehorning, or along the back after heavy summer rains. Blowfly strike is treated by applying an insecticide; clipping of the wool is not absolutely necessary.

Warble-fly larvae

Warble-fly larvae (*Hypoderma bovis* and *H. lineatum*) cause skin lesions on the back of cattle when they emerge from soft, painful lumps after a lengthy period of migration that has taken them from the hairs of the legs through the skin to the oesophagus or around the spinal cord, and then back to the skin. The adult flies are active in the warmer months and the larvae migrate inside cattle during the colder months, so treatment is usually in autumn using organophosphates, such as phosmet (a single 20 mg/kg pour-on dose) or the avermectins and milbemycins, such as doramectin, ivermectin and moxidectin (each 500 μg/kg as a pour-on). Treating infected cattle in summer can cause problems because killing migrating larvae could damage the oesophagus and spinal cord. In addition to having skin lesions, some animals may become paralysed in the back legs due to spinal cord damage, and heavy infestations may cause loss of weight. In many countries eradication programmes have been successful.

Screw-worm larvae

Larvae of screw-worms (*Cochliomyia hominovorax* and *Chrysomyia bezziana*) cause significant skin lesions in some parts of the world due to the cavernous and exudative lesions caused when they infest pre-existing wounds. Secondary bacterial infections and infestation by other blowfly larvae exacerbate the problem. The flies have been eradicated from some countries but still cause problems in Central and South America and in Africa, India and Asia. Subcutaneous ivermectin (200 μg/kg) and topical organophosphates are used to kill larvae.

A number of other flies, midges and mosquitoes irritate cattle and, to a lesser extent, sheep and goats. Some also transmit disease, such as pink-eye, bluetongue, ephemeral fever and onchocerciasis. Despite the diverse nature of these insects, the common approach taken with all of them is the use of repellents formulated into tags or pour-ons. Cypermethrin and permethrin are commonly used for this purpose.

Lice

Lice are host-specific ectoparasites. Two types infest cattle: sucking lice (*Haematopinus* spp., *Linognathus* spp. and *Solenopotes* spp.); and biting lice *(Damalinia (Bovicola) bovis)*. There are also two types in sheep (*Linognathus* spp. and *Damalinia ovis*) and goats (*Linognathus* spp. and *Damalinia caprae)*. Lice are transmitted from animal to animal: there are no intermediate hosts and contamination of the animals' environment is not a factor. Affected animals are severely irritated by these parasites, much as head lice irritate humans, so the main symptoms of infestation are itching and rubbing, particularly in winter, when parasite numbers are the highest. Not surprisingly, lice are of greatest economic importance in sheep. Treatment with pour-on formulations is convenient and effective, using synthetic pyrethrins, such as cypermethrin and deltamethrin, and triflumuron (see Table 10.2).

Ticks and mites

Many species of tick can infest ruminants but seldom do any of them cause significant skin lesions. Instead, ticks are important vectors of disease, such as babesiosis, anaplasmosis, theileriosis, heartwater, louping ill, tick-borne fever and Lyme disease. Some cause anaemia, and heavy infestations may cause loss of production. Tick paralysis associated with infestations of *Ixodes* spp. and some other ticks can occur in young ruminants. The various ticks are classified according to their life cycle: one-host ticks (e.g. *Boophilus* spp.); two-host ticks (e.g. some *Rhipicephalus* spp.) and three-host ticks (e.g. *Haemophysalis* spp. and *Amblyomma* spp.). Most of the pour-on treatments suitable for treating lice will also kill ticks. However, complete control is often impossible because of wildlife reservoirs.

Mites are another distinct group of ectoparasites, and the diseases they cause are called 'mange'. Psoroptic mange (sheep scab) looks like mycotic dermatitis because of the exudate and scabs, which are caused by the mite *Psoroptes ovis* burrowing in the skin to cause severe itching and irritation, probably of an allergic nature. Other external parasites and scrapie can cause similar clinical signs. Psoroptic mange also occurs in cattle and goats but is relatively unimportant in these animals, and may be associated with a different subspecies of the parasite. Sheep scab has been eradicated from many countries but still occurs in the UK, where it has a seasonal occurrence and is the subject of *The Sheep Scab Order 1997*, published by The Stationery Office, London. Infected animals develop scabs in the wool and other parts of the body, and many lose weight. A single topical treatment with diazinon (0.01%), flumethrin (0.05%) and propetamphos (0.0125%) will treat sheep scab, and two doses of ivermectin (0.2 mg/kg) given 7 days apart or doramectin (300 mg/kg) as a single dose by subcutaneous injection are also effective (see Table 10.2).

Photosensitisation

Cattle, sheep and goats can develop inflamed and necrotic lesions on areas of lightly pigmented skin and mucous membranes exposed to direct sunlight due to primary or hepatogenous photosensitisation.

Photosensitisation is a major problem of sheep in many parts of the world, where plants such as *Hypericum perforatum* (St John's wort), *Fagopyrum esculentum* (buckwheat), *Cymopterus* spp. (wild carrot) and *Brassica* spp. (rape, kale, etc) contain photodynamic agents, and plants such as *Narthecium ossifragum* (bog asphodel), *Tribulus terrestris* (puncture vine), *Lantana camara* (lantana) and *Panicum* spp. (panic and millet grasses) contain hepatotoxins. The infection of lupins with a fungus, *Phomopsis leptostomiformis*, and ryegrass and other pasture plants with the saprophytic fungus *Pithomyces chatarum* can lead to liver damage, resulting in lupinosis (see above) and facial eczema.

Hepatogenous photosensitisation is always associated with the retention, due to liver and biliary damage, of phylloerythrin, a metabolic breakdown product of chlorophyll. Phylloerythrin in the skin is activated by light, particularly in non-pigmented areas, to cause necrosis of cells in the skin followed by inflammation and localised discomfort. Oedema is often present and may lead to swelling around the face, head and ears. Animals affected with any form of photosensitisation should be put in shady areas and treated symptomatically.

Facial eczema can affect cattle, sheep and goats. It is a severe problem of sheep in parts of New Zealand, occurring when climatic conditions favour growth of the fungus on dead plants, particularly ryegrass. Sporidesmin, the hepatotoxin released by the fungus, causes acute liver and biliary damage, resulting in the sudden onset of lethargy, jaundice and photosensitisation. There can be a high mortality rate of affected animals. Treatment is limited to moving affected and susceptible animals off contaminated pastures, whereas control is achieved by monitoring for fungal spores, by spraying with fungicides at times of highest risk of excessive fungal growth, and by the daily administration of zinc (30 mg/kg) as a drench, in drinking water, as an intraruminal bolus, or sprayed onto pastures.

Bacterial infections

Caseous lymphadenitis

Caseous lymphadenitis is caused by *Corynebacterium pseudotuberculosis*. It is included here because some vaccines for sheep on the market today include a component to immunise against the occurrence of cheesy gland. The disease is due to chronic infection of lymph nodes by *C. pseudotuberculosis*, resulting in lumps under the skin that are ruptured during shearing. When ruptured, thick yellow-green pus is released. The condition is a cause of economic loss because lamb carcasses can be affected.

Mycotic dermatitis

Mycotic dermatitis is a bacterial infection of damaged skin in cattle, sheep and goats, particularly in tropical and subtropical areas, and in temperate areas at times of high rainfall. Damage to the skin can be caused by prolonged wetting of the fleece and shearing cuts in sheep, and by skin abrasions in cattle. Tick infestations can exacerbate mycotic dermatitis (cutaneous streptotrichosis) in cattle. Damage to fleece causes significant economic losses and predisposes to blowfly strike, and cattle losses from mycotic dermatitis can be significant in Africa. *Dermatophilus congolensis* is also associated with strawberry foot rot in sheep, a condition characterised by scabs above the coronet that reveal red granulomatous tissue when removed. Mycotic dermatitis and strawberry foot rot are best treated with procaine penicillin (10 mg/kg) or oxytetracycline (20 mg/kg) given intramuscularly as a single dose. Sheep should be kept dry, if possible, and inspected regularly for blowfly infestation. Spraying or dipping sheep with 1% zinc sulfate solution after shearing will provide long-lasting protection. In areas where cattle are prone to mycotic dermatitis there should be adequate tick control.

Viral infections

One of the diseases that can be transmitted from sheep to humans is a condition known as pustular dermatitis or orf. It is also called scabby mouth. Goats can also be infected by the orf virus, a poxvirus that causes this skin infection. There are several orf virus strains, all of them related to pseudocowpox virus and bovine papular stomatitis virus. Scabby mouth spreads rapidly amongst susceptible animals, entering the skin through cuts and scratches caused by shearing, barbed wire and the thorns and burrs of plants. An outbreak of sores covered by scabs on the face of sheep is a reasonably common occurrence in countries and regions where the disease is endemic. Secondary bacterial infection of the lesions is common, and the lesions may also occur in the perineal region. Affected animals may lose body weight because of a reluctance to feed but it is seldom of major economic importance because it is a self-limiting disease that results in solid resistance to reinfection.

Humans are infected with the orf virus through the handling of infected sheep or sheepdogs (see chapter 13), resulting in lesions on the hands and forearms. Touching the face and lips may also cause lesions here (see Figure 13.10, page 391).

There is no specific treatment, so the best approach is the adoption of modern wound management principles, particularly the control of secondary bacterial infections and the use of dressings to promote moist wound healing. Vaccination is possible in order to prevent, and perhaps control, outbreaks of scabby mouth in sheep. The vaccines used are avirulent live viruses that are applied to scarified skin to provide around 6 months of protection, but must be used with caution because the viruses can infect cuts and scratches to cause mild skin lesions.

Sheep pox

Sheep pox causes lesions that look like those of orf, but it has a somewhat different geographical distribution, being present in Africa, the

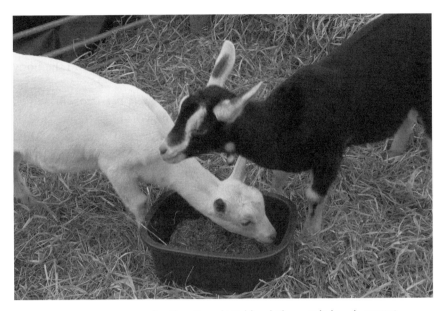

Figure 10.3   Young goats feeding (Royal Highland Show, Edinburgh, 2003).

Indian subcontinent, the Middle East and Central Asia but not in the UK, Australia or New Zealand. Infected animals develop fever and lethargy, then typical lesions on the skin and mucous membranes. In the later stages of the disease the pox lesions are covered in scabs, and some develop into nodules. There can be a high mortality rate among lambs. Goat pox looks like sheep pox and occurs in the same parts of the world. There are no specific treatments for sheep pox or goat pox, but there are attenuated live virus vaccines available to control the disease in endemic areas.

Cowpox

Cowpox infections of cattle are very rare but rodents can be infected with the virus, whereas pseudocowpox is very common and widespread, causing lesions on the teats of cows. The pseudocowpox virus is similar to the viruses that cause infectious papular stomatitis and contagious ecthyma (scabby mouth, orf), so the teat lesions follow a course similar to those of scabby mouth in sheep: acute erythema and pain followed by the development of pustules that rupture and are then covered with thick scabs. The scabs fall off about 10 days later to leave granulomatous tissue.

Ringworm

Ringworm occurs on the head, neck and perineum of cattle, and occasionally all over the body, and rarely on the head of sheep and the body of goats.

The usual cause is *Trichophyton* spp., often *T. verrucosum*, which can also infect humans to cause severe ringworm. Extreme care is needed when handling stock infected with ringworm, especially when brushing off scabs (see below).

The fungus is spread by contact with infected animals, some of which will be asymptomatic carriers. The lesions are typical of ringworm in that there are hairless areas that may be covered with thick scabs and can be confused with cases of mange or dermatophilosis (mycotic dermatitis and lumpy wool), a more deep-seated skin condition caused by *Dermatophilus congolensis*. Many cases of ringworm resolve spontaneously. If treatment is required, the scabs should be removed using a firm brush, and this should be followed by daily or less frequent topical applications of 10% povidone–iodine solution (1% available iodine), 0.2% enilconazole solution or 5% lime sulfur solution. Bordeaux mixture and Whitfield's ointment can be used. The intravenous administration of several daily doses of a 10% sodium iodide solution (70 mg/kg) is an

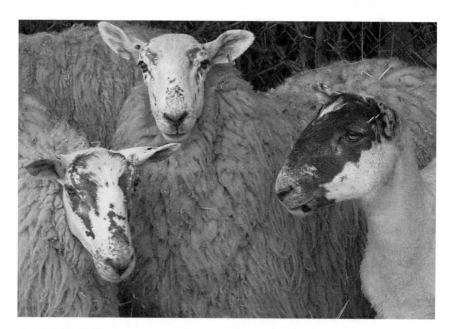

Figure 10.4 Sheep.

alternative to topical solutions, sprays and ointments. An effective vaccine against *T. verrucosum* is available in Europe.

Jaundice

The yellow staining of tissues that occurs in jaundice is best seen in the eyes of cattle, sheep and goats. Other mucous membranes may also be discolored, but visible changes to the colour of skin are less common. Jaundice is due to an accumulation of bilirubin due either to excessive breakdown of red blood cells (haemolytic jaundice) or to liver disease, such as bile duct obstruction (obstructive jaundice) or damage to hepatocytes (hepatocellular jaundice). Several of the diseases in which jaundice occurs have already been discussed: bacillary haemoglobinuria, liver fluke disease, blue-green algal poisoning, toxaemic jaundice due to pyrrolidizine alkaloid poisoning, chronic copper poisoning, lupinosis, and eperythrozoonosis. Other causes include babesiosis and leptospirosis, which are discussed below in the section on urinary tact disorders.

Skin cancers

Bovine ocular squamous cell carcinoma (cancer eye) occurs in non-pigmented areas around the eyes of mature Hereford and Simmental cattle. It has considerable economic significance because there is condemnation at slaughter and a shortened productive life. It is a neoplasm that seldom metastasises but can invade locally, so surgical excision is often worthwhile.

Pink-eye

Pink-eye in cattle is usually caused by *Moraxella bovis*, a Gram-negative bacterium, although other microorganisms can be involved. In sheep, *Chlamydia psittaci* is the most common cause. In both species, the disease has a sudden onset and rapid spread. The clinical signs are photophobia, excessive lacrimation and conjunctivitis. A characteristic lesion is the corneal opacity (pink-eye) that develops, along with some corneal ulceration. Diagnosis is based on the outbreak of eye infections in a mob or herd. Treatment is by the parenteral administration of tetracyclines and by topical administration of amoxicillin, in conjunction with the quarantine of infected animals (the herd) to prevent further spread.

Teat lesions

Teat lesions can be caused by other microorganisms, particularly bovine herpesvirus-2, which is associated with bovine ulcerative mamillitis, and *Staphylococcus aureus*, which causes udder impetigo and black spot. Bovine ulcerative mamillitis has a seasonal incidence and predisposes to mastitis. Some cows can develop severe lesions that are very sore, and this makes milking difficult. Udder impetigo manifests as small pustules that can coalesce and extend into the underlying skin to cause boils, and black spot is a form of hyperkeratosis that affects the tip of the teats, usually because of poor milking practices. Both conditions also predispose to mastitis and make milking difficult.

The treatment of all teat lesions in cows is based on infection control in conjunction with the removal of scabs and wound management. Even when there are no lesions, there should be washing then disinfection before milking, and further disinfection after milking. When lesions are present, additional antiseptic preparations should be applied after milking and emollients used if necessary. The correction of milking errors is also necessary on many occasions. The antiseptic and emollients that can be used, often in combination, are cetrimide (2% cream), chlorhexidine gluconate (0.5% solution), zinc oxide (ointment), glutaraldehyde (1.5% solution), iodine (0.5% solution), dodecyl benzene sulfonic acid (2% solution) and sodium hypochlorite (4% solution) (see chapter 3).

Reproductive disorders

There are two major groups of disorders of reproduction in ruminants: infertility and abortion. Sometimes the causes will be clearly evident, such as when individual animals have traumatic or congenital lesions of the reproductive tract, or when there is the pre-term delivery of a dead fetus following a known disease. On other occasions the actual problem will not be evident until the reproductive history of an entire herd or flock has been examined to determine if reasonable levels of reproductive performance are being achieved, as measured by, for example, the inter-calving intervals, calving, lambing and kidding percentages, the percentage of young animals weaned, and the ratio of males to females required in breeding groups. Some of the measures will indicate problems in the neonatal period rather than at conception or during pregnancy.

In many countries there are well-established herd and flock health programmes which are structured around the measurement of reproductive performance and also include components that seek to maximise productivity and minimise the impact of a number of diseases, such as intestinal parasitic infections and mastitis. Many of these programmes seek to prevent diseases from occurring in the first place.

 A number of infectious agents have a propensity to cause reproductive disorders: *Brucella* spp.; *Toxoplasma gondii*; *Listeria monocytogenes*; *Leptospira* spp.; *Campylobacter* spp.; *Trichomonas* spp.; *Chlamydia psittaci*; and bovine herpesvirus type 1. Some of these agents have the potential to be zoonotic (see chapter 2).

There are also several non-infectious causes of abortion, such as heat stress and plant poisons. Locoweed, broomweed and red salvia are among the plants incriminated.

Brucellosis

Brucellosis occurs in cattle, sheep and goats: *Brucella abortus* is the cause in cattle, *B. ovis* and *B. melitensis* in sheep and *B. melitensis* in goats. Brucellosis can also occur in humans after infection with either *B. abortus* or *B. melitensis*, resulting in undulant fever or Malta fever, respectively. Ovine brucellosis causes infertility in rams and occasionally causes abortions in ewes and neonatal deaths of lambs. The organism is transmitted from ram to ram primarily by homosexual activity. The reason infertility occurs is that epididymitis often results from the infection, and this is difficult to treat. Intramuscular oxytetracycline (20 mg/kg) every 3 days for 3–4 weeks may eliminate the infection but will probably not overcome the infertility.

 Brucellosis in cattle (Bang's disease) has been controlled or eradicated in many countries by vaccination and testing programmes. Before this it was a major cause of abortions in heifers and it was a significant zoonosis for farmers and veterinary surgeons who came into contact with aborted fetuses and uterine discharges from infected animals (see chapter 2).

Brucellosis in goats has a limited geographical distribution, being confined to the Mediterranean region, central and South America, parts of Africa and in central Asia. It is not found in Australia, New Zealand, the USA or most of Europe. Where it does occur, *B. melitensis* causes abortions in goats and sheep. Rams can develop epididymitis after infection with organisms other than *B. ovis*: *Actinobacillus seminis* and *Histophilus ovis* have both been incriminated.

Toxoplasmosis

Ruminants, particularly sheep and goats, can be infected with *Toxoplasma gondii* oocysts passed in the feces of young cats, the definitive host for this protozoan parasite. Animals infected during pregnancy may have late-term abortions or give birth to weak offspring due to placentitis and infection of the fetus. Ewes and does develop good resistance to reinfection so will not suffer further abortions due to the parasite. Pregnant animals at risk of exposure to *T. gondii* can be treated with oral or injectable formulations of combinations of trimethoprim and related drugs (5–10 mg/kg) with sulfonamides, such as sulfadimidine (200 mg/kg) and sulfamethazine (220 mg/kg). Chemoprophylaxis is also possible with decoquinate (2 mg/kg) in the feed (50 g/tonne) during pregnancy. A vaccine is available in some countries to control the disease.

Toxoplasmosis is a significant disease of humans. Even though oocysts from cat feces are the major source of infection in humans, meat from infected sheep or goats is also a source. A related parasite, *Neospora caninum*, appears to be a significant cause of late-term abortion of cattle in some parts of the world. For this parasite the definitive host is the dog, but its pathogenesis and treatment are the same as for toxoplasmosis (see chapter 13).

Listeriosis

One of the manifestations of listeriosis in ruminants, particularly sheep, is abortion in the last trimester of pregnancy, often as an outbreak in a flock or herd. The other common manifestation is a neurological disorder (circling disease), which was discussed earlier in this chapter.

Leptospirosis

Leptospirosis can also cause abortion. It is a zoonosis (see also chapter 13). There are many serovars of the one pathogenic species of leptospire, *Leptospira interrogans*, and most infections are subclinical. However, fetal death can occur several weeks after an infection occurs, particularly in cattle. Leptospirosis is rare in sheep but has been associated with abortions. Vaccination of cattle and pigs is possible but does not always eliminate the carrier state.

Campylobacteriosis

There are several species of the bacterial genus *Campylobacter*, one of which is *C. fetus* var. *venerealis*, the cause of infertility and abortion in cattle, and there are two others, *C. fetus* ssp. *fetus* and *C. jejuni*, that may occasionally cause abortion in cattle, sheep and goats. Bovine genital campylobacteriosis is a disease transmitted by ingestion but which is principally associated with early embryonic death and protracted calving seasons, and it has many features in common with trichomoniasis. Once in a herd, bovine genital campylobacteriosis usually causes problems only in heifers because the older animals develop protective immunity. Vaccines are available to control the disease, and are best administered just before the breeding season. The use of artificial insemination will also prevent and control the spread of the disease. In sheep, campylobacteriosis (vibriosis) is different: the major problem is late-term abortion. However, the epidemiology, pathogenesis and control with vaccines and even artificial insemination are the same as for cattle. Ewes at risk can be treated with intramuscular oxytetracycline (10 mg/kg). See also chapter 2.

Trichomoniasis

A disease which also causes infertility and prolonged calving intervals is trichomoniasis caused by a protozoan parasite, *Trichomonas foetus*. This organism lives in the genital tract of both cows and bulls, and is transmitted venereally. Bulls can remain infected for long periods but cows usually do not, so treatment is therefore directed at the bulls. Treatment has limited success, and control can be achieved by using artificial insemination. The history and clinical signs of trichomoniasis are almost identical to those of bovine genital campylobacteriosis.

Salmonellosis

Salmonellosis is usually considered a severe disease, and it causes abdominal discomfort, diarrhoea and often a generalised septicaemia. It has been discussed above in this context, and mention has been made that pregnant sheep and cattle may abort after the septicaemic phase. There is also a sheep-adapted serotype, *S. abortus ovis*, that primarily causes mid- to late-term abortion in sheep and the birth of sick lambs. Ewes that abort may become sick, something not seen to any extent with the other causes of abortion. When outbreaks occur with any of the *Salmonella* serotypes, the approach usually taken is to isolate the aborted animals and to administer intramuscular oxytetracycline (20 mg/kg) for 10 days to all animals at risk. There are vaccines available in some countries that give some protection (see also chapter 2).

Q fever

The organism responsible for Q fever, *Coxiella burnetii*, can occasionally cause late-term abortion in ewes. However, although many ruminants are infected, few exhibit clinical signs or suffer abortion. When this does happen, the usual approach is taken when abortions occur: isolation of aborted animals and antibiotic treatment.

The most important aspect of Q fever in animals is probably its zoonotic potential (see chapter 2). It joins salmonellosis, leptospirosis and listeriosis as a disease that can readily be contracted from aborted ruminant fetuses and uterine discharges.

Chlamydiosis

Chlamydial late-term abortions are common in sheep and goats in the UK and USA. There are a few reports of chlamydial abortions in cattle too. The animals are infected orally by contact with uterine discharges and placentas passed by infected ewes, does or cows.

Infected animals will abort dead, moribund or weak offspring, and should be isolated from the rest of the flock or herd. Intramuscular oxytetracycline (20 mg/kg) every 10 days will eliminate *C. psittaci* from those animals that are still pregnant but will not prevent them from aborting. After chlamydial abortions, most animals are able to breed again normally and do not have further abortions. Control is best achieved by good quarantine and hygiene practices, and there are vaccines available for use in the pre-breeding period.

Humans can also be infected with this subtype of *C. psittaci* (see chapter 14).

Viral diseases

Abortion outbreaks in cattle can occur some weeks after infection with bovine herpesvirus type 1, the same virus that causes infectious bovine rhinotracheitis (red nose): abortion rates can be around 50% in non-vaccinated herds. The bovine virus diarrhoea virus, which is related to the border disease virus, can also cause infertility and abortion in susceptible herds. For both viral diseases there are vaccines available to assist in the control of the various diseases they cause.

Infertility

Infertility associated with the ingestion of plants containing oestrogenic substances occurs in sheep, and occasionally in cattle. This is quite a different situation to infertility associated with infectious organisms, where early fetal death is the cause. Phytoestrogens are found in soybean (*Glycine max*), lucerne (*Medicago sativa*), various clovers (*Trifolium* species) and mouldy feed containing *Fusarium roseum*. Phytoestrogen poisoning (clover disease and ringwomb) in sheep is usually evident as a significant fall in fertility, which can be transient or permanent, and lambing difficulties in pregnant ewes. Ringwomb, or failure of the cervix to dilate, may have other causes. There is no treatment, although testosterone could be used, so the best approach is to avoid dangerous pastures or provide additional feed.

Infertility is not associated just with problems in cows, ewes and does: the male can suffer a sudden and substantial fall in fertility after an episode of stress, such as any acute disease or injury, and after infection of the genital tract, such as occurs in rams with ovine brucellosis and after infection with *Actinobacillus seminis*.

Pizzle rot

Pizzle rot (enzootic posthitis) is a condition in which there are lesions on and in the prepuce of rams. Ewes can also be affected by sexual transmission. Pizzle rot is seen most commonly in Australia, South Africa and South America, particularly under conditions where high concentrations of ammonia are generated in the prepuce, such as when the animals are on high-protein diets, and the presence in the prepuce of *Corynebacterium* spp. Lesions can begin on the outside of the prepuce and then extend internally and ulcerate. Affected wethers are restless and kick at their bellies, and the prepuce is highly susceptible to blowfly strike. Treatment should begin with removal of the sheep from high-protein pastures and diets, irrigation of the prepuce with 20% cetrimide in water, and surgery if necessary. Prevention for up to 3 months can be achieved by a single subcutaneous implant of testosterone propionate (60–90 mg).

Mastitis

'Mastitis' is a term which means inflammation of the mammary gland. There are many causes, although in dairy cattle these can be subdivided into common and uncommon pathogens, and into contagious and environmental pathogens (Radostits *et al.*, 2000). The changes associated with mastitis can range from being so mild as to remain subclinical to severe and life-threatening. A common feature of mastitis, whatever the severity, is the presence of white blood cells (leucocytes) in the milk.

Mastitis assumes greatest importance in dairy cows because of productivity considerations. The major pathogens in cows are those that can be transmitted from animal to animal during milking, such as *Streptococcus agalactiae*, *Staphylococcus aureus* and *Mycoplasma bovis*, and environmental pathogens that are acquired between milkings, such as *S. uberis*, *S. dysgalactiae*, *Escherichia coli*, *Pseudomonas* spp. and *Proteus* spp. There are other minor and uncommon pathogens that can be troublesome in some circumstances.

Poor management of dairy cows, particularly in early lactation and particularly of high-producing cows, predisposes to mastitis in herds.

The diagnosis of mastitis should be straightforward in clinical cases, although the exact cause and best treatment will depend on bacterial culture results and antibiotic sensitivity testing. Subclinical mastitis is detected by the somatic cell count, in which leucocytes in milk are detected and counted. Treatment is of two types: clinical cases of mastitis are treated with antibiotics given parenterally or by intramammary infusion; and dry cow therapy, in which a long-acting antibiotic is administered into the teat canal when a cow is dried off at the end of a milking season. In both cases only the infected quarter or all four quarters are treated.

Control of mastitis is usually by way of a comprehensive programme, which should include proper management of the milking process and machinery, dry cow therapy, treatment of clinical cases, good record-keeping, and the removal of chronically infected cows from the milking herd.

Pharmacists should be familiar with the treatment options and disinfectants used to treat and control mastitis, and the various dose forms available. The major precautions to be observed when using intramammary products are absolute cleanliness and hygiene when using these products, and care in ensuring that the products are placed in the teat canal and not further into the mammary gland. The teats to be treated must be cleaned (see chapter 3), the medication carefully administered, the teat massaged to disperse the medication, and the teat treated with a disinfectant.

Urinary tract disorders

The main features of urinary tract disorders are discolored urine, dysuria, abdominal pain, and variations in urine output. Red or red/brown urine can arise in three ways: haematuria (blood in urine); haemoglobinuria (haemoglobin in urine); and myoglobinuria (myoglobin released from muscles that passes into the urine). Bracken fern poisoning, contagious bovine pyelonephritis, bacillary haemoglobinuria and chronic copper poisoning all result in red urine being passed by affected animals, and have already been discussed. Other common causes are babesiosis and leptospirosis, both caused by infectious organisms, and postparturient haemoglobinuria. There are abnormal constituents of urine in addition to blood haemoglobin and myoglobin, but they are not visible and have to be detected by simple tests: protein, glucose, ketone bodies, crystals and white blood cells. Dysuria and abdominal discomfort can be associated with contagious bovine pyelonephritis (discussed above in the section on abdominal discomfort) and urolithiasis. Variations in urine output certainly occur but are very difficult to detect in cattle, sheep and goats unless individual animals are closely observed.

Urolithiasis

Urolithiasis is an important disease in wethers and steers fed on concentrated diets or kept on pastures high in chalk. Affected animals kick at their bellies and their condition progressively gets worse. If there is partial blockage some urine will dribble. Treatment involves surgery.

Babesiosis

Cattle, sheep and goats can be infected by *Babesia* spp., a group of protozoan parasites transmitted by ticks. The parasites are species-specific, except that *B. motasi* and *B. ovis* can infect both sheep and goats. After infection by tick bites the parasites enter red blood cells, and this leads to haemolysis as the parasites undergo multiplication cycles in the bloodstream. Then, depending on the level of infection, there will be signs of fever, jaundice and haemoglobinuria. Severely affected animals may die, and those that recover do so gradually and usually lose a lot of weight. Treatment is with an aromatic diamidine (Diminazine) given by intramuscular injection. Imidocarb dipropionate is available in Australia, Eire and the USA. Vaccines are available and eradication programmes are under way.

Plant poisoning

Plants of the *Brassica* spp., such as turnips, rape, canola and cauliflower, contain S-methyl-L-cysteine, which is converted in the rumen to dimethyl sulfoxide, which in turn leads to haemolysis, haemoglobinuria, weakness and diarrhoea. Fortunately, these plants are not uniformly toxic. It would be usual to find several animals in a group affected. There is no treatment other than supportive therapy, such as blood transfusion should it be warranted, and the removal of animals from the toxic plants.

Reference

Radostits O M, Gay C C, Blood D C, Hinchcliff K W (2000). *Veterinary Medicine*, 9th edn. London: Baillière Tindall.

Further reading

Aiello S E, ed. (2000). *The Merck Veterinary Manual*, 8th edn. Rahway: Merck and Co.
Bishop Y, ed. (2001). *The Veterinary Formulary*, 5th edn. London: Pharmaceutical Press.
Hungerford T G (2002). *Diseases of Livestock*, 9th edn. Sydney: McGraw-Hill.
Martin W B, Aitken I D, eds (2000). *Diseases of Sheep*, 3rd edn. Oxford: Blackwell Science.

11

Pigs

Tom Alexander

Involvement with the pig industry is unlikely to be at the forefront of veterinary pharmacy practice unless one of the few remaining pig farms happens to be nearby. In this chapter the common diseases are discussed so that pharmacists have a source of information if required. A bacterial and treatment approach has been principally used here rather than cataloguing symptoms.

The UK pig industry

The pig industry has undergone greater changes during the last forty years of the last century than it did in the previous four hundred. It is safe to predict that it will undergo even more fundamental changes in the first 20 years of this one.

What is likely to happen? The surplus of pig meat products in Europe in the nineties led to the worst economic downturn in pig production in living memory. Early in 2001 swine fever struck and caused further direct and indirect damage followed by foot-and-mouth disease. Many pig farmers and pig organisations were forced out of business and many more will go out of business. At the time of writing, the future of pig production in the UK looks bleak.

What is likely to happen? The increase in average herd size and decrease in herd numbers, which has been going on for over 40 years, will continue. A much greater proportion of sows in the UK are kept out of doors than in other countries and many of their piglets are reared in semi-outdoor systems. This is likely to continue. Few independent pig farmers will survive unless they join vertically integrated operations run by slaughterers and/or supermarkets. The number of sows under the control of individual organisations will increase. The number of practising pig vets will decrease and veterinary work will be even more devoted to preventative rather than therapeutic medicine than it is now. The use of antibacterial drugs is likely to be restricted and vets will be looking for alternative measures. The number of organic herds, which are voluntarily restricted in their use of drugs, is likely to increase. The terms used in this chapter are explained in Box 11.1.

Box 11.1 Glossary of terms used in this chapter

- Sows and boars – mature adults. Pregnant sows and weaned sows are called dry sows.
- Gilts – maiden females or females during their first pregnancy.
- Sucking piglets – piglets being suckled by the sow. They are usually weaned at three to four weeks old into nurseries, which often have perforated floors or solid floors with straw bedding.
- Weaners – young weaned pigs, which are reared in the nurseries until about eight weeks of age when they have reached a weight of about 25–30 kg.
- Growers – pigs after they leave the nurseries; finishers (or fatteners) are pigs being finished for slaughter.
- Farrowing – giving birth.
- Colostrum – the first milk to be produced by the sow at farrowing. It largely comprises antibodies against the full array of pathogenic organisms that have infected the sow but have not necessarily caused disease. They are absorbed undigested through the lining (mucosa) of the piglets' small intestines during the first few hours of life. One of the first instincts of newborn piglets is to find a teat to suck. Unlike human mothers, no antibodies cross the placenta of the pregnant sow into the unborn piglets' circulation. Colostrum is also rich in white blood cells which probably provide additional protection for the mucosa. The sow's milk that is secreted after the piglets have drunk the colostrum also contains antibodies, but at a low level. The important one is secretory IgA. It is similar to IgA in the bloodstream, but on passing through the mammary gland into the milk it acquires a secretory component which prevents it being digested and allows it to be absorbed into the mucus lining the intestines. This antibody prevents pathogens from adhering to the mucosal epithelial cells and thus entering the body. It also helps to destroy them.
- Creep feed – highly digestible food provided in small quantities for sucking piglets in a part of the pen where the sow cannot reach it.
- Scour – a common term used by farmers for diarrhoea.
- Toxoids – formalinised toxins that are no longer toxic and can be used in vaccination.

Anatomy and physiology of the pig

The anatomy and physiology of the pig are more similar to the human than any other domesticated animal. Pigs are monogastric omnivores with a similar digestive tract to humans except that pigs have a relatively large caecum which acts as a fermentation vat, hence they can probably

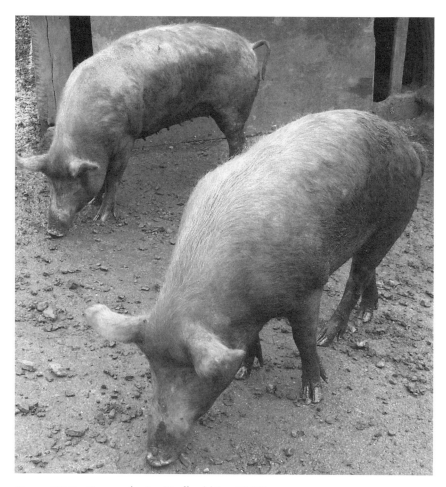

Figure 11.1 Tamworth pigs (Staffordshire, 2002).

digest vegetable matter more efficiently than we can. Another difference is that sows have long horns to their uterus and produce large litters more than twice a year, often rearing well over 20 pigs per sow per year for up to about 7 years. They are then slaughtered which, of course, humans are not. Another difference is that individual piglets are much smaller relative to their dams than babies and consequently there are fewer problems giving birth. They also grow much faster than babies reaching slaughter weight of, say, 90 kg in 16–20 weeks. Most of their other body systems are similar to those of the human and it is not surprising that they are subject to similar types of disease which respond to similar treatments.

Notifiable diseases

These are diseases not normally present in the UK which, if suspected, must be reported to the authorities. In most cases livestock 'standstill' orders will be applied, the disease investigated and, if confirmed, the affected pigs, or more often the herd, will be destroyed. In pigs such diseases include foot-and-mouth disease (FMD), classical swine fever (CSF), African swine fever (ASF), Aujeszky's disease (AD), swine vesicular disease (SVD) and brucellosis. Other diseases, which are not present in this country, such as leptospirosis caused by *Leptospira pomona*, are not notifiable.

Clearly, notifiable diseases, when they occur, are not treated and are therefore not relevant to this chapter.

Vaccines

Several vaccines are routinely used in pig herds. These include vaccines against erysipelas, *Escherichia coli*, clostridial diseases, porcine parvovirus (PPV), enzootic pneumonia (EP), atrophic rhinitis (AR), and porcine reproductive and respiratory disease (PRRS). The most common vaccines are set out in Table 11.1. About half the products are presently classified as pharmacy and merchant supplies (PML).

In general, inactivated vaccines are preferred to attenuated ones because, although the immunity stimulated may be shorter, they are safer and easier to store without loss of potency (see chapter 4). Bacterial diseases are dealt with below but viral diseases are not because treatment is limited and they are of no relevance to pharmacists. The two viral vaccines which are used in the UK are therefore dealt with briefly here.

Parvoviruses replicate mainly in rapidly multiplying cells. In the dog, these are the cells in the crypts of the intestines. In pigs, they are the cells of the embryos. This causes expensive reproductive losses called collectively the SMEDI syndrome (stillbirths, mummies, embryonic death and infertility). The PPV is endemic in virtually all herds. Sows pass specific antibodies against it in their colostrum (first milk) to their newborn piglets, which protects them against PPV until the pigs are 4–5 months old during which time vaccination would be ineffective. Maiden gilts are bred at 6 months or older and therefore there is a narrow window in which vaccination should be carried out. Some pig farmers revaccinate every year. Others rely on reinforcement by natural infection.

PRRS virus (PRRSV) is common in UK herds. It causes reproductive problems when it first infects a herd but when it becomes endemic it tends to exacerbate other common diseases, such as piglet diarrhoea

Table 11.1 Porcine vaccination products

Disease	Vaccine	Type	Legal category	Manufacturer
Atrophic rhinitis (AR)	Porcilis AR-T	Vaccine (I) (toxoid)	PML	Intervet
Clostridial infections	Lambisan	Antitoxin	PML	Intervet
Combination vaccines	Gletvax 6	Vaccine	PML	Schering-Plough
	Heptavac	Vaccine	PML	Intervet
	Lambivac	Vaccine	PML	Intervet
E. coli infections	Intagen	Vaccine (I)	MFS (Premix)	Alpharma
	Neocolipor	Vaccine (I)	POM	Merial
	Porcilis Porcol 5	Vaccine (I)	PML	Intervet
Erysipelas	Erysorb Plus	Vaccine (I)	PML	Intervet
	Porcillis Ery	Vaccine (I)	PML	Intervet
	Navaxyn Erysip	Vaccine (I)	PML	Fort Dodge
Parvo (PPV)	Suvaxyn parvo	Vaccine (I)	POM	Fort Dodge
Pneumonia				
Enzootic (EP)	Hyoresp	Vaccine (I)	POM	Merial
	Stellamune	Vaccine (I)	POM	Pfizer
	Suvaxyn M.hypo	Vaccine (I)	POM	Fort Dodge
Pasteurellosis	Pastacidin	Vaccine (I)	POM	Intervet
Pleuropneumonia	Suvaxyn APP	Vaccine (I)	POM	Fort Dodge
PRRS	Porcilis PRRS	Vaccine (L)	POM	Intervet
Combination vaccines				
E. coli, + Erysipelas	Colisorb	Vaccine (I)	POM	Intervet
EP + PPV	Erysorb Parvo	Vaccine (I)	POM	Intervet
	Porcillis Ery + Parvo	Vaccine (I)	POM	Intervet
EP + Glassers	Suvaxyn M hyo + Parvo	Vaccine (I)	POM	Fort Dodge

(I) inactivated vaccine; (L) living vaccine; POM prescription-only medicine; PML pharmacy and merchant supplies; MFS medicated feedingstuff.

(scours), meningitis and pneumonia, in growing pigs. An inactivated vaccine has come on the market recently and farmers with affected herds hope that it will help to control these secondary conditions and also protect incoming breeding stock which is PRRSV-free. Attenuated PRRS vaccines have been available in Europe and the USA for some time but these are thought to make matters worse in some herds, particularly in the USA, by recombining with wild virus to produce new types. They have been largely avoided in the UK.

Influenza is relatively common in the UK. The same serotypes affect pigs as affect people, who may catch it from them, but vaccination is not used nor is any treatment given.

Bacterial diseases

Actinobacillus pleuropneumonia (APP)

Causative organism

This is a common acute and often fatal necrotic pneumonia of growing pigs. It is caused by virulent strains of a bacterium, *Actinobacillus pleuropneumoniae*, which lives subclinically in the upper respiratory tract until triggered by physical stress, water deprivation or other infections such as PRRS.

Diagnosis

Diagnosis of APP has traditionally been by the typical lung lesions at postmortem examination and the isolation of the causal organism.

Treatment/prophylaxis

APP is sensitive to a wide range of antibacterial drugs but they are not very effective when given in food or water because of loss of appetite and thirst. Injection of individual pigs is more effective.

Vaccines are available commercially. They are inactivated, whole culture, preparations harvested young to obtain maximum capsular and extracellular materials. They are effective in reducing mortality and improving growth rates but they do not stop lesions being formed. There are 12 serotypes of the bacterium and since vaccination only protects against the homologous serotype, vaccines usually contain about four of the most common ones.

Anthrax

Causative organism

The anthrax bacillus does not multiply in the soil of the UK. It multiplies in certain types of soils in warmer climates, for example, the so-called anthrax incubator areas of the USA, Africa and Australia. It is brought into this country in hides, hair and bone-meal.

The bacillus produces spores which are highly resistant and can survive in soil almost indefinitely. The disease is rare and occurs mainly in individual animals or small groups of cattle or sometimes sheep. It usually occurs following flooding of pastures or where digging has been carried out. Although the bacillus is fully sensitive to antibiotics, most affected animals die too rapidly to be treated. Being a notifiable disease, the ministry vets burn the carcasses.

Treatment/prophylaxis

Anthrax is extremely rare in pigs. Only one case has been reported in recent years. The problem was that although few affected pigs died, the farm became bedded down with spores. Since there was no slaughter and compensation policy for anthrax, cases kept occurring. Understandably, slaughter houses would not accept the infected pigs so the farm became increasingly overcrowded. Finally, the herd had to be slaughtered. There is a vaccine for this disease but none was available. Since then the Central Veterinary Laboratory has prepared more stocks but this is not available commercially. This disease is therefore of no commercial interest to pharmacists but is described briefly here because of the public alarm it raises (erroneously) when it is reported.

 There is a zoonotic risk with this disease.

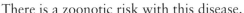

Arthritis

Causative organism

Arthritis is common in sucking pigs, weaners, growers and finishers. It has a variety of infectious and non-infectious causes. Among the bacteria that commonly cause it are *Erysipelothrix rhusiopathiae*, *E. coli*, various streptococci, *Haemophilus* and *Mycoplasma*.

Treatment/prophylaxis

All are sensitive to antibacterial drugs; these are generally given by injection. Depending on the type of joint lesion (e.g. purulent) the drug may take time to be effective and the joint may take time to heal. Vaccines are available against some of these agents but are not as effective as they are against other conditions caused by these bacteria. They are not generally used to prevent arthritis.

Atrophic rhinitis (progressive)

Causative organism

Non-toxigenic strains of *Pasteurella* are common in pigs and are often involved as secondary opportunists in pneumonia. Toxigenic strains of *Pasteurella multocida* are uncommon but when present in a herd can cause serious economically damaging upper respiratory disease in weaners, growers and finishers.

The bacteria adhere to the mucosa of the nose and produce a toxin which disrupts bone growth and damages other organs, but it has the most striking effect on the delicate scroll bones of the nose. The overall effect on the pig is to reduce growth rates directly and indirectly by making it difficult for the pig to eat.

The disease is diagnosed clinically and pathologically by observing changes to the nose and confirming the initial diagnosis by culture and serology.

Treatment/prophylaxis

The bacterium is susceptible to antibacterial drugs such as trimethoprim sulphonamide, e.g. sulfadiazine and trimethoprim (Delvoprim, Intervet). These can be given in feed strategically at times in advance of the anticipated start of the disease. However, the bacterium tends to develop resistance, so this method of control should be regarded as temporary.

A toxoid vaccine is available commercially for sows (Porcilis, AR-T, Intervet). The passive immunity passed to their piglets through the colostrum reduces the clinical signs.

Brucellosis

Little need be said about this here because although *Brucella suis* exists in pigs and wild hares in parts of Northern Europe, it does not occur in the UK and is unlikely ever to gain entry. It should not be confused with *B. abortus* which used to occur here in cattle but which does not infect pigs (see chapter 10).

Clostridial diseases

Causative organism

Occasionally sudden deaths occur in liquid-fed heavy finishing pigs and sows, particularly sows kept out of doors. This may be due to several causes, one of which is *Clostridium novyi* (*oedematiens* type B). If the number of cases warrant it, the pigs at risk can be protected with *C. novyi* vaccine. Also, bacitracin is sometimes given in the sow feed.

Treatment/prophylaxis

More commonly, clostridia are involved in outbreaks of piglet dysentery. This is an acute fatal disease of newborn piglets caused by *C. perfringens* type C. In the short term, it can be partly prevented by dosing all newborn piglets with penicillin. In the long term it should be prevented by vaccination of the pregnant sow with toxoids of *C. perfringens* type C, two doses being given 10–14 days apart, the second a few days prior to the anticipated farrowing date. If a sheep vaccine is used, a double dose should be given.

Diarrhoea (scours) in piglets and weaners

Causative organism

Diarrhoea is very common in sucking piglets and fairly common in recently weaned pigs. The commonest cause in both sucking piglets and weaners is pig-specific serotypes of enterotoxigenic *E. coli*. Natural protection is by passively acquired colostral antibodies and secretory IgA (see Box 11.1). When these are deficient, or if the animal is overwhelmed by large doses of *E. coli*, diarrhoea results. This rapidly leads to dehydration and electrolyte imbalance and death.

Treatment/prophylaxis

E. coli are susceptible to many antibacterial drugs, but strains resistant to individual drugs or groups of drugs occur. It is common practice, therefore, to culture *E. coli* from diarrhoeic feces and test their drug sensitivity.

Drugs commonly used parenterally, or preferably orally, include ceftiofur, semisynthetic penicillins, neomycin, streptomycin, spectinomycin, apramycin, lincomycin, cephalosporins, fluoroquinolones and trimethoprim sulphonamide. Antibacterial therapy is often supplemented by providing hypotonic electrolyte solutions which piglets drink spontaneously and which reverse the dehydration and restore electrolyte balance.

Killed vaccines are commercially available and may contain several serotypes along with toxin antigens. These are used particularly in pregnant gilts whose litters tend to be more prone to diarrhoea than sows' litters but also in pregnant sows when outbreaks occur. Some farmers deliberately expose gilts, and sometimes sows, to diarrhoeic feces from piglets and weaners to enhance natural immunisation.

Attention should also be paid to farrowing house and nursery hygiene and management practices.

Enzootic pneumonia (EP)

Causative organism

This is very common and a constant source of economic loss. The most common primary cause is *Mycoplasma hyopneumoniae* which affects pigs from about 6 weeks of age to slaughter. More mature animals become immune and throw off the infection. PRRS (see below) exacerbates the clinical signs. Opportunist invaders, such as *Pasteurella* spp., are almost always involved. *A. pleuropneumoniae* (see above), which is a primary pathogen in its own right, may also cause complications.

Treatment/prophylaxis

The first approach to control is often to inject the worst affected pigs with, for example, tiamulin and to medicate the feed or water with tetracycline, tiamulin, lincomycin and spectinomycin, spiromycin or tylosin, particularly for those age groups in which the disease starts. Fluorinated quinolones, such as enrofloxin, given orally or parenterally, are also useful. Effective commercial vaccines against *M. hyopneumoniae* are available.

Medication and vaccination must be reinforced by improvements in housing and management, such as reduction in stocking density, reduction of dust and gases and in improvements to ventilation and temperature control.

There are a number of techniques for producing EP-free herds but, but since the *Mycoplasma* can be wind-borne over several kilometres, these are only effective long-term if the pigs are housed in farms well away from other pigs.

Eperythrozoonosis

Causative organism

Eperythrozoon suis is a tiny organism adherent to the red cells of the blood. It is associated with anaemia, fever and jaundice in newborn piglets and in weaners and abortion in sows. Cause and effect are difficult to establish and some people question its significance. The organism is widespread in healthy herds.

Treatment/prophylaxis

Pigs can be treated with tetracyclines given by injection or in the feed.

Erysipelas

Causative organism

This is a relatively common disease of pigs caused by *Erysipelothrix insidiosa* (syn. *E. rhusiopathiae*) and is endemic in virtually all herds, is often found in soil and is shed in the droppings of birds. It causes disease in poultry.

It usually affects growing and finishing pigs but can affect gilts and sows or, rarely, sucking litters. It takes several forms; in the skin form raised red areas called diamond markings, because of their shape, appear on the skin of the body. It can cause septicaemia, which if untreated may be fatal or in pregnant sows result in abortion. It can cause lesions on the heart valves and can also cause arthritis.

Treatment/prophylaxis

E. insidiosa has never developed drug resistance and is still fully susceptible to penicillin which is given by injection. Killed vaccines are available and are given routinely on some farms to growers and breeding stock. Like most killed bacterial vaccines, the immunity provided is not strong and only lasts about 6 months.

Exudative epidermitis (greasy pig disease)

Causative organism

Staphylococcus hyicus is part of the normal flora of pigs and is endemic in virtually all pig herds. It tends to multiply in the vagina of sows prior to farrowing and infects the piglets during birth. It also survives well in the environment which can contaminate piglets. It does not, however, cause clinical disease in every herd, probably because there are non-virulent as well as virulent strains. The presence of non-virulent strains on the skin may suppress virulent strains. Furthermore, immune sows pass immunity to their piglets through colostrum which may not prevent lesions altogether, but which may restrict them to small harmless patches on the skin. Similarly, in older pigs, skin lesions tend to be mild and localised.

Signs and symptoms

In susceptible sucking piglets and weaners, usually between 1 and 5 weeks of age, the disease can be acute and severe. The bacterium gains entry through scratches and abrasions on the skin caused by biting particularly on the cheeks (piglets have sharp teeth), scrabbling with the knees on rough floors while sucking the dam, and sharp constituents of the bedding. The first clinical signs are listlessness and brown scabs on the skin. Within several days these spread diffusely all over the body and legs, covering them with a greasy exudate. There is no pruritus. In addition to the skin lesions, virulent strains produce toxins that seriously damage the kidneys. Affected piglets lose weight and most die from the effects of the toxins within 5–10 days, unless treated promptly. In sucking piglets, outbreaks tend to be sporadic affecting a few litters, but extensive outbreaks can occur repeatedly in weaners housed in humid nurseries with abrasive walls or floors or in weaners that are already suffering from sarcoptic mange.

Treatment/prophylaxis

The bacterium is sensitive to a range of antibacterial drugs but tends to develop resistance. It is therefore necessary in any new outbreak to determine its sensitivity to antibacterial drugs either by culture and testing in a laboratory or by trial and error in affected piglets. Affected piglets should then be injected daily for 5 days or on alternate days with the drug of choice. This may commonly be amoxicillin, oxytetracycline, ceftiofur, cefalexin, gentamicin, penicillin or lincomycin. The latter is the drug of choice for many vets. Topical applications of antibacterial drugs in ointment or oil, such as mastitis preparations used for dairy cows, may be effective. Small piglets can become dehydrated and may be given electrolytes orally.

No commercial vaccines are available. In any case, they would only be effective against homologous serotypes. Autogenous vaccines are sometimes prepared for severe persistent cases.

Glasser's disease

Causative organisms

Glasser's disease is similar clinically and pathologically to the disease produced by *Haemophilus influenzae* infection in infants. It affects weaned pigs, usually of about 5–7 weeks of age. The bacterium is ubiquitous. Normally sows are repeatedly stimulated immunologically. They then pass their immunity to their offspring in their colostrum. The passive immunity in the piglet is strong and prevents natural infection until it starts to wane after weaning when subclinical infection occurs, stimulating an active immunity. However, in some circumstances, such as sows kept out of doors, the level of infection in the environment is too low to stimulate an adequate immunity in the sows to provide full passive protection in their piglets. Thus, when they are weaned into nurseries and exposed to *H. parasuis* they come down with septicaemia, polyserositis, polyarthritis and meningitis. Co-infection with PRRS (see below) exacerbates the disease. Also, in rare cases, in very high health status herds which are free from *H. parasuis* infection, the disease can be acute and fatal in all age groups.

Treatment/prophylaxis

The bacterium is susceptible to a range of antibiotics (e.g. penicillin, tetracycline, ceftiofur, enrofloxacin and trimethoprim sulphonamide) which, if injected early enough, will save affected pigs but not if treatment is delayed. Feed medication over the period of risk will prevent the disease. An inactivated vaccine is available commercially but is only used in herds with persistent problems. It is only effective if it contains the same serotypes as those present in the nurseries. Natural immunisation can be achieved by placing affected untreated pigs or parts of dead pigs in with the pregnant sows.

Meningitis

Causative organism

A number of common bacteria can cause sporadic cases of meningitis in sucking pigs, weaners or growers. The most serious is that caused by *Streptococcus suis* type 2 which also, uncommonly, causes meningitis in humans. *S. suis* type 2 is the most serious because once virulent strains have gained entry to a herd, 2–5% of weaners or growers may develop meningitis.

Most meningitis bacteria in pigs are endemic in the herd and are opportunist invaders requiring another factor to trigger them off, including moving and mixing of pigs, overcrowding or PRRS (see below). They generally gain entry through lymphoid tissue, such as the tonsils, and get engulfed by monocytes which migrate into the brain and joints, releasing the bacteria which cause acute meningitis and arthritis.

Treatment/prophylaxis

Depending on the bacterium, prompt injections with the appropriate antibacterial drug are effective. Penicillin is usually the drug of choice for treating meningitis caused by *S. suis* type 2 but some strains are resistant to it. Antibacterial drugs (e.g. phenoxymethylpenicillin which survives pelleting of feed) given in feed through the period of risk may prevent disease. For most meningitic bacteria there is no effective vaccine.

Neonatal septicaemia

Causative organism

This tends to occur when newborn piglets have failed to take in any or sufficient sows' colostrum (see Box 11.1) or when they ingest overwhelming doses of bacteria, particularly before they have had a chance to suck their dam. It may also occur when the sow has not produced specific antibody in her colostrum. Common causes of septicaemia are *E. coli, Klebsiella*, and *Streptococci*.

Treatment/prophylaxis

These are susceptible to antibacterial drugs given parenterally such as semisynthetic penicillins, streptomycin and trimethoprim sulphonamide. Treatment is largely by guesswork or based on trial and error because there is usually no time to identify the causal organism or to test its drug sensitivity; treatment must be prompt to be effective. Vaccines are not used. Farrowing-house practices should be attended to.

Oedema disease (*syn.* gut oedema)

Causative organism

This disease, caused by *E. coli*, is rarer than it used to be but tends to be persistent in the few herds that are affected. However, it has no commercial relevance to pharmacists. It generally occurs about 10 days after weaning. Its name derives from the marked subcutaneous oedema of the face which gives affected pigs a sleepy appearance. There is also oedema of internal organs.

Serotypes of *E. coli* which produce certain verotoxins adhere to the wall of the anterior small intestine and multiply. The toxin is absorbed into the bloodstream and damages the walls of the small arterioles including those of the brain. The pigs become depressed, partially paralysed and die.

Treatment/prophylaxis

Treatment with antibacterial drugs, to which the *E. coli* may be sensitive, has no effect because by the time the pigs become ill the damage has already been done. Antibacterial medication of feed or water through the period of risk often gives disappointing results. Changes in feed and the quantity fed after weaning may help. There are no vaccines.

Porcine intestinal adenometosis (PIA) complex (*syn.* porcine enteropathy or ileitis)

Causative organism

This is a very common group of related conditions. The causal bacterium is in virtually all herds and is difficult to keep out.

PIA itself occurs in growing pigs. It is caused by *Lawsonia intestinalis* which can only multiply intracellularly and which is endemic in virtually all herds. It multiplies in the gut epithelium causing diffuse cellular multiplication and thickening from which it gets its name. The epithelium may become necrotic (necrotis enteritis) and/or the intestinal wall may become permanently thickened losing its flexibility ('hosepipe gut'). These conditions lead to diarrhoea and poor growth rate. Older pigs, particularly breeding gilts, which have been moved from one farm to another, may develop diffuse intestinal haemorrhage, acute anaemia or die.

Treatment/prophylaxis

L. intestinalis is susceptible to penicillin, enrofloxacin, erythromycin, tetracyclines, spiromycin, tiamulin, tilmycosin and tylosin. Tetracyclines and tylosin are probably the commonest drugs used. The latter is widely available in oral and injectable forms in the UK from several manufacturers. Treatment may be given parenterally, preferably using long-acting products (e.g. Norotyl LA Depot, Norbrook), to badly affected individuals or on a group basis in water or feed (e.g. Tylan Soluble, Elanco, (POM), and Tylan premixes, Elanco (MFS)). Some growth promoters in the feed may reduce the severity of the condition, so if these are banned in the future a rise in this disease can be expected. Improvements in hygiene may help. To prevent the haemorrhagic form in gilts, feed medication with tetracycline for a few weeks after arrival on the new farm usually prevents clinical signs. Field trials of a vaccine are under way at the time of writing.

Salmonellosis

Causative organism

Virtually all herds in the UK have endemic salmonella. Of the 2000–3000 serotypes of salmonella most herds will have less than ten, reflecting the environment, the feed and wildlife on the farm, including rodents and birds. In spite of that, clinical salmonellosis is relatively uncommon. When it occurs it usually takes the form of mild scours in weaners.

There are two host-adapted serotypes in pigs, *S. choleraesuis*, which is rare in the UK, and *S. derby*. The former can cause severe disease in pigs and people. The latter generally doesn't. Host-adapted serotypes are not host specific but they tend to persist in individual pigs for long periods and are difficult to eliminate.

The most common serotypes in pigs are *S. derby* and *S. typhimurium*, including some drug-resistant phage types. The latter poses a food-poisoning threat to humans (see chapter 2). Fortunately, most people cook pork and pork products well, which removes the risk.

Treatment/prophylaxis

If salmonella scours occurs in a herd, the hygiene in the affected areas must be improved and the pig density in pens reduced. There is a wide-spread view that clinical salmonellosis should not be treated with antibacterial drugs, but there is a pig welfare problem to be considered and most vets would apply treatment.

The more severely affected pigs should be treated parenterally. The rest can be treated orally, with drugs delivered in feed or water. Tetracyclines, streptomycin, apramycin (Apralan, Elanco), neomycin, semisynthetic penicillins, trimethoprim sulphonamide, enrofloxacin (Baytril, Bayer), danofloxacin (Advocin, Pfizer) and ceftiofur (Excenel, Pharmacia & Upjohn) may be effective. The salmonella will almost certainly have been cultured to make a diagnosis in which case its drug sensitivity should be tested.

Killed and live attenuated vaccines are available, particularly against *S. typhimurium*, and have some effect but they are not routinely used in most herds.

Swine dysentery

Causative agent

Brachyspira hyodysenteriae is a large *Spirochaeta*, similar to a *Treponema*, and is a specific pathogen of the pig. It multiplies in the mature colon and caecum, burrowing into the cells of the mucosa and destroying them, thus causing leakage of fluid and blood and chronic mucoid diarrhoea, which leads to dysentery.

The disease occurs most commonly in growers and finishers. It starts mildly in one or two pigs in a pen and slowly spreads to other pigs and other pens. The appetite of the pigs is decreased and they rapidly lose condition, appearing thin and hollow in the flanks. It also occurs sometimes in sows in which it tends to take a more acute form.

Treatment/prophylaxis

The spirochaete is sensitive to tylosin, tiamulin, valnemulin, lincomycin and nitroimidazole drugs but strains slowly become resistant to one or more of these. The drug of choice in most cases is tiamulin (Tiamutin, Leo). Severely affected pigs may be dosed parenterally but most are dosed orally in drinking water (POM) or via a dietary premix (MFS). Initially, because the pigs' appetites are reduced, medication is best given in water but when all are eating adequately again it can be given in the feed.

Blanket herd medication, which is expensive, combined with thorough removal of feces, and good hygiene sometimes succeeds in eradicating the infection altogether. It can usually be kept out fairly easily by introducing pigs only from herds with no history of the disease and preventing pig feces being brought in from other herds (e.g. from dirty pig lorries).

Tuberculosis

Causative organism

Although this infection with members of a complex mycobacterium is relatively common in pigs, no treatment is ever used. Hence, it has no direct commercial relevance to pharmacists but may be of interest nevertheless.

The *Mycobacterium avium/intracellulare* complex comprises a group of bacteria, many of which multiply saprophytically. *M. avium* is itself very variable depending on which species of bird it is derived from. Infected wild birds are common in the UK. Growers and finishers are usually infected by oral ingestion of contaminated materials such as peat bedding in which the organism may multiply or water from header tanks in which the organism is multiplying or pig feed contaminated by bird droppings. Birds are attracted to the feed stored in pig farms particularly in winter.

Signs and symptoms

The lesions are small, persistent, infected nodules in the lymph nodes of the neck or mesentery which do not progress. They go undiagnosed in living pigs but may be detected in pigs at slaughter. The infected part is condemned. In fact, such dormant lesions pose no more disease threat to normal healthy people. At most they are only likely to cause small non-progressive undetected lesions similar to those in the pig. Unfortunately, they can cause serious progressive disease in immunologically-suppressed people and people with diseases such as acquired immune deficiency syndrome (AIDS).

Treatment/prophylaxis

No treatment is used for tuberculosis in the pig. If it is causing problems with condemnations at slaughter the source of infection has to be found and eliminated.

Fungal diseases

Ringworm

Pigs are susceptible to all pathogenic species of ringworm which appear as variable sized patches on the relatively hairless skin of the back, sides and abdomen. It is derived from other pigs, rodents, other wild animals and the environment; it is common in pigs kept out of doors. It does not worry the affected pig, which seems to be oblivious to its presence, and it has no effect on growth rate. It resolves spontaneously without treatment. Farmers are not willing to spend money on treatment. They generally ignore it.

Ringworm in pigs (as in other farm and pet animals) is zoonotic.

Pigs can also suffer from ingesting fungal toxins in feed but the effect is delayed, specific diagnosis is often not possible and no treatment is used.

Parasite diseases

Parasites are common in pigs but under modern conditions of pig management are relatively easy to control and generally do little economic damage. Nevertheless, treatment is often applied.

Mange (scabies)

Causative organisms

Over 60% of herds in the UK have endemic mange caused by *Sarcoptes scabei*. The most common and serious form in pigs is that caused by *S. scabei* which burrows down in the skin causing intense pruritus which, when widespread over the body, causes loss of condition. On welfare grounds alone it should be suppressed or eradicated.

Signs and symptoms

The pruritus makes the pig scratch itself on gate posts, etc. The burrowing mite causes the release of serum which coagulates on the skin causing crusts. Hyperkeratinisation (thickening of the skin) also occurs. Following treatment, the mites are likely to survive indefinitely in the ears, occasionally flaring up again. They can be detected in carrier pigs in ear scrapings.

Treatment/prophylaxis

Mange can be treated with ivermectin, doramectin, amitraz, or phosmet. Subcutaneous injection of ivermectin or doramectin kills mites in ears and skin in 7–14 days. Pigs with crusty ears should be treated a second time within 14 days. Alternatively, the disease can be controlled by in-feed medication. Amitraz solution can be sprayed all over the pig's skin and in the ears. Because of the life cycle of the mite, this should be repeated in 7–10 days. Phosmet can be poured over the skin and into the ears. A single treatment usually suffices. Whatever treatment is used, farmers must be advised to observe the required withdrawal period before sending pigs to slaughter.

Various control regimens have been applied. For example, boars are treated three or four times a year, sows and gilts before farrowing and piglets in the nursery. Replacement breeding stock should be treated on arrival if they have not come from a mange-free herd. Mange can be eliminated from herds by repopulating with mange-free stock, widely available from breeding companies. This, however, is too radical and expensive a procedure for eradicating mange alone. Mange can also be eradicated by treating all the pigs in a herd on at least two occasions and, because the mange eggs can survive in the environment, on wood for example, after treatment the pigs should be moved into accommodation that has been cleaned and rested. Before starting eradication a control programme should be carried out until mange is at its lowest endemic level.

Since mange spreads from herd to herd with the movement of carrier pigs, if replacement stock is only obtained from mange-free herds or is isolated and well treated on arrival, a mange-free herd can remain free indefinitely.

Diarrhoea in piglets

Causative organisms

Diarrhoea can be caused by non-infectious factors as well as infectious ones. The infectious ones include clostridia, viruses and parasites. Clostridia are dealt with above. Viruses are not relevant to this chapter because they are untreatable and no vaccines are available in the UK.

Treatment/prophylaxis

The parasites which cause diarrhoea in the UK are coccidia (*Eimeria, Isospora* and *Cryptosporidia*). These are intracellular in the sucking piglets' intestines and cause damage to the mucosa, diarrhoea and dehydration between 7 and 21 days of age. The diarrhoea does not respond well to antibacterial therapy. Coccidia are shed in the sows' feces. To eliminate this sows are fed rations medicated with amprolium (Coxoid, Harkers general sales list (GSL)) or sulfadimidine from the time they enter the farrowing house until they are weaned. Monensin sodium, normally given to poultry and cattle (PML or zootechnical feed additives (ZFA)) has also been used. Each litter is injected with long-acting sulphonamide at 6 days of age. Also small amounts of milk powder medicated with a coccidiostat such as amprolium, or salinomycin, are provided for piglets to eat with their creep feed (see Box 11.1). Because salinomycin improves feed conversion rate, products are generally classified as ZFA (see chapter 1) although one product is in fact PML. This feed is given daily from 3 days of age until weaning. Toltrazuril mixed in glycerol and water is given daily at 4, 5 and 6 days of age. In addition, sow and piglet feces should be removed daily. Attention should be given to the cleaning of the farrowing crate and pen floors.

Worms

Causative organism

A variety of species of worm can multiply in the pig's alimentary tract.

Under modern conditions of housing and management worms are rarely a problem and generally do not cause clinical disease; however, a more wary approach has to be taken to outdoor herds because of the possible build-up in paddocks that are used over long periods. Paddocks that are regularly rotated and rested, particularly if sheep or cattle graze them after or before the pigs, are likely to give less trouble. Cattle and sheep will reduce the worm egg burden.

Hyostrongylus spp. (stomach worms) may produce signs of anaemia, inappetance and loss of condition in sows kept in poor conditions on dirty straw or in permanent paddocks or, rarely, in grower-finishers.

Oesophagostomum spp. occur in the colon and caecum of sows but have to reach exceptionally high numbers to cause loss of weight and perhaps diarrhoea. If the sows are suckling litters, this may result in reduced milk yield and reduced piglet growth rate.

Ascaris suum is a common large roundworm multiplying in small intestines of growing and finishing pigs. The adult worm in the intestines rarely causes clinical disease, but the larvae migrate through the liver causing scarring, the so-called milk spot liver. These do not harm the pig but, if a lot of livers are affected, the slaughter house is likely to complain and the farmer will have to take action. Also, a massive dose of larvae migrating through the lungs may cause acute coughing which may alarm the farmer.

Metastrongylus spp. (lungworms) invade the bronchioles of the lung and in heavy infections cause coughing and breathing difficulty and sometimes reduction in growth rate.

Trichuris suis infects the crypts of the large intestine of growers and finishers causing colitis and sometimes haemorrhage if the infestation is heavy.

Infection of pigs' muscle with *Trichinella* or of pigs' livers with *Cysticercus cellulosae*, both of which pose public health risks, have not been reported in the UK for many years.

Treatment and prophylaxis (see Table 10.1, pages 266, 267)

Treatment needs to be carried out routinely if the pigs are heavily infected or in situations where a build-up of worms is anticipated. A variety of anthelmintics are available and the choice depends on the species of worm, whether it has developed drug resistance, age of pig, ease of dosing and cost. They can be given as pour-ons, by injection or most commonly by feed medication.

Further reading

Muirhead M R, Alexander T J L (1997). *Managing pig health and the treatment of disease. A reference for the farm.* Sheffield: 5M Enterprises. (Online version can be accessed through ThePigSite.com)

Muirhead M R, Alexander T J L (1998). *Recognising and treating pig diseases*. Sheffield: 5M Enterprises.
Muirhead M R, Alexander T J L (1998). *Recognising and treating pig infertility*. Sheffield: 5M Enterprises.
Taylor D J (1999). *Pig diseases*. Bury St Edmunds: St Edmundsbury Press.

Useful website

http://www.ThePigSite.com

12

The diseases and healthcare of bees

Michael H Jepson

Invertebrates, such as bees, are remarkably similar in some respects to vertebrates as far as their susceptibility to viral, bacterial, protozoal, fungal and mite (acarine) infections are concerned. The extent to which adult bees are susceptible to the diseases caused will depend upon the vigour of the colony, such that disease may only be apparent in colonies that are in a poor condition. Large thriving colonies appear capable of suppressing or containing many diseases. As is no less true with much animal or livestock husbandry, the most assured way of keeping bees healthy is by following good beekeeping practices. Knowledge of the most important diseases and their treatment and prevention are of value to those, such as pharmacists, who can supply treatment products, as well as to responsible beekeepers.

There are relatively few preparations that have been granted marketing authorisation in the UK for administration to bees. This is because they are a potential source of problems due to the fact that most bees are kept as food producers of honey. Consequently, there is a possibility of residue contamination in honey, especially from the use of unauthorised products. Appropriate medication can be administered to bees as powder, in syrup, by aerosol, in smoke or by contact with a medicated strip. Traditionally it has been common practice to use a variety of chemical substances to aid disease prevention and contribute to healthcare, but there is limited information generally available regarding dosage, residue levels and the relative risks of contamination. Veterinary surgeons, and pharmacists in particular, have been helped considerably in recent years by the publication of authoritative information in the several editions of the *The Veterinary Formulary*. This complements, and is in addition to, the admirable information leaflets covering a wide range of relevant topics and produced by the National Bee Unit (NBU) of the Central Science Laboratory (CSL), an executive agency of the Department for Environment, Food, and Rural Affairs (DEFRA). It should be emphasised that certain diseases are notifiable in the UK and the national British Beekeepers' Association (BBA) and local associations play an important part in containing disease outbreaks and maintaining the health of very many colonies of honeybees throughout the country.

Honey is the most significant product produced by honeybees, but there is also the production and importance of beeswax, royal jelly and venom. The contribution of honeybees to pollination in agricultural and horticultural crop production, as well as in the domestic garden, is enormous and often crucial. Replacement stock of new colonies, propagation of queen bees and research applications are all matters of particular importance, not only to beekeepers but also to the entire agricultural and horticultural environment and industries. Some background knowledge of how a honeybee colony functions can be of help to those who may be asked to supply items for use with bees, especially if related to the health of a bee colony.

The honeybee colony

During the summer there may be as many as 50 000 bees in a strong colony. A colony will consist of a queen, who alone is capable of laying over 2000 eggs each day. She is supported by several hundred drones, or male bees, from unfertilised eggs, whose only known function is to mate with the queen. All the rest are worker bees from fertilised eggs. They live together as a community upon double-sided combs containing brood and stores of honey and pollen. Figure 12.1 shows bees in the comb.

Fertilised eggs laid by the queen in worker cells hatch after 3 days when the tiny grubs or larvae are fed by nurse bees and grow rapidly to reach full size in 5 days. Their cells are then sealed with porous wax cappings and the larvae pupate before emerging as young worker bees 12–14 days later, having chewed their way through the cappings and thereby joining the older workers on their comb. Drones take a few days longer to develop. The role of the worker bees changes during their adult life, from initially tending and feeding larvae, cleaning or constructing the wax comb cells, then serving as guards at the hive entrance before progressing to finding water and foraging for nectar, pollen and propolis from plants. Propolis is a red resinous substance, a mixture of natural resins from buds, used by the bees to stop up crevices and strengthen and waterproof the hive. The plant nectar is converted into honey and the pollen is either used to feed the larvae or stored. After a colony reaches its maximum size of up to 50 000 or more bees by

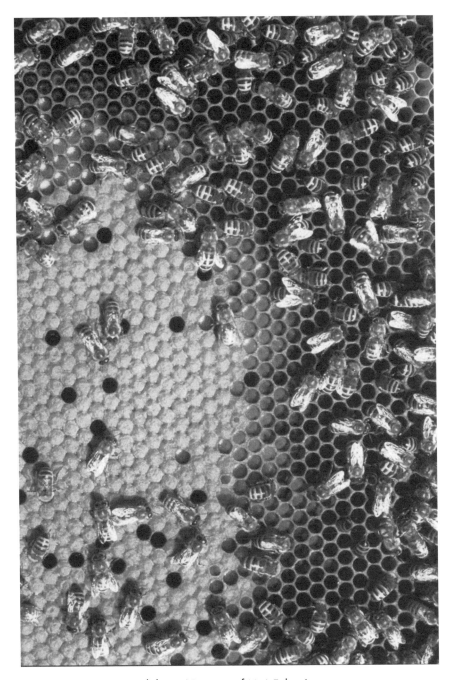

Figure 12.1 Honeycomb bees. (Courtesy of Mr L Faber.)

midsummer, the population of workers will start to decline. In early autumn, all the drones will have died and the queen will remain with a reduced number of worker bees to survive through the winter. In the UK, breeding will slowly start again in January or February and depending upon conditions will reach a peak by May or June, 4 months later. Beekeepers have to be alert to the possibility of swarming, especially in May, June or July, which is an important part of beekeeping husbandry, as swarming can seriously deplete the productivity of a hive at the height of the season. The triggers that cause swarming are not fully understood, but overcrowding of a hive is considered to be a factor. If a beekeeper takes a swarm, it can be the means of establishing an additional colony rather than leaving the swarming bees and queen to fly off and start a new colony elsewhere. The brood combs in the hive with the remaining bees will include some characteristic queen cells, which are fed on a special diet of 'royal jelly' produced by the nurse bees. The cells, which contain larvae from normal fertilised eggs, are relatively large, acorn shaped, and hang mouth down. It is from these cells that new queens will develop, one of which will become the new queen of the colony after mating successively in the air with several drones.

A honeybee colony acts as a unit and, while not domesticated in the way that farm animals are, in a modern hive the beekeeper is enabled to manipulate the colony and observe and assess the varied needs of the colony. Experience is most important, as prompt action may be necessary due to a variety of reasons including dramatic changes in weather, temperature, environmental conditions and spread of disease threats.

The beekeeper needs to follow a seasonal management programme if a colony of honeybees is to maximise honey production during the summer season.

Thus autumn preparations for wintering include the need to ensure that the queen, up to 2 years old, and colony are healthy with adequate supplies of food in the combs and that the hive is in good condition, affording good protection from the weather and possible disturbance from such animals as mice. Providing no serious disturbance takes place, November to February should involve little attention being given to the colony. After the bees start to fly more actively in March, a first brief inspection to check that the queen and brood are healthy is timely on, for example, a warm day in early April. Checking the brood should ensure that the queen is 'queenright' and producing worker brood and that there is no evidence of disease, such as 'foul brood'. It also provides an opportunity to check the adequacy of food store remaining in the combs. A second and more thorough spring examination is considered

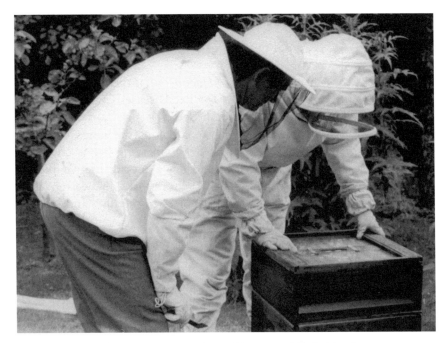

Figure 12.2 Beekeepers managing hives. (Courtesy of Mr L Faber.)

advisable in late April or early May and will consist primarily of removing unserviceable combs, cleaning, providing a source of water and the possible uniting of two small colonies.

Good beekeeping practice and the natural control of disease

Before detailing some of the more important diseases affecting bees it is relevant to note some of the major factors that will help to ensure a healthy and thriving colony:

- It is important, and essential, to examine colonies at regular intervals throughout the active season. The entire brood must be examined at least every spring and autumn for signs of the two serious bacterial diseases, European and American foul brood.
- Bees must be well fed.
- Colonies must be headed by fertile queens from good stock and normally only up to 2 years old.
- Bees must be generally healthy and free from foul brood diseases.
- A colony needs adequate comb space for expansion and food storage.
- The swarming instinct needs to be controlled.

Common diseases affecting honeybees

Varroosis

Infestation by the acarine mite, *Varroa jacobsoni*, is the causative organism and is a notifiable disease under the Bee Diseases Control Order in the UK. At high concentration in the brood, the mite causes abnormal and deformed development of the larvae, affecting the wings, abdomen and salivary glands. As a consequence, the emerging bee is unable to perform its normal roles in the hive and has a shorter life. Unlike the Asian honeybee (*Apis cerana*), the mite's natural host, the western honeybee, *Apis mellifera*, has no natural defences to the mite and infested colonies are eventually killed.

The need to control *V. jacobsoni* mites has increased considerably, as they have spread northwards from mainland Europe as far as Scotland. The first report of *varroa* in the UK was in Devon in 1992 and it has spread rapidly since, reaching southern Scotland in 1997. During the 1960s, the first honeybee colony losses reportedly caused by the *varroa* mite occurred in the Far East. In temperate climates, honeybee colonies can collapse within 1–3 years. It has been reported that in Poland 2 000 000 colonies have been lost; 300 000 colonies have been lost in Spain. The mite is present on all continents except Australasia. As the mite cannot be eradicated, it is essential that all beekeepers practise effective control to keep the mite population below the critical level at all times. The NBU provides detailed information on the types of treatment available; these can be grouped under the headings 'biotechnical' and 'varroacides'.

- Biotechnical treatments focus on the use of husbandry methods to reduce the mite population, taking advantage of aspects of the mite life cycle. Mites trapped in brood combs, once sealed, are removed from the colony before the emergence of the young bees or mites. Such methods require experience to be successful and can be time consuming.
- Varroacide treatments involve the use of chemicals to kill the mites and may be applied in feed, topically on adult bees, as fumigants, as contact strips or by evaporation. Authorised varroacides have proven safety, quality and efficacy, are convenient to use and can often be used alone in accordance with the manufacturer's product data sheet and package insert. Unauthorised varroacides are often considered to be 'natural' products and relatively cheap, but their efficacy is likely to be variable. If misused, such compounds can be harmful to both the beekeeper and the bees. Problems of resistance and of residues, if misused, can apply to varroacides.

Authorised varroacides

Flumethrin impregnated strips – 3.6 mg per strip – are licensed in the UK as Bayvarol (Bayer) and were reclassified as general sale list medications (GSL), formerly pharmacy and merchant supplies medicines (PML), to facilitate concerted administration by beekeepers in a wide area. Unfortunately, resistance has been reported and can be aggravated by failure to remove exhausted strips from hives. Pharmacists will recognise the guidance given in the manufacturer's data sheet, where the strips may be used for 24 hours to diagnose or for a maximum of 6 weeks for therapy. It should be obvious that fresh strips must be used for each application. As a means of diagnosis, after 24 hours, an estimate of the number of dead mites on the floor tray is indicative of the level of infestation. It is essential to protect the tray with a mesh or screen to prevent the bees from removing the dead mites. Several factors will need to be taken into account in assessing the significance of the estimate, including the size and condition of the colony, the time of year and level of breeding activity, as well as previous treatment.

Fluvalinate as 'Apistan' (Vita – formerly a Sandoz product available only in Europe) is now authorised for use in the UK as impregnated strips containing 10% fluvalinate. For both of these authorised products, the withdrawal period for honey is nil and they can be used safely during a honey flow if necessary, though not during comb honey production. This can be particularly advantageous if the nature of local flora does not allow a sufficient honey-free interval for treatment or if an infestation is serious. However, other bee produce intended for human consumption should not be taken until the spring following treatment. It must be emphasised that it is illegal for beekeepers to purchase and import products into the UK, which may be authorised in mainland Europe, for treating varroa. There is the added risk that such illegal use could exacerbate the problems of resistance.

Guidelines for controlling and minimising mite invasions

Treatment with a varroacide will never eliminate the possibility of mites entering a treated colony from a locally infested colony. However, a number of measures can be taken to minimise the risk of infection:

- All colonies must be treated at the same time.
- Treatment time should normally and best be coordinated in a local area with other beekeepers and the local beekeepers' association.

- If emergency treatment is necessary, do not delay the start of treatment which can be overlapped with treatment by other beekeepers.
- Feral colonies of bees lost by swarming are a good potential source for breeding mites. Prevent losing swarms and where necessary find and remove feral colonies.

Common varroacides are summarised in Table 12.1.

Mite resistance The two authorised GSL products, flumethrin (Bayvarol, Bayer) and fluvalinate (Apistan, Vita), utilise synthetic pyrethroids as their active constituents. Consequently, the possibility of minimising the development of resistance will not be offset by alternating these products on an annual basis. The development of resistance can be delayed and minimised by:

- Only applying treatments when needed.
- Strict adherence to the manufacturer's instructions and always using the recommended dose of the varroacide product.
- Under no circumstances leave varroacide strips in hives at the end of the recommended treatment time; promptly remove and destroy them.
- Varroacide strips must not be considered for reuse, as they will not release a full and effective dose of the active ingredient.
- Where possible use chemically unrelated alternate treatments.

Integrated pest management (IPM) is a principle increasingly and widely used in agriculture. It involves keeping a pest species at as harmless a level as possible by using a combination of control methods, each working in different ways and often at different times of the year. Such an approach can ensure that pest numbers are prevented from reaching a critical and damaging level requiring more drastic treatment. For the integrated control of varroa this could include the use of biotechnical methods during the summer months, a varroacide treatment in the autumn and a second treatment, preferably with a different treatment product, in the following spring.

Traditionally, various other chemical substances have been used to maintain the health of bees in a hive. Various mites have been controlled by lactic acid, formic acid, menthol and methyl salicylate. Wax moths and their larvae have been controlled by acetic acid, formaldehyde solution and paradichlorbenzene. These substances are not licensed for these indications. The concern of the BBA, with regard to the enforcement of the 1997 Residue Regulations which may prohibit the supply or sale of animal products (including honey) that contain detectable unauthorised substances, is most understandable. Pharmacists supplying chemicals should be aware of any relevant problems of administration.

Table 12.1 Varroacides used by beekeepers

Active constituent	Product name	Application	Effect	When to use	Warnings
Authorised products					
Flumethrin (synthetic pyrethroid[a])	Bayvarol (Bayer)	Plastic strips hung between brood combs	Contact	Autumn or early spring for 6 weeks	>95% effective; can use during honey flow
Fluvalinate, (synthetic pyrethroid[a])	Apistan (Vita)	Plastic strips hung between brood combs	Contact	Autumn or early spring for 6 weeks	>95% effective; can use during honey flow
Non-authorised generic substances					
Formic acid, 60–85% solution		By vaporiser	Evaporation	Late summer and autumn; temperature dependent	Kills mites in sealed brood cells; highly corrosive
Lactic acid solution		Sprayed over beecombs	Contact	Winter and broodless periods	Skin burns; respiratory irritant
Oxalic acid solution 3.2–4.2% solution in 60% sucrose		2.5 mL trickled over each brood comb	Contact	Winter and broodless periods	Toxic by inhalation, ingestion or percutaneous absorption
Essential oils (terpenes)		Various systems	Evaporation or sublimation, temperature dependent	Spring or late summer, 6–8 weeks	Respiratory irritant to skin and eyes

[a] Particular care should be taken when disposing of strips, as synthetic pyrethroids are dangerous to fish. Do not contaminate ponds, waterways or ditches with the strips or used packaging.

Note: It is important to ascertain details of any safety warnings and the need to use protective clothing when considering the use of any chemicals.

Principal sources: NBU leaflets and *Veterinary Data Sheet Compendium*.

The Veterinary Formulary is again a most useful source of information together with the DEFRA publications previously referred to, many of which are free.

European foul brood/American foul brood

European Foul Brood (EFB) caused by *Melissococcus pluton* and American Foul Brood (AFB) caused by *Paenibacillus larvae* are of bacterial origin and both are serious notifiable diseases. Nurse bees transmit the infection to newly hatched larvae and the build up of bacteria is influenced by the oxygen to carbon dioxide ratio. Both infections are fatal, EFB does not sporalate and is less persistent than AFB. However, EFB can appear in a colony unexpectedly and it may be that it persists at a subclinical level. The remains of AFB-infected larvae and bacterial spores are difficult to remove from the comb and could present an extended source of recurrent infection. As a consequence, it is required that any infected material, including frames and combs, should be destroyed by burning.

It is relevant to refer to the NBU, which manages an inspection service on behalf of DEFRA in England, and the National Assembly of Wales. Several full-time regional bee inspectors manage teams of seasonally employed bee inspectors and organise training for beekeepers in disease control. The NBU inspectors have powers to enter an apiary at any time to inspect colonies, especially if disease is thought to be present. Details of the statutory procedures for controlling foul brood are given in one of the leaflets published by DEFRA.

Nosema

Nosema is a disease spread in the feces of infected bees. It is caused by *Nosema apis* Zander, a microscopic spore-forming parasite, which invades the digestive cells lining the midgut of the bee and produces huge numbers of spores. Bees normally defecate away from the hive during the warmer time of the year and there is little if any risk to the colony. Adverse weather conditions may result in fecal contamination within the hive, and the young bees responsible for cleaning soiled frames are prone to being infected with the organism. Infection may also be spread by beekeepers placing infected combs contaminated with *N. apis* spores into healthy colonies.

Nosema shortens the lifespan of bees and adversely affects the number of eggs laid by an infected queen. Serious damage to colonies is relatively uncommon and infection in a large thriving colony rarely reaches a level requiring control treatment. Where required, treatment with 20 mg/g fumagillin powder (Fumidil B, Thorne, UK) is administered in the sugar syrup for winter stores at the rate of 8 g per colony. Nosema infection is suppressed for the following spring.

Formaldehyde solution (BP) with potassium permanganate as a fumigant is also used to control *N. apis* but should only be applied to empty combs and hive bodies. 240 g of potassium permanganate in 500 mL formaldehyde solution is sufficient for 30 m^3 and should be left in contact with empty combs or hive bodies for 14–17 days. Care should be taken to avoid inhaling the fumes. This fumigant is also used to control *Malpighamoeba mellificae* (see below), EFB and wax moths (see later).

Amoeba disease

Amoeba disease is caused by the protozoa *M. mellificae* which encysts in the malpighian tubules. Bees can be infected by ingesting dormant cysts from infected bee feces. The cysts germinate and continue their life cycle of 22–24 days before being expelled with the feces. It has been estimated that 2% of colonies in England and Wales are affected, but the effect on a colony is uncertain. There is no known drug treatment. Combs can be sterilised for reuse with acetic acid as a fumigant. For this purpose, pads of cotton wool are soaked in 150 mL acetic acid (80%) and placed between hive bodies full of combs in winter storage for 1 week. The combs must be ventilated before offering them to bees. This treatment may also serve for *N. apis*. The honey or pollen stored in the combs is unharmed. As the acid will corrode, care should be taken of any exposed metal surfaces and metal end-spacers are best removed. These may be subsequently scalded with hot water containing washing soda or detergent.

Acarine

Acarine is an infestation of the trachea of the adult honeybee by a parasitic mite – *Acarapis woodi* Rennie. All castes of bees: queen, workers and drones can be affected, although during the active season little effect on the activity of workers is observed. However, the lives of over-wintering bees are shortened. If over 30% of bees are infested in the autumn, the colony may dwindle to the point of extinction in early spring, with few adults surviving to support brood rearing. Several chemical substances have been effectively used for the control of mites as indicated below.

Mites may be controlled using formic acid (60–80%) delivered by vaporiser. Treatment can be applied at any time of year if ambient temperature is high enough to achieve adequate vaporisation and the bees are not clustered. A few bees may be killed especially those emerging from sealed cells.

Although methyl salicylate does not kill mites, it can be used to prevent migration from infested bees to healthy bees. For use as a fumigant, a gauze pad should be moistened with 2.5 mL methyl salicylate and applied over frames daily for 6 days. Alternatively, a small bottle of methyl salicylate, fitted with a wick, should be placed at the back of the hive, allowing natural evaporation. The use of methyl salicylate should be avoided when honey spurs are present, as the honey may become tainted.

Thymol (25%) in a gel formulation (Apiguard, Vita, UK) may be used to control mites, either by contact or as a fumigant, by following the manufacturer's instructions.

Vegetable oils and light paraffin oils have also been used to control mites when vegetable oils are added to sugar patty or by fine nozzle spray. The mites are not killed directly but the attractiveness of host bees is markedly diminished.

Other treatments used to repel mites

These include the use of inert powders which have been found to control mites, including varroa. Sprinkling, using a sugar or flour dredger containing chalk, glucose, corn starch, icing sugar, milk powder, talc or flour, for example, causes the mites to lose their grip on their host bees. The mites can then be collected from the hive floor trays. Such treatment can be repeated at 4-day intervals as required. Excessive amounts of powder can present a risk to uncapped brood and too fine a powder could block bee spiracles. All bees on each side of combs in the brood chamber should be lightly covered with powder before closing the hive entrance for 20–30 minutes. Mites should then be collected from the hive floor tray.

Essential oils, including citronella oil, cinnamon oil and sandalwood oil act by repelling mites from beeswax that has oil incorporated. Some oils, including cinnamon oil, are toxic to many mites.

Paralysis

Paralysis can result from chronic bee paralysis virus (CBPV) which is widely distributed in the UK and often present in seemingly healthy colonies. Visual symptoms, which are fairly reliable in diagnosing the disease, include bees crawling on the ground outside the hive, trembling wings and hairless or bloated bodies. It is thought that overcrowding may help the disease to spread or to a lesser extent it may spread by transmission from infected worker bees. The disease rarely causes severe problems and the only control is to re-queen a colony with a less susceptible queen.

Several other virus infections affecting bees only do so to a modest extent and are not easy to detect or diagnose. In some cases, they can increase to lethal levels when in combination with other infections such as *V. jacobsoni*.

Chalkbrood

Chalkbrood is caused by the fungus *Ascosphaera apis*. Most hives have a few cells with infected larvae, but the condition can spread if other factors, such as chilling, weaken the brood. Thymol applied as a fumigant or by contact, as previously described, can be used to control chalkbrood.

Wax moths' larvae

Wax moths' larvae of either the greater wax moth – *Galleria mellonella* – or the lesser wax moth – *Achroia grisella* – will feed on larval skins, pupal remains and wax in brood combs, causing the bees to abandon areas of comb. Extensive damage can ensue. Control can be achieved by the use of acetic acid as fumigant, formic acid as vaporiser, formaldehyde solution with potassium permanganate as fumigant (all as described previously) or with paradichlorbenzene (PDB), which is effective against adults and larvae. PDB crystals should be sprinkled throughout stored stacks of comb and is the same as the treatment for clothes moths often used domestically. PDB crystals may not kill wax moth eggs and combs should be aired before replacing in the hive. A warning is also given that it may be carcinogenic.

A biological larvicide containing *Bacillus thuringiensis*, marketed as 'Certan' (Swarm/Thorne, UK), is available for treating comb infestations affected by the larvae of the greater wax moth – also known as the honeybee moth. A diluted solution is thoroughly sprayed on each comb surface in the autumn before storing the combs or in spring prior to placing in the hive.

Methods of administering drugs and chemicals

A crucial matter is to ensure that any treatment is put in place immediately and that a drug or chemical is not stored with the added risk of contamination of the honey. For the administration of medicated sugar syrup, it is important to use a slow-feeder from which the medication is taken over a period of 2–3 days. If a rapid-feeder was used, the bees would be able to take maybe several litres of syrup overnight, which would then be likely to be put into the honey super. It should be emphasised that under normal circumstances, medication should not be given with honey supers still on the hive.

Some drugs present a risk of accumulating in the wax of the comb and not breaking down for a considerable time, which is one reason why manufacturers will recommend that bee products, other than honey, are left until the spring following treatment, if intended for human consumption.

The stability of formulations is likely to be affected by conditions within a hive and the ambient temperature will have a direct bearing on the rate of vaporisation of some chemicals and may require monitoring to ensure an effective but safe concentration of active substance.

As previously stated, there are few medicinal product preparations which have UK marketing authorisations, but it is possible for a veterinarian to obtain a product available in another country, under a Special Treatment Authorisation available from the Veterinary Medicines Directorate (VMD). The VMD is the UK government and DEFRA agency responsible for the safety, quality and efficacy of veterinary medicines. Regulations otherwise prohibit personal imports of such products into the UK. Reassuringly, as bees are considered as food-producing animals, the VMD has indicated that a number of non-medicinal substances may be used by beekeepers where such substances are unlikely to be harmful to human health. These substances include formic acid, lactic acid, oxalic acid, talc, thymol, oil of wintergreen, some essential oils, liquid paraffin and homeopathic treatments.

Diagnostic services

Diagnostic services are available from the NBU of the CSL based in York, which provides a fast and reliable service to identify any likely infection and monitor the health of honeybee colonies. For this purpose, a sample of not less than 30 bees which have recently died and been taken from a hive should be despatched promptly in a stout cardboard box. The sample bees will be individually examined for acarine, nosema and amoeba and a report, including advisory notes as appropriate, is normally sent by return to the beekeeper.

Agricultural chemicals

Bees are and have been adversely affected by some of the chemicals utilised in modern agricultural practice, particularly by crop protection products which include pesticides. The listing of Approved Products for Farmers and Growers (Stationery Office) classifies approved chemicals according to their relative toxicity to bees. Where relevant, the classification includes categories which may be 'dangerous' or 'harmful'. The BBA publish an advisory leaflet on the protection of bees from certain pesticides.

Further reading

Bailey L (1963). *Infectious Diseases of the Honey-bee*. London: Land Books.

Bishop Y, ed. (2001). *The Veterinary Formulary*, 5th edn. London: Pharmaceutical Press.

Morse R A, ed. (1978). *Honey-bee Pests, Predators and Diseases*. Ithica: Cornell University Press.

UK government publications/websites

DEFRA (1991). *Common Diseases of the Adult Honey Bee*. London: DEFRA.

DEFRA (1999). *Statutory Procedures for Controlling Foul Brood*. London: DEFRA (available free from CSL and online at http://agrifor.ac.uk/whatsnew/detail/3010016.htm).

DEFRA (2000). *Managing Varroa*. London: DEFRA (available free from CSL or online at http://www.csl.gov.uk/prodserv/cons/bee/factsheets/Managing_Varroa.pdf also see http://www.csl.gov.uk/prodserv/cons/bee/resistance/vrtp.cfm).

DEFRA (2003). *Diseases of Bees*. London: Stationery Office.

DEFRA (2003). Bee health. http://www.defra.gov.uk/hort/bees.htm (accessed 8 July 2003).

Varroa jacobsoni. For current information about monitoring and forecasting mite populations within honey bee colonies in Britain see the following websites: http://www.csl.gov.uk; http://www.defra.gov.uk http://www.csl.gov.uk/prodserv/cons/bee/

Useful addresses/websites

British Beekeepers' Association, National Agricultural Centre, Stoneleigh, Warwickshire CV8 2LZ, UK (http://www.bbka.org.uk).

International Bee Research Association, Cardiff, CF10 3DT, UK (http://www.ibra.org.uk).

National Bee Unit (NBU), Central Science Laboratory, Sand Hutton, York YO41 1LZ, UK (http://www.csl.gov.uk/prodserv/cons/bee/).

Part 4

Companion animals

13

Cats and dogs

Steven B Kayne

There are 6.9 million owned dogs (pets and working) and 8 million cats in the UK, giving a total of 14.9 million (Pet Food Manufacturers' Association, 1999). This takes no account of stray or feral animals.

Under normal circumstances there is little problem in keeping these pets, but the potential for zoonotic infection is very real and pharmacists may keep a valuable watching brief on the situation. Further, ensuring a healthy pet involves regular use of prophylactic measures, and here again pharmacists are well placed to be involved.

In this chapter, zoonotic and other diseases of cats and dogs are discussed, together with measures to ensure that the animals and their owners remain healthy.

History

Cats

More than 50 million years ago, a small, weasel-like animal called *Miacis* roamed the Earth. Most scientists now believe that this animal was the ancestor of today's domestic cats, as well as the ancestor for other mammals including raccoons, dogs and bears. It was about 40 million years ago that actual members of the cat family first appeared. The domestication process began about 3000 BC in Egypt, when cats were enlisted to protect grain silos from rodents. These felines became so valuable that they were regarded as gods. The basic domestic cat descended from this Egyptian stock. The concept of breeds began in the mid-nineteenth century, when the idea of cat shows was invented. Pedigrees were developed by breeders from natural cat breeds that had been in existence for thousands of years. People took the cats with traits that they most favoured and then bred them to continue and enhance the desirable characteristics. Domestic cats then spread throughout Asia, where they were used to protect the silkworm cocoons from rodents, which was vital to the silk industry. The people of the Orient greatly admired the mystery and beauty of the cat, and many writers and artists in Japan and China celebrated these animals in their art. Cats first came to Europe and the Middle East about 1000 BC, most likely from Greek and Phoenician traders. The ancient Greeks and Romans also valued cats highly for their ability to control undesirable rodents. The cat was considered the guardian spirit of a household, and the symbol of liberty in Rome. Traders, explorers and colonists began to realise the important role cats played in controlling rodents, and took domestic cats with them to the New World during the 1600s and 1700s. The first cat show was held in London in 1871 and the first cat association, The National Cat Club of Great Britain, was formed in 1887.

Dogs

The history of domestic dogs began 20 000 years ago, when Mesolithic Man first began to use dogs while hunting. When livestock became domesticated 7000–9000 years ago, dogs were important as protectors and guards. Skeletal remains indicate that five diverse types of dog existed in the Bronze Age (about 4500 BC) – mastiffs, wolf-type dogs, greyhounds, pointing dogs and shepherding dogs – and cave paintings show dogs working alongside human hunters. In the fifth century BC, the Greeks used dogs as guards. In 350 BC Aristotle made a list of the known breeds, discussing the merits of some. The Romans took their dogs with them on their European conquests. After the fall of the Roman Empire, dog breeding and care was less important that eating and war. Packs of abandoned dogs formed and terrorised the towns and villages of the Dark Ages. Frightened, invaded and uneducated, peasants blamed dogs for much of the horror around them and superstitions about dogs arose – werewolves, monsters with fangs and curled lips, and many other evil creatures were based on dogs. What saved the dog was its continued skill at hunting, and feudal nobility began to reconstruct lost breeds. Monasteries recognised dog breeding as a good source of revenue, and turned to creating breeds to sell to wealthy nobles. From these breeds came the hunting dogs of France, notably bloodhounds. Dogs soon became expensive, and hunting was reserved as the right of the rich. The random-bred dogs of the poor were required to wear large blocks around their necks to prevent them from mating with the prized breeds of the aristocracy. During the Crusades, European knights took their dogs to the Holy Land, where they discovered different breeds. The resulting crossbreeding gave us the ancestors of today's hounds and spaniels. Speciality breeds really took off in the Middle Ages. The Renaissance saw a further refinement of breeds. A wealthy merchant class had both spare cash and spare time, and dogs bred strictly as companions became popular. Speciality breeds found themselves in trouble once again after the French Revolution. With their aristocratic owners mostly headless, many of these breeds went into decline. Although peasants could now hunt, their needs were different, and so different breeds emerged. Gundogs were now popular, and by crossing greyhounds with braques a variety of pointers was developed. In the 19th century many new breeds were created. This process was driven both by people recreating lost ancient breeds and by the requirement for yet more specific traits for working dogs. Breeds once again were refined for hunting, ratting, coursing, retrieving and as companions. With the advent of the first dog show in 1859, the continued success of the most popular breeds was assured.

Anatomy

Cat

Size

An adult domestic cat is about 20–25 cm high. The length from the tip of the nose to the base of the tail averages around 50 cm and the tail is about 30 cm long. Females usually weigh from 2.7 to 4.5 kg and males from 4.5 to 6.8 kg depending on skeletal size (see chapter 8, Figure 8.1).

Head

The head is large compared with the rest of the body. The nose and jaws are short, so the face seems flat when compared with the faces of many other kinds of animals. The ears are large and they flare at the base. They taper to rounded or pointed tips and stand erect in almost all breeds. A cat has keen hearing and can detect many sounds that humans cannot hear. A cat usually turns its head, not only its eyes, in the direction of a sound. This aids both hearing and vision. In the cat, as in the human, the inner ear – a bony structure of fluid-filled semicircular canals – contains a complicated mechanism for maintaining body balance. It is this mechanism that enables the animal to land on its feet when it falls.

Eyes

The cat's large and prominent eyes are placed well forward on the head and, like the eyes of humans, they face forward. The cat comes closer than does any other animal except the owl and the ape to having binocular vision similar to that of humans. The size and position of the eyes permit as much light as possible to enter them and ensure an extensive field of vision – important factors in hunting and nocturnal prowling. A cat cannot see in total darkness, but it can see better in dim light than can most other kinds of animals. In bright light a cat's pupils contract to narrow vertical slits, but in the dark these slits enlarge to round openings that admit the maximum amount of light. The eyes seem to shine in the dark. This shininess results when even the smallest amount of light strikes the reflective area of iridescent green or yellow crystalline needles in the inner lining of the eye. The eyes of the Siamese cat appear red in the dark; the retinas lack pigment and the colour is provided by blood vessels. A cat is very alert to any movement, but it probably cannot distinguish colour. For these reasons, it will pounce when a victim moves but may not attack prey that remains still.

Nose and whiskers

The tip of a cat's nose, the leather, may be black, reddish or pink and is usually cool and moist. All cats have an acute sense of smell, scenting prey or their favourite delicacies at surprising distances. A cat's whiskers, or vibrissae, serve as delicate sense organs of touch. Four rows of stiff whiskers grow on the upper lip on each side of the nose. Small groups of whiskers are also situated on other parts of the body, including above each eye, on both cheeks and on the backs of the forepaws. Cutting off the whiskers not only detracts from the animal's appearance but also impairs its ability to feel its way about.

Teeth

A cat's teeth serve primarily as weapons as well as for tearing food. The animal has 30 permanent teeth. The strongest and sharpest are the four large, curved, pointed fangs (canines). With these teeth the cat grasps and tears its food or an enemy. The small front teeth (upper and lower incisors) function chiefly as grooming aids. The cat has fewer side teeth (premolars and molars) than do most other mammals. In most mammals the side teeth are used for grinding food. The cat uses these teeth only for cutting.

Tongue

The tongue of a domestic cat feels much like coarse sandpaper. Its surface is covered with rasp-like projections or barbs that face backward into the throat. All cats use their tongue as a major grooming tool to clean and comb the fur, but they also use it as an efficient tool to strip flesh off the bones of prey.

Jaws

Although a cat's jaws are short, they are extremely strong. They clamp down upon prey with enough power to crush the bones. The lower jaw is attached to the upper by means of a simple hinge. This arrangement permits only up-and-down motion. A cat cannot move its lower jaw sideways, nor can it grind its teeth. When a cat clamps its jaws shut, the teeth mesh side by side, somewhat like the meshing of gears. Cats tear and crush their food, but they do not chew it. Much of the food is swallowed whole, and digestive juices break it down for use.

Sounds

All cats – domestic and wild – purr. The sound may be very loud or so soft as to be inaudible to the human ear. Kittens may begin to purr a few days after birth. In all animals, vocal sounds come from vibrations of the vocal cords, which are in the voice box in the throat. No one knows exactly how the cat uses these to produce purring nor why no other kind of animal purrs. In addition to purring, cats make several different kinds of sounds, including meowing, chirping, hissing, yowling, and even growling.

Limbs

The legs appear short when compared with the length of the body, but they are powerful. Strong muscles produce instant power for leaping upon prey or for great bursts of speed to catch prey on the run. The sharp angles of the knee and 'heel' of the hind legs also contribute to the power for sudden sprints, for climbing and for jumping. The front legs are also powerful and extremely flexible. A cat can stretch its forelegs wide apart to hug the body of an enemy and hold it close. The forepaws can be tucked under the chest when the animal crouches, can be curved around the head when the animal washes behind the ears, and can be turned palm up for washing under and between the toes. Most cats have five toes in the forepaws and four in the hind paws. Some domestic cats, especially in the north-eastern USA, have extra toes on the inner sides of the front feet or of all feet. This oddity, called polydactylism, is an inherited dominant trait. Cats with this trait are prized by many owners.

Movement

Perhaps among the most striking things about a cat are its litheness and grace of movement and the amazing flexibility of its body. It can with ease roll up into a ball, double up sideways, stretch the back into almost a straight line, or arch it until the front and back legs are only a few inches apart. It can turn its body easily so that its tongue can reach the fur on the centre of its back for grooming.

Spaying

Female cats come into heat repeatedly and may become nervous or ill-tempered and lose weight if not permitted to mate. Males wander restlessly, cry loudly to get out, and spray strong-smelling urine about the premises. To prevent the birth of undesired kittens, females may be spayed after 5 or 6 months of age. Males may be neutered after 8–10 months to keep them from spraying or wandering. Neutered cats may need to have their food intake reduced to keep them from gaining weight.

Dog

Size

While the Irish wolfhound, for example, stands about 80 cm high at the top of the shoulders (withers), the diminutive Chihuahua struggles to reach 15 cm. The colour of a dog's coat, and the hair cover, also ranges widely, even within a breed. Three major structures determine the shape of a dog: the head, the body and the legs.

Head

There are two basic head shapes – a narrow skull with a long face and a wide skull with a short face – plus several intermediate head shapes. Long-faced dogs, such as the German shepherd and the cocker spaniel, may have jaws around 20 cm long. By contrast, the nose of small-faced dogs, such as the Pekingese and the pug, may be only 2–3 cm from the eyes.

Teeth   Dogs have 42 teeth. Six pairs of sharp incisor teeth are in front of the mouth, flanked by two pairs of large canine teeth. The other teeth are premolars and molars. The incisors and the canines are very important because the dog bites and tears at its food with these teeth.

Nose   Air breathed in through the dog's nose passes on its way to the lungs through the two nasal cavities behind the nose. These cavities are lined by a mucous membrane containing many nerve endings stimulated by odours. Smell is the dog's most acute sense. A dog continually sniffs the air, the ground and nearby objects to learn what is happening around it. The indentation in the dog's forehead just above eye level is called the stop. The stop in some dogs is deeper than that in others.

Tongue   The fairly thin tongue of the dog is used mainly for guiding food to the throat, for licking the coat clean, and for perspiration. When a dog is overheated, it cools off by hanging its tongue out and panting. As it pants, the evaporation of perspiration from its tongue cools the animal. The dog also sweats through the pads on its paws and, to a lesser extent, through its skin.

Ears   A dog's ears either stick up or hang down. The earliest dogs prob-ably had erect ears, but the ears began to droop in smaller, later breeds because of excessive ear skin. Dogs have a fine sense of hearing. They can hear sounds at frequencies too high for people to hear. This is why dogs can respond to 'silent' whistles.

Eyes   Each eye of a dog has three eyelids, the main upper and lower lids and a third lid hidden between them in the inner corner of the eye. The third eyelid can sweep across the transparent cornea of the eye and clean it like a windscreen wiper.

Body

The head and body of a dog are connected by its neck. The neck may be long or short, depending on the size of the seven bones that support it. The length of the vocal cords in the neck is a factor influencing the pitch and loudness of a dog's voice – its barks, grunts and howls.

The body may be covered with straight or with wavy hair. Hair shafts emerge from tiny follicles in the skin. The shafts are connected to tiny muscles that cause the dog's hair to stand up, or bristle, when they contract.

During times of stress, a dog raises its hackles – the hair along the neck and spine. Special sensory hairs called whiskers are near the nose, but their usefulness is doubtful because a dog rarely relies on the sense of touch.

Limbs

The front legs and back legs of a dog are also called the forelimbs and hind limbs, respectively. A dog uses its legs for movement, for scratching, and, in some breeds, for digging.

Each of the forelimbs is connected to the body by a long, narrow scapula, or shoulder blade. Its lower part, in turn, forms a shoulder joint with the humerus, the upper forelimb bone. The lower forelimb bones, the radius and the ulna, are fused at two points and act as a single bone.

The foot, or paw, has five toes. One of them – the dewclaw – is too high to be of any use. It is a vestigial part and is often surgically removed from puppies. The toes of the foot are composed of a number of bones. A toenail, or claw, emerges from the end of each toe. The foot also has cushiony pads for each toe and two larger pads farther up the paw. Dogs perspire through their pads.

Each of the two hind limbs is connected to the body at the pelvic bone. The upper portion of the femur, or thighbone, fits into a socket in the pelvic bone to form the hip joint. The tibia and the fibula are beneath. They make up the lower thigh. The joint where their upper portions link with the femur is called the stifle. The joint where their lower portions link with the foot bones of the hind limbs is called the hock. Like the forefeet, the hind feet have pads and four functional toes, although a dewclaw is sometimes present.

Risks to human health associated with keeping cats and dogs

The potential risks to human health of keeping pets in general were discussed in chapter 1. Specific risks applicable to keeping cats and dogs are outlined below. These include:

- Allergies.
- Zoonotic transfer of disease.
- Injuries and infections from bites and scratches.

Allergies

Allergic symptoms resulting from contact with cat and dog hair (dander) can range from acute rhinitis and lacrimation to urticarial skin eruptions. More serious effects, including eczema and asthma, have also been reported. The cat flea, *Ctenocephalides felis*, has been shown to be responsible for papular urticaria in humans (Naimer *et al.*, 2002).

Contact dermatitis may erupt in some owners after contact with commercially available flea collars, especially if the collar is wet. Allergic symptoms may prove difficult to treat because of the continuing presence of the stimulus. It is not unusual for owners to self-medicate with antihistamines and then allow the family pet to sleep on their bed at night! Getting people to change this habit can be extremely difficult.

Simple allergic reactions may be treated symptomatically with calamine lotion, topical corticosteroids, oral antihistamines or antibiotics. Eliminating the source of infestation is of prime importance in preventing reinfection. There is some evidence that installing air cleaners in the homes of adult asthma patients who are sensitised and exposed to cats and/or dogs may be beneficial (Francis *et al.*, 2003).

Parents are sometimes wary of keeping pets when they have a new baby, and indeed domestic cats are often said to be particularly implicated in childhood allergies. However, research has suggested that children who are exposed to two or more cats and dogs in their first year of life have a reduced risk of allergy. It could lead to boys having better lung function. The study was carried out by scientists at the Medical College of Georgia in Augusta, USA, and the Henry Ford Health System in Detroit, Michigan, USA, and involved 473 children (241 girls and 232 boys), some of whom had pets until they were about 7 years old (Henry Ford Health System Report, 2002).

Zoonotic diseases in cats and dogs

General signs and symptoms of disease

Cats and dogs suffering from disease or acting as a pool of infection are potentially a risk to human health. As with all companion animals, identifying disease in cats and dogs may often depend on astute observation by the owner. The following signs may indicate all is not well:

- Eating or drinking less than normal.
- Restless or lethargic, or a crouched, huddled appearance.
- Coat that looks dull or is soiled or itchy.
- Discharge from the eyes, ears or nose.

- Soiling around the vent with urine or feces.
- Feces abnormal in colour or texture.
- More or less urine being produced, or urine unusual in colour.
- Offensive odour from the ears, mouth or vent.
- Difficulty in eating, drinking or moving.
- Difficulty in breathing or raspy noises from the chest.
- Visible signs of stress.

It is important that owners are vigilant for the benefit of not only their animals' welfare but to minimise any risk to human health.

In this section the main cat and dog diseases that have potentially important implications for human health are discussed in some detail. As described in chapter 1, zoonoses are infectious animal-associated diseases that may be transmitted to humans from vertebrate animals by a variety of routes.

Ectoparasitic infection

The sources of ectoparasitic infection include fleas, lice, mites and ticks.

Fleas

Causative organism　There are about 2000 species of flea that exist on every continent on the globe. They are wingless, with laterally compressed bodies from 1.5 to 4 mm in length. The thick and chitinous covering is dark brown; some species have large or simple eyes. The long legs are strong and adapted to leaping: the flea can jump more than 100 times its own body length. Cat and dog fleas (*Ctenocephalides felis* and *C. canis*) are even more impressive, being able to execute a leap from standing of up to 33 cm. More than one species of flea may be present on an animal. These variants are not identical in habit, action or antigen. At any one time, *C. felis*, *C. canis* or *Pulex irritans* (the human flea) may be dominant on a dog. Studies have shown that *C. felis* is most common on dogs in London (Beresford-Jones, 1981) and Denmark (Guzman, 1984); *C. canis* is more prevalent in Dublin (Baker and Mulcahy, 1986). A 1999 survey of dogs in the London area found that almost half were infested mostly with the cat flea, double the number found in a similar survey in 1981. Cat fleas on cats had increased from 56% to 63% over the same period. Cat fleas are much less host-specific than dog fleas but tend to be the only species found on cats. Both cats and dogs pick up fleas from rabbits, hedgehogs and squirrels, but these fleas tend to be host-specific and do not remain on the animal for long.

Life cycle The flea life cycle is illustrated in Figure 13.1. Adult fleas must obtain a blood meal to become sexually mature and reproduce. At the anterior end of their body, fleas have two pairs of palps to feel the skin surface and two lance-like blades bearing rows of 'teeth' with which they can puncture the skin. Once punctured, saliva is injected to prevent blood-clotting, and it is this saliva that causes hypersensitivity in animals. The female flea lays up to 20 eggs at one time and 400–500 eggs over a lifetime. The oval, glistening ova measure about 0.5 mm and are pearly white in colour; they are dropped in dust or dirt or deposited directly on the host. As the eggs are not sticky, they soon drop off the host. The rate of development varies greatly, and depends on the ambient humidity and temperature. The creamy yellow-coloured larvae may hatch in 2–16 days. The main source of dried blood that is necessary for larval development is the adult parasites' feces, often present on pets' bedding. In fact, over 99% of fleas live in the bedding and other soft furnishings around the house. Comfortable furnishings, increased living temperatures, and draught-free conditions in modern houses offer suitable conditions for the development of virulent strains. Fleas breed in warm weather, and the pupae hatch simultaneously when stimulated by vibration (which is good news for fleas, indicating that there is a meal about). So, on return from holiday, a room that has been the favoured

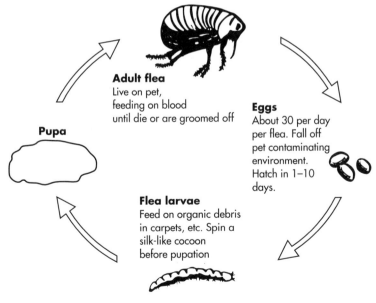

Adult flea
Live on pet,
feeding on blood
until die or are groomed off

Eggs
About 30 per day
per flea. Fall off
pet contaminating
environment.
Hatch in 1–10
days.

Pupa

Flea larvae
Feed on organic debris
in carpets, etc. Spin a
silk-like cocoon
before pupation

Figure 13.1 The flea life cycle.

snoozing place for pets can suddenly appear to be alive with infestation (Williamson, 1995). There is evidence that some fleas are developing increasing resistance to the common organophosphate anti-flea preparations. Even non-pet-owning households can become infected as a result of people unwittingly transferring the insect's eggs after patting a neighbour's pet. Fleas may also be obtained from hedgehogs, except in New Zealand, where the species of hedgehog present is parasite-free.

Signs and symptoms of flea infestation   Figure 13.2 shows the results of flea infestation in a cat. The most usual clinical signs for the presence of fleas include:

- Alopecia.
- Bloody inflammation and other skin conditions brought on by hypersensitivity to the flea saliva during warm weather and the animal's response.
- Excessive grooming.
- Pruritis.
- Scratching.
- Visual evidence (e.g. fleas and flea feces in the fur).

 Zoonotic risk   Fleas can cause a range of allergies and skin conditions (including eczema) in humans. When infestation gets out of control,

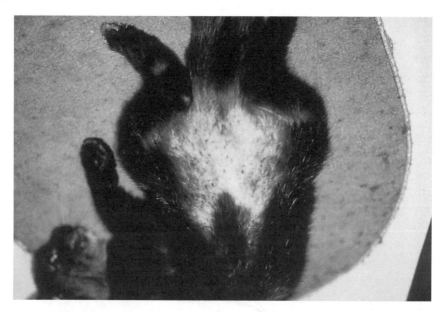

Figure 13.2   Flea infestation on a cat. (Courtesy of the University of Glasgow Veterinary School.)

hungry fleas may even bite pet owners. Further, fleas can often act as intermediaries in endoparasitic life cycles, facilitating the transfer of worm infestation between animals.

Lice

Causative organism   These small wingless insects lay eggs on the host body and these become glued to a hair or feather. The emergent louse is a miniature form of the adult.

Two distinct families of louse exist on domestic animals. The Siphunculata have compressed heads and strong claws with pointed sucking mouth parts. The Mallophaga have mouthparts that comprise a set of mandibles to facilitate biting.

Signs and symptoms   Symptoms include skin conditions and allergic responses. Important species in the cat and dog include a sucking louse (*Linognathus setosus*) and a biting louse (*Trichodectes canis*). The latter acts as an intermediary in the life cycle of *Dipylidium caninum*, the canine tapeworm.

Treatment   Treatment is by application of a suitable insecticide and associated procedures.

Zoonotic risks   They are generally host-specific, so cannot live for longer than a few days if transferred to humans. Nevertheless, their appearance can cause considerable anxiety and requests for help from pharmacy staff in whispered tones.

Mites

Causative organism   Demodex mites in small quantities are normal inhabitants of dog skin. Generalised demodicosis occurs when the immune system is compromised, allowing the mites to multiply and cause demodectic mange. This condition is most likely to occur in puppies or older dogs with an underlying problem such as malnutrition, diabetes or hypothyroidism.

Signs and symptoms   The canine strain of the mite *Sarcoptes scabei* causes the highly contagious sarcoptic mange, characterised by scaling, crust formation and hair loss. It is extremely uncomfortable and stressful for the infested animal. *Notoedres cati* from the cat (and *S. equi* from the horse) can occasionally affect humans too. The condition produced in humans has been termed 'Cavalryman's itch'.

Treatment   Treatment of sarcoptic mange is similar to that for demodectic mange described above, except that the Amitraz solution is half the strength, i.e. 0.025%. The environment should also be treated.

Zoonotic risks   The mite may be transferred to humans, causing scabies, and care should be taken while treating an infected animal. The disease usually appears on the skin between the fingers, in the groin or below the breasts, but it may spread to other sites. Eggs deposited in the epidermis hatch after 3–4 days and the resulting larvae provoke intense irritation. Treatment is with topical benzyl benzoate, benzyl hexachloride or monosulfiram.

Ticks

Causative organisms   Ticks may be seen in dogs that have visited commercial kennels or have been exercised in rural settings. They are subject to infestation with dog ticks (*Ixodes canisuga*) and hedgehog ticks (*I. hexagonus*).

Signs and symptoms   The reaction to tick bites is similar to the reaction to other ectoparasites.

Treatment   Usually involves physical removal and application of an organophosphate acaricide (see below).

Zoonotic risks   There is an important zoonotic implication from Lyme disease from dogs infected with ticks.

Lyme disease

Lyme disease is a tick-borne disease, endemic to the northern states of the USA but also present in the UK, particularly in the southern counties of England (Goddard, 1997).

Causative organism   It is caused by the spirochaete *Borrelia burgdorferi*, of which at least 10 genospecies are known. Between 10 and 20% of sheep in the New Forest area of southern England are infected with *B. garinii*. This is the most widely occurring of the four variants found in the UK.

Life cycle   The disease is transmitted to humans through the bite of infected sheep ticks: *Ixodes ricinus* in Europe, *I. scapularis* (formerly called *I. dammini*) in the eastern USA and *I. pacificus* in the western USA. The sheep tick feeds on a variety of wildlife, including mice, voles, hedgehogs, hares, blackbirds, deer, rabbits and rodents. Pheasants are thought to be particularly important in the epidemiology of Lyme disease in the UK. In England, approximately 20 million farm-reared pheasants are released into woodlands each year to increase numbers for shooting. In some areas, they may provide a larger reservoir of infection than other species. Dogs can also be infected and act as carriers for ticks.

   I. ricinus has three development stages: larva, nymph and adult. Apart from the adult male, each life stage feeds once on a host. The two motile stages must attach to a host, feed, and fall off before transforming into the next stage. If no blood-providing host is available, the ticks perish; therefore, an important aspect of a successful life cycle is host availability and diversity. The entire life cycle may extend over 2–3 years, depending on the geographic region. Ticks ingest *Borrelia* during their blood meals on an infected animal. The bacterium migrates from the gut to the salivary glands. After moulting to the next development stage, the tick may transmit the bacterium to another animal when it next feeds.

Signs and symptoms   Typically, redness of skin expands from the bite area, often producing a large erythematous ring within 3 days to several weeks; smaller rings may appear on other parts of the body and last for several days. Dogs that are affected may show fever and arthritis-like symptoms.

Zoonotic risk   The risk of humans developing Lyme disease after being bitten by an infected tick has been estimated at around 20%; thus, pet owners should be advised to take care when walking in areas likely to harbour ticks. The disease may be long-term, with symptoms ranging from mild to severely debilitating (possibly including chronic fatigue syndrome). Cardiac, neurological and joint involvement may also develop.

   From personal experience, the symptom most frequently presented in the pharmacy is a swelling of the elbow joint. This is often treated with a non-steroidal anti-inflammatory agent, but does not improve. Patients seek a pharmacist's opinion as to what can be done about this annoying condition when a cortisone injection has been suggested by the physician. The first thing to ascertain is whether the person has been in an environment where they could have been bitten by a tick. Typically, this might be while exercising a dog in long grass in the vicinity of wild deer, perhaps in a large parkland area. The patient may be unaware that a bite has been inflicted. A positive response would lead one to suspect Lyme disease. Early-stage Lyme disease responds well to oral antibiotics, including doxycycline and amoxicillin, which are generally prescribed for 2–3 weeks. Later-stage disease may be more difficult to treat, and the choice of drugs and treatment is the subject of considerable discussion. Tetracycline and ampicillin have been used in dogs, with topical organophosphate lotions.

A vaccine is available to guard against the US strains of *Borrelia* but, due to considerable genetic divergence, no such prophylactic exists in Europe.

Treatment of ectoparasite infestation in cats and dogs

Pet owners who seek advice from pharmacists about flea infestation should be advised that cats act as a greater source of infection than dogs. In some cases, a cat living in the same household as a dog may provide a reservoir of fleas for the latter, but is apparently unaffected itself.

General guidelines Initially, the animal should be clipped and washed with an insecticidal shampoo to remove debris and clean up the animal's hair coat. Ticks should be removed. A topical agent should then be applied. Sprays are the most popular form, probably because of their ease of use; powders are the second preference of animal owners. Flea collars are useful but, whilst providing insecticidal protection, they can invoke an allergic reaction due to continual contact with the skin. The ingredients are mainly based on pyrethrum and permethrin, although there are also some 'natural' products (e.g. oil of citronella and oil of lime). Care must be taken to avoid toxicity with pregnant and nursing bitches. Many agents should not be used on young kittens and puppies. Most owners recognise the importance of minimising the risk of transfer of diseases between animals. As a result, insecticidal products have become very popular, and a wide range of different formulations are available, including some herbal varieties. Animals should be treated according to the instructions on the product chosen. To obtain effective flea control, an animal and its surroundings must be treated. Careful attention should be given to an animal's bedding, which may need to be destroyed to prevent reinfection.

For some products it is required that owners should not be in close contact with their animal for 6–8 hours and, more specifically, should not allow it to sleep on their bed.

Types of ectoparasiticides

A large number of ectoparasiticides are available for treating cats and dogs.

There are two main groups of ectoparasiticides, characterised by their route of action. They should not be used concurrently.

Topical preparations include collars, dips, lotions, powders, sprays and washes.

Systemic parasiticides are administered orally e.g. Lufenuron suspension for cats (Program, Novartis) or by subcutaneous injection e.g. Lufenuron Injectable (10 mg/kg for cats; Program, Novartis). They are also available as a 'pour-on', a liquid that is poured along the dorsal midline of the animal, or as a 'spot-on', a liquid applied in a small amount to an area on the head or back. Active material is absorbed through the skin and passes into the circulation and then into the ectoparasite. Most of these preparations for companion animal use are prescription-only medicines. This systemic group includes the growth regulators (see below).

The choice between the above types of preparation depends on the wishes of the animal owner, the circumstances, the species and breed of animal, and environmental considerations. The sections below discuss the main ectoparasiticides available on the UK market.

Amitraz   Chemically, amitraz is an amidine and is used in dips or washes for the elimination of flea, tick and mite infestations. It is a monoamine oxidase inhibitor, and also inhibits insulin release, causing an increased blood glucose level. It is contraindicated in cats or dogs suffering from heat stress, puppies less than 12 weeks old or pregnant and lactating bitches. Amitraz 0.05% solution (Aludex, Intervet) should be applied to dogs as a wash, principally for the treatment of demodectic and sarcoptic mange. The treatment should be repeated every 14 days as recommended by the veterinary surgeon.

Fipronil   Fipronil (Frontline, Merial) is another spot-on chemical interfering with neurotransmission. Adult fleas are killed rapidly before laying eggs. It should not normally be used in dogs less than 10 weeks old or cats less than 12 weeks old. Fipronil also exists as a spray that may be of use in the control of lice and mites.

Imidacloprid Imidacloprid (Advantage, Bayer) is chemically a nitroguanidine. Applied as a spot-on preparation for cats and dogs, it acts by binding to nicotinic acetylcholine receptors in the insect central nervous system, causing an interruption of cholinergic transmission, paralysis and death. The chemical prevents reinfestation for up to four weeks and should not be used on kittens and puppies less than 8 weeks old.

Ivermectin Ivermectin is not authorised for use in cats and dogs in the UK. However, it is administered to cats by subcutaneous injection and to dogs by mouth for the treatment of mites. Collies and collie-cross dogs are reported to have had adverse reactions to this drug.

Organophosphates Concerns over the use of organophosphates has been explained in chapter 3, and they are not used so widely in the UK for domestic animals as they once were. In Australia, New Zealand and the USA many variants still exist.

Dimpylate In liquid form diazinon is used to dip sheep; it is active against blowflies, keds, lice and ticks. In cats and dogs it treats infestation with fleas on cats and fleas and ticks on dogs. It is presented as a collar containing 15% active ingredient by several manufacturers (e.g. Bob Martin, Johnson's, Sherley's) in which form it is classified as a General Sales List (GSL) item. The collar may cause localised skin irritation.

Dichlorvos Nuvan Top (Novartis) combines the organophosphates dichlorvos (0.2%) and fenitrothion (0.8%) as an aerosol, and is classified as a pharmacy and merchant supplies medicine (PML).

Fenthion Fenthion (Tiguvon, Bayer) is available as a spot-on to treat flea infestation on cats and dogs. It should not be used on dogs less than 6 months old or whose body weight is less than 3 kg, or cats less than a year old weighing 2 kg or under. Cats may show some signs of excitement after treatment. The usual restrictions for pregnant animals apply.

Care should be taken not to handle animals within 8 hours of treatment or to allow treated animals to sleep on owners' beds.

Pyrethrins and synthetic pyrethroids

Fenvalerate Fenvalerate (Deosan Flyaway, Fort Dodge) is used to control ticks and fleas on cats and dogs as a spray or dip. Dogs less than

3 months of age, cats less than 6 months as well as pregnant and nursing animals should not be treated with fenvalerate. This product is classified PML (see chapter 4).

Permethrin Permethrin is active against fleas, ticks and possibly lice on cats and dogs. There is a wide range of GSL pour-ons, spot-ons, powders and shampoos and collars available. Cats may become excitable after application. Flea collars may cause localised irritation.

Products include Canovel (Pfizer) spot-on and powder for dogs, Catovel (Pfizer) insecticidal powder for cats, Defencat Insecticidal Foam (Virbac), applied to cats as a ball of foam according to animal's body weight, Vetzyme JDS Insecticidal Shampoo (Seven Seas), and various collars.

Permethrin pour-on and spot-on products should be applied to dogs in the evening and the animals should not be handled for up to 6 hours or allowed to sleep with humans, especially children. Children should not be allowed to play with flea collars impregnated with permethrin.

Pyrethrins Most usually offered in an aerosol or non-aerosol spray, dusting powder, shampoo and even a mousse, pyrethrins are used against fleas and lice on cats and dogs. Pyrethrins extracted from pyrethrum flowers contain about 25% pyrethroids. Many products also contain piperonyl butoxide, with which pyrethrins are synergistic. Puppies and kittens below 12 weeks old or pregnant and nursing animals should not be treated with pyrethrins. Examples include Canovel Insecticidal Spray (Pfizer), Cat Flea Dusting Powder and Non-aerosol Spray (Johnson's) and Flea Killing Mousse (Bob Martin).

Pyrethrins (extracted from pyrethrum flowers) and synthetic pyrethroids act on the sodium channels of the parasites' nerve axons, causing initial excitement, then paralysis and death. Synthetic pyrethroids are often present in formulations as mixtures of *cis* and *trans* isomers. For example, in a spot-on the proportion of *cis* to *trans* might be 80 : 20, in a shampoo and collar 40 : 60 and in a powder 75 : 25.

A selection of topical ectoparasiticides is shown in Table 13.1.

Growth regulators

Lufenuron Lufenuron is a prescription-only insect growth regulator. It does not kill the parasite directly but interferes with its ability to

Table 13.1 Selection of topical ectoparasiticides for cats and dogs (not exhaustive)

Ectoparasiticides	Legal	Parasite	Animal	Manufacturer
Powders				
Permethrin	GSL	Fleas, ticks, possibly lice	Cats and dogs	BHB Pfizer[a] Schering-Plough Sinclair
Pyrethrins (with piperonyl butoxide)	GSL	Fleas and lice	Cats and dogs	Bob Martin
Shampoos				
Permethrin	GSL	Fleas, ticks, possibly lice	Dogs	Pfizer Vetzyme (Seven Seas) Virbac
	GSL	Fleas, ticks, possibly lice	Cats and dogs	BHB Johnson's
Pyrethrins (with piperonyl butoxide)	GSL	Fleas and lice	Dogs	Bob Martin
Others				
Foam	GSL	Fleas and ticks, possibly lice	Cats	Virbac
Mousse	GSL	Fleas and lice	Cats	Bob Martin
Flea collars				
Carbaril	GSL	Fleas	Cats and dogs	Johnson's Secto (Sinclair)
Dimpylate (Diazinon)	GSL	Fleas	Cats	Armitage Bob Martin Johnson's Virbac
	GSL	Fleas and ticks Ticks	Dogs	Armitage Bob Martin Johnson's Sherley's Virbac

(continued)

Table 13.1 *Continued*

Ectoparasiticides	Legal	Parasite	Animal	Manufacturer
Dimpylate and EFO esters	GSL	Fleas and ticks	Cats and dogs	Pfizer[a]
Permethrin	GSL	Fleas, ticks, lice	Cats	Sherley's Sinclair Virbac[a]
	GSL	Fleas, ticks, lice	Dogs	Virbac
Permethrin + EFOs	GSL	Fleas, ticks, lice	Cats and dogs	Virbac[a]
Pour-on and spot-on				
Fenthion	POM	Fleas	Cats and dogs	Bayer
Fipronil	POM	Fleas, ticks, lice and mites	Cats and dogs	Merial
Permethrin	GSL	Fleas, ticks, lice	Dogs	Bob Martin Pfizer Schering-Plough
Sprays				
Dichlorvos and fenitrothion	PML	Fleas	Cats and dogs	Novartis
Fenvalerate	PML	Fleas and ticks	Cats and dogs	Fort Dodge
Fipronil 0.25%	POM	Fleas, ticks and possibly other ectoparasites	Cats and dogs	Merial
Pyrethrins	GSL	Fleas and lice	Cats and dogs	Johnson's
	GSL	Fleas and lice	Dogs	Pfizer

[a] denotes separate versions available for cats and dogs

develop. The drug acts mainly on immature stages and is therefore unsuitable for the rapid removal of a large infestation, for which reason it may be initially combined with other parasiticides. Lufenuron accumulates in fat tissue, allowing subsequent slow release. Fleas ingest the drug with blood and transfer it to their eggs, where it interferes with the formation of chitin structures and larval development. No viable eggs are produced 24 hours after administration. Dogs are given lufenuron orally by addition to the feed (10 mg/kg) and to cats by subcutaneous injection or addition to the feed (Program, Novartis). The dose for cats is dependent on body weight. The drug should not be given to unweaned animals.

Methoprene Methoprene is another insect growth regulator. This juvenile hormone analogue mimics the activity of naturally occurring hormones and prevents metamorphosis from the larva to the adult stage. In the UK it is included in several sprays for the environmental control of ectoparasites (see Table 13.2). The drug is available in flea collars in Australia and New Zealand.

Combined ectoparasiticides There is just one combined ectoparasiticide for cats and dogs on the UK market (see the PML product 'Nuvan Top' (Novartis) under Organophosphates, above). In Australia and New Zealand there are several products available for both working dogs and pets.

Environmental procedures for dealing with infestation

Household furnishings should be treated as if they are suspected of being infested. Box 13.1 can act as a framework.

A sample of suitable environmental products is given in Table 13.2 and pictured in Figure 13.3.

Endoparasitic infection in cats and dogs

Endoparasitic infection in farm animals (cattle, sheep and pigs) has important welfare implications and can lead to economic loss. In the companion animal, public health issues are also involved. Worm species are usually specific to an animal species, and many different species can infest one animal at the same time.

There are two main groups of endoparasites: the roundworms or nematodes and the tapeworms or cestodes. Flukes are also a problem in

Table 13.2 Selection of environmental parasiticides (not exhaustive)

Contents	Formulation	Trade name	Manufacturer
Amitraz	Liquid conc. for dilution, spray (mites)	Taktic Buildings Spray	Intervet
Bioallethrin + methoprene + permethrin	Spray	Arrest	Arnolds
Bioallethrin + permethrin	Aerosol spray	Defest II	Sherley's
Malathion	Solution	Ban Mite	Johnson's
Methoprene + permethrin	Aerosol spray	Acclaim Plus	Ceva
Methoprene + piperonyl + permethrin	Aerosol spray	Canovel Pet Bedding & Household Spray	Pfizer
Permethrin	Powder (carpets)	Carpet Flea Guard	Johnson's
Permethrin	Powder	Rug-de-Bug	Sherley's
Permethrin + pyrethrins	Aerosol spray	Household Flea Spray	Johnson's
Pyrethrins	Solution	Alfadex	Novartis

Box 13.1 Measures to eliminate environmental infestation

- Thoroughly vacuum the house with a new dust bag in place, ensuring thorough disposal afterwards. Concentrate on those areas where fleas and photophobic larvae are known to hide (e.g. dusty corners, under furniture, and between sofa cushions).
- If necessary, wash carpets. This will raise the carpet's pile, facilitating more complete penetration of the insecticidal product.
- Apply a suitable anti-flea spray to all floors, carpets and indoor rugs.
- Do not vacuum the house for at least 7–10 days after application of the insecticidal product.
- Repeat the procedure twice, at two-weekly intervals; subsequent once-monthly application should be continued for as long as necessary.
- Repeat the procedure more frequently in warm weather, and alternate products to prevent resistance developing.
- If severe infestation is present, it may be necessary to obtain help from local Environmental Health Safety Officers.

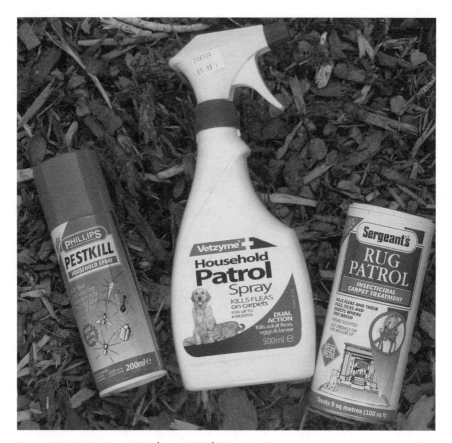

Figure 13.3   Environmental parasiticide treatments.

farm animals, but are rarely seen in companion animals, except perhaps sheep dogs.

Roundworms

Roundworms usually have a direct life cycle, with a free-living development phase in the animal environment, a parasitic development phase, and an adult phase in the host. Infection of the host generally occurs by ingestion of the larval stage of the parasite. Typical roundworm life cycles in the cat and dog are illustrated in Figures 13.4 and 13.5.

Strongyloidiasis   This is a chronic roundworm infection transmitted by direct contact with feces (Bell *et al.*, 1988).

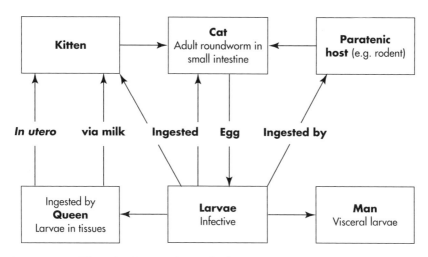

Figure 13.4   Life cycle of a roundworm (cat).

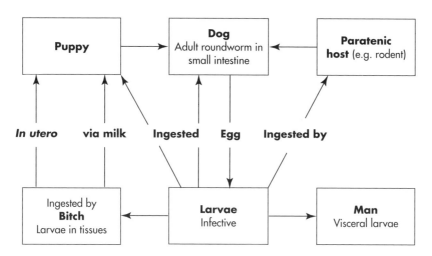

Figure 13.5   Life cycle of a roundworm (dog).

Causative organisms   The causative agents are *Strongyloides sterco-ralis cata* (affecting dogs) and *S. fuellebotni* (affecting non-human primates). The helminth is usually sited in the duodenum, from where eggs are shed in the feces; they later develop into larvae. Young cats and dogs have thin skins that allow large quantities of larvae to penetrate.

Signs and symptoms These include skin inflammation and pruritis at the site of entry, followed by bronchial symptoms, fever, diarrhoea and abdominal pain. In animals there is often severe dermatitis accompanied by coughing and vomiting.

Treatment Both humans (see below) and animals may be treated with tiabendazole or its more recent derivatives.

Zoonotic risk Humans may be infected by penetration of larvae. On entering the body, they migrate to the lungs and gastrointestinal tract.

Toxocariasis

Causative organisms There are several orders of roundworm, but the one that concerns the domestic animal most is from the order Ascaridida. Ascarids are amongst the largest and most common of nematodes, and the adults are host-specific: *Toxocara canis* infects dogs, *Toxocara cati* infects cats and *Parascaris equorum* infects horses. *Ascaris suum* infection, specific to pigs, is considered only occasionally to be a zoonosis. Dogs and cats also share a second ascarid, *Toxocara leonina*. *Toxocara cati* has a similar life cycle to *T. canis*, but is rarely involved in human disease. Over 80% of puppies under 1 year old are thought to be infected with *T. canis*. Most infection is acquired pre-natally from the mother; some animals are infected through maternal milk. About 2% of the UK's total human population and 15% of dog breeders are thought to be seropositive. Figure 13.6 shows a dog intestine infected with *T. canis*.

　　T. cati is the most common roundworm of cats. It has a wide geographical distribution, and adult forms have been recorded in man.

Life cycle Effective control of *T. canis* depends upon a proper under-standing of its highly complex life cycle. Eggs excreted in feces (up to 15 000 eggs/g puppy feces) enter the animal after a period of matura-tion in the soil. Survival of the eggs depends upon weather conditions. Dry conditions cause desiccation; in moist humid climates, however, the eggs can remain viable for several years. After becoming infective (usually within about 2–6 weeks) and their ingestion, the eggs hatch in the small intestine. In puppies less than 5 weeks old, second-stage larvae penetrate the intestine wall to enter the blood vessels, migrating through the liver, lungs and kidneys to the trachea, where a third larval stage develops. These can be coughed up and swallowed, returning to the small intestine and stomach. The adult parasite then develops in the

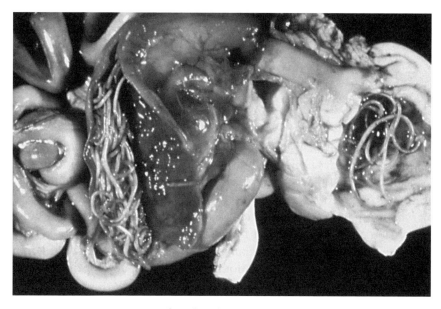

Figure 13.6 Dog intestine infested with *T canis*. (Courtesy of the University of Glasgow Veterinary School.)

intestine 3–6 weeks after ingestion of the eggs. Any larvae excreted by the puppies may mature in the bitch once ingested.

In older dogs, development ceases at the second larval stage, and these larvae undergo somatic migration into the tissues where they persist for long periods. These dormant larvae reactivate during pregnancy, possibly due to hormonal changes, and migrate to the placenta to mature in the unborn puppies. Perinatal transmission appears to be highly efficient, as almost all puppies are infected by the time of whelping.

The life cycle of *T. cati* is similar to that of *T. canis*, except there is no placental transfer of larvae.

Zoonotic risk

- Dogs. Although puppies and nursing bitches are an important source of human infection, a more significant public health risk comes from embryonated *Toxocara* eggs in the soil. Freshly voided feces are not a problem because the eggs need 14–21 days under optimal conditions to become infective. The animals may develop substantial worm burdens and pass large numbers of eggs in their feces, leading to heavy contamination, especially in densely populated urban areas where dog owners walk their pets in public areas. In the UK, a quarter of soil samples have been shown to contain eggs of

T. canis (Borg and Woodruff, 1974). In central USA, 16% of samples were positive (Paul, 1988). Humans are infected when eggs from contaminated soil and grass are ingested.

- Cats. Although there is less chance of human infection from cat worms than from dog worms, the habit of cats burying their feces can cause children to acquire infections from contaminated soil; sandpits may also be a source of infection.

Human infection   This is frequently subclinical. The disease has two forms: visceral larva migrans affects children of 1–4 years of age, who develop fever, asthmatic attacks, acute bronchiolitis, nausea and vomiting, and enlarged liver and spleen; sometimes the heart and central nervous system become involved. Second-stage larvae migrate through the tissues and usually present typically in a young child with a history of pica. The second form, ocular larva migrans, affects older children and occasionally adults. Granulomatous nodules develop in the eye, causing severe ocular inflammation and loss of vision.

Actions to minimise risk of zoonotic infection   The UK Pet Council have stressed that there are only about two new cases of illness annually due to *Toxocara* per million of population (Miles, 1994). There is evidence that people can take active steps to minimise the risk of contracting toxocariasis by regular worming of their pets and 'pooper scooping'. The most recent studies on soil in parks show lower levels of *Toxocara* eggs than previously recorded, and a study conducted through the University of Glasgow's Department of Parasitology, in cooperation with Canine Control Scotland, found considerably reduced incidence of *T. canis* than in previous studies.

Most infections are self-limiting because the host inflammatory response kills many larvae. Products containing diethylcarbamazine and tiabendazole are effective as treatment. Corticosteroids may be used to control allergic symptoms, especially in the eye. Guidelines for the control and prevention of the disease are:

- Worm both young and adult animals routinely (see below).
- Remove and destroy all voided feces ('pooper-scooping').
- Train dogs to defecate in gutters or on ground not used by children.
- Wash the hands after handling animals and before eating food.
- Do not allow nursing bitches to lick children's faces and hands.

Tapeworms

Tapeworms are most numerous in adult dogs and cats, about 10% of animals being infected. Tapeworms require a two-host system: the developmental stages occur in the intermediate host; final development and adult stages occur in the definitive host. Infection is by ingestion, and transmission relates to the carnivorous eating habits of dogs and cats; rabbits, mice, birds, and large herbivores (cattle and sheep) provide for completion of the life cycle. The main vector is the flea, especially in the urban family pet. The main tapeworms in the UK are *Dipylidium caninum* and *Echinococcus granulosus*. A typical tapeworm life cycle is illustrated in Figure 13.7.

Dipylidiasis Definitive hosts for the infective organism of this disease are cats and dogs. The intermediate hosts are the fleas *Ctenocephalides canis* and *C. felis*. Gravid proglottids, the first stage of a complex life cycle, are passed in the pet feces. This permits release of the eggs into the environment, where they are ingested by fleas and lice. Infection of cats and dogs is caused by ingestion of the ectoparasites in which cysticercoids have developed; these further develop into adult worms in the cat or dog gut.

Accidental human ingestion of fleas infected with *Dipylidium caninum* results in the appearance of diarrhoea and abdominal pain; there may also be anal itching, and there is the characteristic appearance of melon-shaped proglottids in the feces. Children are most frequently affected. Prevention is by control of fleas on the animal and regular worming. Treatment of humans is with niclosamide and praziquantel.

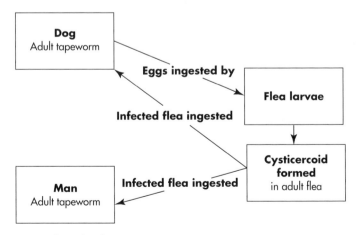

Figure 13.7 Life cycle of a tapeworm.

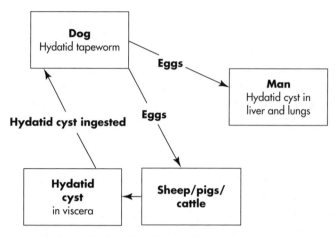

Figure 13.8 The life cycle of a canine hydatid tapeworm.

Echinococcosis (hydatid disease)

Causative organism   Infection is usually caused by the cystic larval form of *Echinococcus granulosus*, the canine tapeworm. Depending on the intermediate host, the bacterium is further differentiated into *E. granulosus granulosus* (sheep and cattle) and *E. granulosus equinus* (horses). Other echinococcal species (e.g. *E. multilocularis*, *E. oligarthus* and *E. vogeli*) are restricted to certain geographical regions. *E. granulosus* is present throughout most of the world in communities where humans, grazing animals and carnivores live in close association; two exceptions are Iceland and Ireland. It is endemic in mid- and south Wales, where the proportion of infected animals is 37% and 15%, respectively in sheep and 26% and 12%, respectively in dogs. In the Western Isles of Scotland, studies have shown that 20% of sheep and 12% dogs are affected. *E. granulosus* is a cestode 3–9 mm in length, with three or four proglottids. The terminal segment becomes gravid and is the broadest and longest. Adult worms may be found in the intestines of dogs, foxes, dingoes and wolves as a result of eating raw offal.

Life cycle   Adult tapeworms shed eggs that pass in the feces of the primary host, often a sheepdog, about 6 weeks after infection (Figure 13.8). Ungulates and humans are infected from these feces by ingestion of eggs that contaminate the environment, dog hairs, or growing vegetables. The larval forms hatch out in the intestine and migrate to the lungs, liver or other organs, via the bloodstream. The embryo grows into a large vesicle 5–10 cm or more in diameter (the echinococcus or hydatid cyst). The cyst comprises an inner germinal layer, which may burst to form daughter cysts, and an outer laminated cyst wall, which may calcify. Eventually, this will interfere with body function. If it ruptures suddenly, instantaneous death can occur or further cysts may develop.

E. granulosus equinus infection is common in hunt kennels throughout the UK, but seems to be of low human pathogenicity for hydatid disease. Apart from the risk to humans, hydatidosis causes condemnation of offal, especially liver and lungs, causing financial loss to the meat industry.

Treatment/prophylaxis   Control begins with education of farmers and their families and workers on the maintenance of strict hygiene. Several other measures are possible:

- Routine worming every 3 months to prevent infection of pastures by tapeworm eggs.
- Denial of access by dogs to infected offal.
- Burning or burying of carcasses, although this may not be possible for hill farmers in winter months.

 Zoonotic risk   Symptoms in humans depend on the site of the cyst and its pressure on surrounding tissues. Commonly, liver cysts cause abdominal pain and sometimes jaundice. Lung cysts cause chest pain, cough and secondary infection. The majority of infected humans are more than 25 years of age. The cysts are removed surgically in humans, although mebendazole and albendazole may be useful.

Other types of worms

Hookworm   Other possible, but extremely rare, sources of helminth infection in the UK include the dog hookworm (*Ancyclostoma caninum* and *A. braziliense*), found in the intestine of cats, dogs and various other carnivores. It is responsible for cutaneous larva migrans (ancylostomiasis).

Human infection results from direct skin contact with larvae in areas contaminated with animal feces. The condition is often asymptomatic, although self-limiting pustular skin eruptions may occur.

The following endoparasitic diseases are included in this section for convenience but do not have zoonotic implications

Heartworm   Dirofilariasis due to infection with the dog heartworm, *Dirofilaris immitis*, is restricted to warmer climates. If the climate warms in the southern UK, it could occur here in the future. The adult worm resides in the pulmonary artery and the right ventricle of its canine host. Mosquitoes are involved in the life cycle. Pulmonary symptoms are extremely rare; the disease is usually self-limiting.

Lungworm Infection with *Olerus, Angiostrongylus* and *Aelurostrongylus* may lead to a persistent husky cough.

Treatment and prophylaxis of endoparasitic infestation

General guidelines Anthelmintics can be used to eliminate adult parasites from the intestine or to kill larvae in the tissues and break the life cycle.

In roundworm infection, piperazine is usually the drug of choice: it is well tolerated by dogs and cats and can be given to young animals either over a period of five days or as a single dose. Adult worms in lactating bitches and puppies are central to the parasite's life cycle. Therefore, an effective control measure is to treat lactating bitches, and then the puppies until 3 months of age, to eliminate the successive waves of prenatal transmission, transmammary transfer of larvae, and the ingestion of infective puppy feces. The bitch is wormed from day 45 to day 50 of pregnancy through to day 21 after whelping, with high daily doses of a broad-spectrum preparation (e.g. fenbendazole 50 mg/kg or mebendazole). This kills migrating larvae in the bitch and minimises transmission of infection to the puppies. To control infection adequately, puppies should be treated at 2, 4, 8 and 12 weeks of age; adult dogs should be wormed every 6 months.

Tapeworm infection is often treated with dichlorophen, but new drugs are being developed to offer a broader spectrum of activity. Regular dosing at 3-month intervals is recommended for the treatment of worms in older animals.

Various factors (e.g. resistance, spectrum of effectiveness, safety in young animals, dosage form (tablets, granules, powders, pastes, or liquids) and cost) should be considered when recommending appropriate anthelmintics to pet owners. For maximal effectiveness in eliminating intestinal worms and preventing the excretion of eggs, the correct therapeutic dose of the selected drug should be given at strategic intervals. If there is uncertainty about which type of helminth is present, or if both are likely to be present, dual-purpose wormers should be used (see Tables 13.3 and 13.4). When calculating the dose, it is important that the manufacturer's instructions are followed carefully. Doses are usually based on the animal's weight, and pet owners may require help in estimating the size of their animal.

In addition to the worming procedures outlined above, owners should minimise the chance of zoonotic infestation by the following means:

- Disposing of dog feces and not leaving them to foul public places.
- Grooming their animals and keeping them free from fleas.
- Avoiding direct contact with feces.

Types of endoparasiticides

There are four main groups of endoparasiticides.

- Drugs to treat roundworms and tapeworms.
- Compound endoparasiticides.
- Drugs for other types of worms.
- Drugs for other endoparasites (e.g. protozoa).

The main route of administration is oral, using tablets, granules, liquids or pastes, but indictable and spot-on preparations are also available.

Drugs for roundworms

Benzimidazoles Benzimidazoles disrupt parasite metabolism by binding to rubilin, a protein required for the uptake of nutrients and other functions. Their activity is directly proportional to the duration and amount of blood content and therefore varies with the species and size of animal. Most benzimidazoles are effective against larval and adult roundworms.

Fenbendazole Fenbendazole is active against roundworm adults, larvae and ova and may be used in pregnant and lactating bitches to reduce roundworm burden in puppies. It can also be used against lungworms and tapeworms. Doses for the various applications vary and owners should read the instructions carefully before administering the medicine. PML products available for cats and dogs include oral granules (Granofen, Virbac and Zerofen), an oral suspension (Panacur 2.5% Liquid, Intervet) and an oral paste (Panacur, Intervet). Worming granules for cats and for dogs (Sherley's) are classified as GSL and should not be used in animals under 6 months old.

Mebendazole Mebendazole treats gastrointestinal roundworms, *Echinococcus* and *Taenia* tapeworms in cats and dogs. It is available as tablets or an oral solution (Telmin, Janssen) and is classified PML. Doses for the various applications vary and owners should read the instructions carefully before administering the medicine.

Nitroscanate This is used in dogs for the treatment of roundworms and tapeworms, principally *Dipylidium* and *Taenia*. It has limited effectiveness against *Echinococcus*. It is administered orally at a dose of 50 mg/kg on an empty stomach or after a light meal. GSL tablets are available in 100 and 500 mg (Lopatol, Novartis; Nitroscanate, Millpledge and Troscan, Chanelle). Sherley's One Dose Wormer is available in 100 mg tablets.

Nitroscanate is irritant and tablets should be given whole (i.e. not crushed or broken). Occasionally vomiting may occur.

Piperazine Piperazine is used against roundworms, including *Toxocara*. It may cause vomiting and diarrhoea in high doses. Owners should follow the manufacturer's recommended doses. There is a wide range of GSL tablets and liquid formulations containing piperazine. Examples include Canovel tablets (Pfizer), Easy Round Wormer tablets for puppies and for kittens and Puppy Easy Worm Syrup (Johnson's) and Sherley's Worming Syrup. Sherley's also have a Worming Cream that is administered with an applicator. This oral paste should not be used on kittens and puppies less than 2 weeks old.

Pyrantel Pyrantel, a tetrahydropyrimidine, interferes with parasitic neurotransmission, causing neuromuscular paralysis. It is effective against adult and larval forms of roundworms in dogs. Strongid Paste for Dogs (Pfizer) is a PML product containing pyrantel as an oral paste. It is given in a 16 g metered dose applicator.

Selamectin Selamectin (Stronghold, Pfizer) is effective against roundworms and in heartworm prophylaxis. It is prescribed as a spot-on (6 mg/kg body weight), and should not be given to kittens and puppies less than 6 weeks old, or when the animal's hair is wet.

Children should be kept away from treated animals until the coat has dried.

Note that ivermectin is widely used to treat roundworm and lungworm infestation in farm animals. It is also used for cats and dogs in Australia but not in the UK.

Drugs to treat roundworm infestation are summarised in Table 13.3.

Table 13.3 Selection of roundwormers for cats and dogs (not exhaustive)

Roundworm anthelmintic	Legal	Animals	Trade name	Form	Manufacturer
Fenbendazole	GSL	Cats and dogs	Easy to Use Wormer	Oral granules	Bob Martin
	PML	Cats and dogs	Granofen	Oral granules	Virbac
	PML	Cats and dogs	Panacur 2.5% & 10%	Oral Suspn	Intervet
	PML	Cats and dogs	Panacur	Oral granules	Intervet
	GSL	Cats and dogs	Worming Granules	Oral granules	Sherley's[a]
	PML	Cats and dogs	Zerofen 22%	Granules (add to feed)	Sherley's
Mebendazole (also against tapeworms)	PML	Cats and dogs	Telmin KH	Granules (add to feed)	Janssen
Nitroscanate (also against tapeworms)	GSL	Dogs	All in One Wormer 100 mg & 500 mg	Tablets	Novartis
	GSL	Dogs (up to 6 kg)	Lopatol 100 mg & 500 mg	Film coated tablets	Novartis
	GSL	Dogs	Nitroscanate 500 mg	Tablets	Millpledge
	GSL	Dogs	One Dose Wormer 100 mg & 500 mg	Film coated tablets	Sherley's
	GSL	Dogs	Troscan 100 mg & 500 mg	Film-coated tablets	Chanelle
Piperazine	GSL	Cats and dogs	Canovel/Catovel Palatable Wormer	Tablets 416 mg	Pfizer[a]
	GSL	Kittens (6 weeks +) & puppies (2 weeks +); cats and dogs	Easy Round Wormer	Tablets 104 mg	Johnson's[a]
	GSL	Cats and dogs	Palatable Worming Tablets	Tablets 220 mg	Sherley's
	GSL	Cats and dogs (1.25 kg +)	Piperazine Citrate Worm Tablets	Tablets 500 mg	Loveridge
	GSL	Puppies (up to 4 weeks)	Puppy Easy Wormer Syrup	Oral syrup	Johnson's

(continued)

Table 13.3 Continued

Roundworm anthelmintic	Legal	Animals	Trade name	Form	Manufacturer
	GSL	Cats and dogs (more than 2 weeks and 1.2 kg +)	Roundworm tablets	Tablets 105 mg	Bob Martin's[a]
	GSL	Cats and dogs	Worming Cream	Oral paste	Sherley's
	GSL	Cats and dogs (2 weeks +)	Worming Syrup	Oral syrup	Sherley's
Selamectin	POM	Dogs	Stronghold	Spot-on	Pfizer

[a] Indicates cat and dog versions available

Drugs for tapeworms

Benzimidazoles   See above for the use of fenbendazole and mebendazole.

Nitroscanate   The use of this chemical against *Dipylidium* and *Taenia* and to a lesser extent against *Echinococcus* is discussed above (under Drugs for roundworms).

Dichlorophen   Dichlorophen is effective against *Dipylidium* and *Taenia* and to a lesser extent against *Echinococcus*. The normal dose is 200 mg/kg body weight. It should not be administered to animals less than 6 months old or to those that are pregnant or nursing. There are also varying restrictions on administration to animals with low body weights (read the manufacturer's recommendations). Apart from a generic form of dichlorophen 500 mg tablets BP (Battle, Hayward and Bower), various brands of the drug are available in strengths from 250 to 750 mg (Easy Tape Wormer, Johnson's; Tapeworm tablets, Bob Martin; Vetzyme Veterinary Tapewormer, Seven Seas). The products are all classified GSL.

Praziquantel   Praziquantel is effective against all tapeworms in cats and dogs. It is particularly useful as it kills all forms of *Echinococcus*. The drug works by increasing the porosity of the parasite's tegument to calcium ions, precipitating muscular spasm. Disruption of the tegument renders the tapeworm more susceptible to enzymic action and thus the segments found in the feces are partially digested. Praziquantel is available as 50 mg tablets (Droncit, Bayer) that are GSL, and as an injection (56.8 mg/mL) that may be given subcutaneously or intramuscularly at a dose of 0.1 mL/kg body weight.

Compound wormers   In domestic animals endoparasitic infection is due to a mixture of organisms rather than one or two in isolation. Thus, the administration of a compound wormer would seem to make sense. Combination products in cats and dogs usually have a wide spectrum of control for both roundworms and tapeworms. Most formulations contain dichlorophen and piperazine but other combinations are available. Owners should read manufacturers' instructions for restrictions on use with respect to age and reproductive status.

Some examples are given below.

- Drontal Cat Tablets (Bayer): praziquantel (20 mg), pyrantel (230 mg). Dose: 1 tablet per 4 kg body weight. Concurrent administration of piperazine and use during pregnancy are contraindicated.
- Drontal Plus (Bayer) for dogs: febantel (150 mg), praziquantel (50 mg), pyrantel (144 mg). Dose: 1 tablet per 10 kg body weight. Concurrent administration of piperazine and use during pregnancy are contraindicated. Febantel is a wide-spectrum endoparasiticide used mainly in large animals.
- Dual Wormer (Bob Martin) for cats: dichlorophen (250 mg), piperazine citrate (297 mg).
- Twin Wormer for Dogs (Johnson's): dichlorophen (500 mg), piperazine phosphate (416 mg).

Drugs for the treatment of tapeworm infestation are summarised in Table 13.4.

Drugs for other types of worms

Lungworm   Fenbendazole may be used to treat lungworm (see above: Drugs for roundworms, Fenbendazole).

Heartworm   Heartworm is not found in animals in the UK. However, treatment may be necessary in dogs being exported or imported to this country, in which case veterinary advice should be sought.

In Australia and the USA, heartworm prophylaxis in dogs is achieved using diethylcarbamazine, a compound similar to piperazine; a number of tablet and syrup formulations are available. Diethylcarbamazine is also active against roundworms. Melarsomine, an arsenical derivative, is used to treat heartworm infection in both countries mentioned above.

Drugs for other endoparasites   Giardasis, a protozoan disease characterised by chronic diarrhoea, is treated with metronidazole or fenbendazole (see above: Drugs for roundworms, Fenbendazole) and oral replacement therapy is necessary.

Table 13.4 Selection of tapeworm anthelmintics (not exhaustive)

Tapeworm anthelmintics	Legal	Effective against	Animals	Trade name	Form	Manufacturer
Dichlorophen	GSL	*Dipylidium, Taenia*	Cats and dogs	Catovel/Canovel Tapewormer	Tablets 750 mg	Pfizer[a]
	GSL		Cats and dogs (6 months +, 1.25 kg+)	Dichlorophen Tablets BP	Tablets 500 mg	Battle Hayward & Bower
	GSL		Cats and dogs	Easy Tape Wormer	Tablets 500 mg	Johnson's[a]
	GSL		Cats and dogs (6 months +)	Flavoured Tapeworm Tablets	Tablets 500 mg	Johnson's
	GSL		Cats (900g+) and dogs (1.75 kg+)	Kitzyme and Vetzyme Veterinary Tapewormer	Tablets 750 mg	Seven Seas
	GSL		Cats (6 months +)	Tapeworm Tablets for Cats	Tablets 250 mg	Bob Martin's
	GSL		Dogs (6 months +)	Tapeworm Tablets	Tablets 500 mg	Bob Martin's
Mebendazole		*Echinococcus, Taenia* (Also against roundworms)	See Table 13.3 for products			Various
Nitroscanate		*Dipylidium, Taenia* (Also against roundworms)	See Table 13.3 for products			Various
Praziquantel	GSL	*Dipylidium, Echinococcus, Taenia*	Cats and dogs (after weaning)	Droncit	Tablets (50 mg) and Injection (POM)	Bayer

[a] Indicates cat and dog versions available

Infections resulting from bites and scratches

Causal organisms

A dog or cat that is teased, frustrated or locked up on its own too much may become a 'biter'. Apart from the obvious physical injury, the risk of bacterial infection after a bite or scratch is high. Infected cat and dog bites have a complex microbiological mix. The normal oral flora of dogs includes *Pasteurella multocida*, which is found in almost half the wounds from dog bites, and *Eikenella corrodens*, found in gingival plaque. Two other bacteria, *Capnocytophaga canimorsus* and *C. cynoodegmi* are also found in the canine oral flora. In immunosuppressed people, these bacteria can cause severe disease. Other bacteria commonly isolated in dog-bite wounds include various species of *Pseudomonas*, *Actinobacillus*, *Streptococcus*, *Staphylococcus* and *Corynebacterium*.

Zoonotic risk

A bite wound that becomes infected with *Clostridium tetani* may lead to tetanus, but this is relatively unusual. Cats also have a number of organisms that are potentially harmful to humans.

Because of the rich array of flora in animals' mouths, bites should be treated promptly, cleaned, and stitched if necessary. Anti-tetanus and antibiotic treatment should be considered. Tips to prevent pets from biting include not disturbing an animal while it is eating or sleeping, not intruding upon the private territory of a confined animal and not teasing it by dangling food. A playful nip can escalate into a painful injury. A potentially dangerous dog has ears raised up and forward, teeth bared in a snarl and hair raised on the shoulder and rump.

Rabies

There are an estimated 15 000 cases of rabies world-wide each year. Because of strict quarantine rules and an extensive animal vaccination programme, rabies has been eradicated in the UK, New Zealand, and several other countries for many years. During 2001, 49 US states and Puerto Rico reported 7437 cases of rabies in non-human animals and one case in a human to the Centers for Disease Control and Prevention, an increase of < 1% in non-human animals from 7364 cases, and five human cases, reported in 2000 (Krebs *et al.*, 2002).

Pharmacists can provide useful information for those intending to visit, or have recently returned from, countries where the disease is endemic. High-risk areas include most of the countries of Africa, Asia (except Taiwan and Japan) and Latin America.

Causal organism Rabies is caused by the Rhabdoviridae, a widespread family of highly infectious viruses (Cockrum, 1997). There are at least 27 different rhabdoviruses in animals; some can infect humans and cause disease. The virus is enveloped and bullet-shaped (70 × 170 nm). Rabies is usually transmitted by saliva containing the virus from the bite of an infected animal.

Signs and symptoms The incubation period in cats and dogs varies from 10 days to more than a year, although usually some symptoms appear within a month of infection. Three separate phases of the disease may be identified.

- Behavioural changes, slight pyrexia, slowing of reflexes and skin irritation at the point of viral entry.
- Increasing behavioural changes characterised by excitability and aggression and lack of muscular coordination. This phase may continue for some weeks, during which viruses may be shed through saliva.
- Progressive general paralysis, frothing at the mouth and death.

If rabies is suspected the animal should be isolated immediately. The disease is notifiable.

Treatment/prophylaxis Some dogs are believed to have recovered from rabies but this is extremely rare; normally the animal cannot be saved.

Cats and dogs may be vaccinated against rabies using an inactivated vaccine (Nobivac, Intervet or Rabisin, Merial) from 4 weeks of age with a further dose at 12 weeks. Cats and dogs more than 12 weeks old require only one shot with a booster every 2 years.

Zoonotic risk Until comparatively recently, most human cases of rabies arose from a dog bite; this is still the case in developing countries. However, since 1990, 74% of human rabies deaths in the USA have been caused by variants of rabies virus associated with bats. Some deaths in the USA have occurred when no animal bite is involved. In such cases, rabies is assumed to be the result of contaminated saliva or other body fluids having entered the person's body through an abrasion, a cut on the skin, or through moist tissues in the lips or eyes. In rare instances, infection may occur by an airborne route (e.g. after exposure to air in caves densely populated with rabid bats). Once in the human host, the virus seeks out a nerve, and then travels to the brain, where it multiplies and leads to full-blown disease.

The incubation period in humans can be from 10 days to 7 years (the usual period is up to 2 months). If immunisation is given within 3 days of the bite, rabies is usually prevented. During this early incubation stage, the condition is reversible. The incubation period becomes shorter the nearer the bite is to the head. Once symptoms appear, death is almost invariably the outcome.

Symptoms include fever, behavioural changes, headaches, spasmodic contractions of the muscles that facilitate swallowing, convulsions, and ultimately death. Rabies is sometimes called 'hydrophobia' because in its terminal stages patients refuse to drink liquids and react violently towards attempts to give them fluids orally.

People travelling to countries where the disease is endemic should avoid stroking seemingly docile pets (especially dogs) and any wild animals. In Western Canadian parks, racoons appear very tempting to feed and pet, particularly if they are in family groups; but racoons can carry rabies. Any person coming into contact with a rabid animal should change all clothing at once and comprehensively disinfect the body. In the case of a bite, assistance should be sought as quickly as possible from local health authorities, to allow tests on the animal to determine the presence of rabies. It is important to gather as much information about the animal as possible. Unfortunately, not all rabies vaccines used abroad meet the levels of safety and efficacy found in UK products. If the risk is considered high, pre-exposure vaccination before departure may be appropriate. The rabies vaccine is an inactivated-virus vaccine and is given as a series of three injections given on days 0, 7 and 21 or 28.

There are three different types, each of which is considered safe during pregnancy:

- RVA rabies vaccine contains thimerosal as preservative.
- HDCV contains small amounts of neomycin.
- PCEC contains no preservative, but it does contain small amounts of neomycin, chlortetracycline and amphotericin B.

These options allow a choice for those people likely to suffer an adverse reaction to one of the vaccines caused by the agents used in its formulation.

Cat scratch disease

Cat scratch disease is associated with contact with a cat (but not necessarily an actual scratch). It is thought to be caused by infection with a rickettsial organism, *Bartonella henselae*. It also occurs occasionally in dogs and cattle.

 Zoonotic risk Symptoms include localised lymph node enlargement near the scratch; sometimes fever and rash are present. Treatment is with neoarsphenamine.

Other zoonotic infections

Bacterial

Campylobacter *Campylobacter jejuni* has been known to cause severe disease in animals for more than 70 years, but it is only comparatively recently that modern culture methods have facilitated more intense study. Its main reservoir is probably wild birds, in which it forms part of the normal fecal flora. Domestic animals may carry the organism for long periods without any symptoms. Surveys carried out in the 1980s showed that around 50% of dogs and cats carry the bacterium. Highest isolation rates are found in animals with diarrhoea.

 Zoonotic risk Infection acquired by humans in the home is confined mainly to close contact with a sick puppy and occasionally a kitten or caged bird. Most human infections are self-limiting but can cause severe abdominal pain and diarrhoea for 2–3 days. Treatment for humans is with fluid replacement to prevent dehydration, and possibly erythromycin. Prevention of infection is effected by prompt disposal of excreta from sick persons and disinfection of contaminated areas. Keeping pets out of the kitchen and dining areas, and frequent handwashing are also important measures, as *C. jejuni* is also acquired by ingesting contaminated raw milk, undercooked chicken or other food contaminated in the kitchen (see chapter 2). Recent indications show that the incidence of *Campylobacter* infection is rising, and the organism is taking over from *Salmonella* as the new food-poisoning villain.

Weil's disease

Causative organism Weil's disease, or leptospirosis, is a zoonotic disease carried by dogs and several other wild and domestic animals.

The causative agent is *Leptospira interrogans*, which has several distinct serovars, the most common in dogs being *L. icterohaemorrhagiae, L. canicola* and *L. grippotyphosa*. *L. icterohaemorrhagiae* is found in rats, and dogs containing this organism have often been in contact with the rodents or swum in slow-moving water. Transmission in animals is accomplished by close direct contact, placental transfer, biting, or ingestion of infected tissues.

Signs and symptoms   The signs of leptospirosis vary greatly depending on the animal's age, immune status, environmental factors and the serovar involved. Severe disease is characterised by acute haemorrhage, hepatitis and jaundice. Less severe disease may be seen as fever, dehydration, anorexia, thirst, vomiting and malaise.

Treatment   Clinical infection in dogs is minimised by the administration of leptospira vaccine, but subclinical infection with excretion of leptospires may still occur. If a case should occur, antibiotics should be given (oral ampicillin 10 mg/kg body weight twice daily or benzylpenicillin by intramuscular or intravenous injection 24 mg/kg twice daily). Once renal function is restored, dogs should be treated for a further 2 weeks with streptomycin (15 mg/kg) to eliminate kidney infection. Environmental disinfection is required.

Zoonotic risk   Leptospirosis can follow contamination of cuts and abrasions, or contact with mucous membranes, with infected urine from dogs and rats (also cattle and pigs). The disease, therefore, is one which is more common amongst certain occupations, most of them in rural areas. The predominant serovars that cause disease in humans are *L. hardjo* and *L. pomona*. Leptospirosis is widely distributed in Australia, with the highest prevalence in Queensland.

Following contact with infected urine, two broad types of disease can develop. A mild form, usually associated with *L. hardjo* and *L. pomona*, is characterised by acute onset of fever, myalgia and headache. A macular rash may also develop. After about a week the symptoms should subside, only to be replaced in some patients with symptoms of meningitis. Infection with *L. copenhageni* can result in a more serious illness, characterised by acute onset with fever, jaundice, headache, myalgia and vomiting. Renal failure may also occur. Diagnosis, like that of most zoonoses, is greatly assisted by something in the history indicating exposure to animals or animal products. Leptospires can be detected in urine about a week after infection. Serological tests are available, but these are ineffective until 7–14 days after infection.

Treatment with doxycycline is usually effective. Control is assisted by the fact that leptospirosis is a notifiable disease, which facilitates the determination of the source of infection. Animals infected with leptospires can develop clinical or subclinical infections. Many recover but continue to excrete leptospires in the urine for prolonged periods; leptospires in kidney tubules are substantially protected from host defences, and can survive under favourable conditions in the environment for several weeks.

Fungal

Ringworm

Causative organism Infection with *Microsporum* causes ringworm. Dogs, cats and kittens (also horses and farm animals) are the main sources of infection. Transmission is by direct contact with the infected individual, or indirectly via blankets and brushes. The infective agent may remain for months in dry, cool, shaded environments. Animals act as reservoirs of infection, generating spores that contaminate the environment.

 Zoonotic risk In humans, ring-shaped scaly papules appear on the scalp and spread peripherally, with loss of hair within 4–14 days of infection; eventually, a scaly erythematous plaque develops. In animals, lesions similar to those in humans appear 1–4 weeks after infection. Cats infected with *M. canis* present a moth-eaten appearance; lesions on dogs are discrete, circular, crusty areas of alopecia. The condition is often self-limiting if untreated, but may last up to 3 months. Oral griseofulvin has been used for many years in association with topical antifungal preparations on both humans and animals. In animals, the skin is usually brushed before application of natamycin or enilconazole. This is when zoonotic infection typically occurs in humans. Control is effected by keeping farm animals well fed and in sunlight. All grooming tools and equipment should be disinfected with formalin. Direct contact with the animal should be avoided as far as possible.

Protozoal

Giardiasis

Causative organism *Giardia lamblia* is a pear-shaped protozoan parasite usually found in the duodenum and occasionally the colon. In cats the parasite is found in the jejunum and ileum. It causes a condition known as giardiasis, characterised by intermittent or persistent chronic diarrhoea in kittens and puppies. The diarrhoea has an oatmeal-like or frothy appearance and is fatty. Symptoms are believed to be due to physical damage to the mucosa resulting in malabsorption and digestive imbalances.

Treatment   About 70% of cases respond to metronidazole; fenbendazole is also licensed for the treatment of giardiasis.

Zoonotic risk   Giardiasis is a zoonotic disease, so strict hygiene standards should be maintained. Giardia cysts can remain viable in a moist environment for several weeks.

Toxoplasmosis

Causative organism   The main protozoal disease seen in the UK (albeit relatively infrequently) is toxoplasmosis, an infection caused by the protozoan parasite *Toxoplasma gondii*. It is common in cats but rarely causes clinical symptoms.

Figure 13.9 shows a representation of the epidemiology of toxoplasmosis.

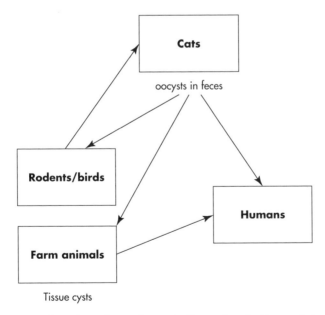

Figure 13.9   Epidemiology of toxoplasmosis. (Reproduced with permission of School of Pharmacy, Queen's University, Belfast.)

Life cycle Cats are infected by eating raw meat, birds or mice containing parasite cysts. The cats excrete oocysts for about 10 days when first infected. Intermediate hosts are rodents and farm animals, which ingest oocysts from infected soil. Farm animals, especially sheep, in which *T. gondii* causes enzootic abortion, are involved in the infective life cycle. Humans have been infected by eating vegetables contaminated by cat feces or by eating undercooked meat containing bradyzoites. Some cases have been associated with drinking raw milk, particularly goat's milk.

Treatment/prophylaxis A living veterinary vaccine (Toxovax, Intervet) is available and licensed for use in sheep.

Zoonotic risk Toxoplasmosis does not pose a significant health risk to most healthy humans, although it can be dangerous in immunocompromised patients and those receiving immunosuppressive therapy after transplantation surgery. It also presents a risk to pregnant women who have not previously encountered the parasite and have not developed an immune response. This can result in transplacental infection, leading to fetal defects.

Ocular toxoplasmosis usually occurs as posterior uveitis and is usually acquired congenitally. The most common symptom in adults is generalised or localised lymphadenopathy; fever and sore throat may also be present. As with *Toxocara*, recent infections may be diagnosed using an enzyme-linked immunosorbent assay.

Steroids and anthelmintics have been used for treatment with varying success.

Preventive measures are particularly important for pregnant women, who should be advised not to handle cat litter trays, to wash vegetables thoroughly before consumption, and to wear gloves whilst gardening to guard against inadvertent contact with buried feces.

Similarly, contamination of animal feedingstuffs with cat feces should be prevented.

Accidental self-injection or oral ingestion of toxoplasmosis vaccine can cause human disease.

Leishmaniasis Leishmaniasis is found in approximately 90 tropical and subtropical countries around the world. More than 90% of the world's cases of visceral leishmaniasis occur in Bangladesh, Brazil, India, Nepal and Sudan. This is a serious protozoal disease that is rarely seen in the UK, only being associated with recently imported animals.

Causative organism The disease that primarily affects dogs is caused by species of the protozoan *Leishmania* and is usually transmitted by sandflies belonging to the genus *Phlebotomus*.

Signs and symptoms The main symptom is a painful ulcer at the site of infection, persisting for several months, with residual scarring.

Treatment Treatment is with approved human drugs – antimony derivatives, e.g. sodium stibogluconate (Pentostam, GlaxoWellcome) and amphotericin B (Fungizone, Squibb). Culling of infected animals is also practised but may not be effective because there is a pool of infection in domestic animals and even in humans (Gavgani *et al.*, 2002).

Zoonotic risk Vaccines and drugs for preventing infections are not currently available. Preventive measures for the individual traveller are aimed at reducing contact with sandflies. Travellers should be advised to avoid outdoor activities when sandflies are most active (dusk to dawn). Contact with sandflies can be reduced by using bed nets and screening on doors and windows.

Viral

Canine distemper

Causative organism Canine distemper is a highly contagious disease caused by canine distemper virus, a virus closely related to the virus causing measles in humans. It is most often transmitted through contact with mucus and watery secretions discharged from the eyes and noses of infected dogs. Contact with the urine and fecal material of infected dogs can also result in infection.

Signs and symptoms The first signs of distemper an owner might notice are squinting, congestion of the eyes and a discharge of pus from the eyes. Weight loss, coughing, vomiting, nasal discharge and diarrhoea are common. In later stages the virus frequently attacks the nervous system, bringing about partial or complete paralysis as well as fits or twitching. Dogs suffering from the disease are usually listless and have a poor appetite. Canine distemper is relatively rare other than in dog rescue homes because of effective immunisation programmes.

Treatment/prophylaxis Supporting treatment for dogs with distemper is important. They should be kept warm, dry and clean with dimmed lighting and given a highly nutritious diet. Hydration must be maintained, either orally or systemically. Broad-spectrum antibiotics, antidiarrhoeals and anti-emetics may be necessary. Unfortunately, at least 50% of patients succumb to the disease or have to be 'put down', usually because of paralysis.

Vaccines for canine distemper virus (CDV) are available in combination with other canine vaccines (Table 13.7). Examples of some multicomponent canine vaccines containing CDV are Canigen DHPP (Virbac), Nobivac DHPPi (Intervet) and Quantum Dog 7 (Schering-Plough). Other products are available. A combination antiserum preparation (Maxagloban, Intervet) is also available and may be used in animals exposed to infection. An antiserum will provide passive immunity for up to 14 days, but to ensure protection the dose is usually repeated at 10-day intervals.

 Zoonotic risk   There has been some discussion about whether canine distemper is implicated in the development of human multiple sclerosis or Paget's disease; there is little evidence to support these theories.

Hardpad disease   Thought at one time to be a separate disease in its own right, hardpad is now considered to be caused by the distemper virus (see previous section).

Orf (contagious pustular dermatitis)   Although orf is mainly considered to be an occupational zoonosis associated with sheep farming, there have been occasional instances of working dogs contracting it. As these animals are often considered to be pets, a brief description is included here (see also chapter 10).

'Orf' was a word used in Scotland to describe a disease of sheep characterised by pustular dermatitis of the mouth and feet. The word is derived from an old Nordic word *hrufa*, meaning a scab or boil.

Causative organism   The strains of virus that cause orf in sheep, goats, dogs, and humans are members of the pox family of viruses, which includes pseudocowpox, true cowpox and smallpox. The infective agent is known as the orf virus. Sheep and goats are the main natural reservoirs of the infective agent. Transmission is by direct or indirect contact with the superficial lesions through skin abrasions. Where animals have injured their mouths by eating gorse or other prickly plants, infection occurs swiftly. Young kids and lambs transfer the virus from their lips to teats and udders.

Signs and symptoms   The animal tends to rub its muzzle on its legs to gain some relief from the painful condition, transmitting the virus to the feet. Pustules may be present at other sites on the body which, after 10–12 days, become thick brownish black scabs that, if lifted, reveal an angry red lesion. If orf affects a flock, the affected animals should be isolated and their lesions painted with crystal violet and covered with an appropriate dressing. Antibiotics may be given. The animals should be kept apart from the healthy flock for about 2 weeks after recovery, when they should be dipped. Any lesions on the feet or lower legs may be treated with a footbath.

Treatment   Anyone treating an infected animal should ensure scrupulous hygiene, scrubbing up with disinfectant, to prevent carrying the virus from one animal to another and to prevent self-infection. A living sheep vaccine (Scabivax, Schering-Plough and Vaxall Orf, Fort Dodge) is available to reduce the chance of animals becoming infected.

Zoonotic risk   Transfer to humans, mainly sheep farmers and their staff and (far less frequently) to working dogs is generally by direct contact in the working environment. In humans, primary lesions are usually on the hands (Figure 13.10) and forearms; the lips may be

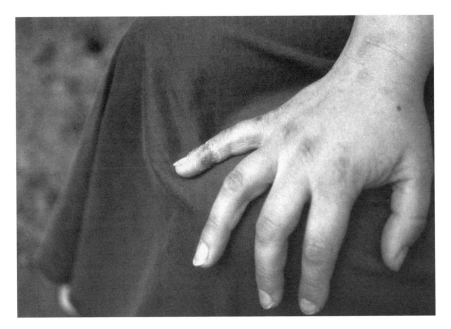

Figure 13.10   The photograph shows orf lesions on the hand.

affected by transference from the hands. Initially, there is a single painful red area at the site of contact, which lasts from 3–6 weeks; this develops to a pustule, from which fluid exudes.

The back may also be involved. In animals, the minor form of the disease is characterised by vesicles, followed by ulcers on the lips, especially at the corner of the mouth. In the severe form, the inside of the mouth is involved. The condition is self-limiting in humans, but antibiotics are often prescribed to contain any potential secondary infection.

Other ailments of cats and dogs

This chapter has been biased towards the human–pet interface so far, but for completeness brief details of cat and dog diseases without zoonotic implications will also be given, so that pharmacists will be able to make informed responses when consulted for information. The conditions have been chosen using my personal experience of questions received from pet owners during a 30-year career in community pharmacy and are not meant to be exhaustive.

Feline conditions

Allergies

Aetiological factors for feline allergies are similar to those for dogs (see below); they include flea allergies, food intolerance mites (*Otodectes cynoctis* and *Notoedres cati*) and atopic dermatitis. A complicated oral and/or dermal condition known as eosinic granuloma complex may also occur in cats as the result of an allergic response.

Signs and symptoms   Pruritis and alopecia, the latter associated with overgrooming, may be seen in allergic responses. Feline miliary dermatitis (also called popular dermatitis) appears as crusted papillae and may be due to flea allergy dermatitis if distributed over the lumbosacral region, or to mites or food allergies if distributed over the head and neck.

Treatment   Treatment is similar to that suggested for dog allergies (see below): removing the source of allergic challenge with parasiticides and environmental disinfection, taking measures to prevent self-injury from biting and scratching, and the use of antihistamines and corticosteroids.

Feline infectious enteritis (panleukopenia)

This intestinal viral infection, which affects domestic cats, other members of the Felidae and certain other animals, including the mink, is highly infectious.

Causative organism The causative organism is a parvovirus resistant to heat and many disinfectants, and it can lie dormant in the environment for many months.

Signs and symptoms Symptoms include diarrhoea in the later stages of the disease, vomiting and rapid dehydration. In young kittens a staggering gait may be seen due to brain damage. The disease may be fatal in young kittens. The virus is spread in saliva, urine and feces.

Treatment/prophylaxis Immunisation using a modified living vaccine (Feliniffa P, Merial) has been extremely effective in preventing the disease, which is now seen almost exclusively in young unvaccinated cats. If an infection should occur, cats should be vaccinated and all living areas disinfected with a bleach solution.

Feline immunodeficiency virus

This virus attacks the immune system in a similar way to human immunodeficiency virus (HIV) and causes immunodeficiency, making the cat susceptible to a wide range of secondary infections. Prevalence is extremely low in domestic cats. No vaccine is available.

Feline infectious peritonitis virus

Until 1991, feline infectious peritonitis (FIP) was one of the few remaining non-preventable diseases of cats – and one of the most important. A vaccine is now available. Twenty-five to 40% of cats in the general feline population (excluding catteries and multiple-cat households) have developed antibodies to coronavirus, the virus group that includes the FIP virus. As the disease advances, abdominal distension occurs as a result of the accumulation of peritoneal fluid. Other symptoms may be seen in the eyes, kidneys and nervous system. No treatment is available and death ensues.

Feline influenza

The primary causal agents are the feline herpesvirus and feline calicivirus, but secondary bacterial infection with *Chlamydia psittaci felis* can occur. Antibiotics can be used against the bacterial infection but there is no treatment for the viral infection. Immunisation with killed or modified live vaccines is recommended, although protection is not always complete and the animal may still exhibit symptoms, albeit of reduced severity. Sneezing, eye and nasal discharges, ulcers on the tongue and absence of appetite are among the most obvious signs of disease.

Feline leukaemia

Infection with the feline leukaemia virus (FeLV) can cause a variety of sequelae, ranging from lymphoid cancer to anaemia and arthritis as well as leukaemia, from which the virus gets its name. The virus may also upset the immunosuppressive mechanism, leading to a number of long-standing chronic conditions. Kittens up to 4 months of age are more likely to become permanently infected with FeLV than older cats. The FeLV is second only to road accidents among the causes of cat mortality. It requires close contact for transmission. Diagnosis is with the aid of a blood antibody test. The spread of the disease may be limited by removing infected cats from the population for euthanasia. Cats with positive blood tests but no clinical signs of the disease are also removed. Routine vaccination is generally recommended, although the degree of protection may not be 100%. Combined vaccines are available that contain FeLV include Fel-o-Vax IV (Fort Dodge) and Fevaxyn Pentofel (Fort Dodge).

Hairballs

Few creatures are as fastidious as cats. They can spend hours licking their coats, and when they have covered every inch they will happily start again. They do not seem to mind swallowing a little hair – it is all part of good grooming. Sometimes, fur that should pass right through the digestive system gets trapped in the stomach. As more and more hair arrives, it begins forming an uncomfortable wad and causing the animal to retch and vomit. While this retching may look wretched, hairballs are rarely a serious problem. Passage of the hairball may be facilitated with a commercial lubricant or light liquid paraffin.

Canine conditions

Genetic factors

Compared with cats, dogs are particularly susceptible to inherited genetic defects, probably because they have been bred much more extensively and selectively. The difference in appearance between modern dog breeds and that of their wild ancestors is much more striking than is the case with cats. Thus certain breeds have problems that can result in a lifetime of discomfort. For example, the poodle can carry a number of defective genes producing abnormally shortened leg bones, a defect in the arteries near the heart, ocular difficulties, epilepsy and bladder stones. Dogs with abnormally short noses and jaws (bulldogs, Pekingese and Boston terriers) often suffer obstructed breathing. Among cats, the Siamese suffers a cleft palate.

Some personal observations on breed-specific problems in dogs are shown in Table 13.5. This information is not exhaustive and is presented merely as an indication of what might be expected by owners of these animals.

A very common condition in many of the larger, fast-growing breeds is hip dysplasia. Dogs are generally born with good hips but the disease often develops in the joint as they grow. Feeding puppies to get

Table 13.5 Common breed-specific problems in dogs

Breed	Recurrent condition
Afghan hound	Eye problems
Beagle	Heart disease, epilepsy, skin conditions
Boxer	Heart disease, digestive problems, bloat
Border terrier	Heart problems
Border collie	Epilepsy, deafness
Bulldog	Heart disease, respiratory problems, skin and eye problems
Cairn terrier	Skin allergies
Cavalier KC	Eye problems
Dachshund	Heart disease, diabetes, skin conditions
English sheepdog	Skin and eye conditions
Golden retriever	Heart problems, skin problems, epilepsy and eye problems
German shepherd	Gastric disorders, bloat, eye disease
Jack Russell	Problems due to characteristic stubby legs
Labrador	Cataracts and other eye problems, bloat
Pekinese	Eye problems, respiratory problems, urinary problems
Poodle	Eye and ear problems
Rottweiler	Eye problems, bloat
Scottish terrier	Skin allergies, leg cramps
Shetland sheepdog	Ear problems, rheumatic problems in legs
Spaniels	Eye problems
W Highland terrier	Skin conditions, liver disease
Yorkshire terrier	Eye infections, teeth and gum problems

maximum growth quickly may be one cause. An incomplete fit between the ball-and-socket components of the joint results in friction and pain. Over time, the friction creates a build-up of calcium and changes the shape of the bones, making the problem even worse. Severely dysplastic dogs may need extensive surgery just to enable them to walk without pain. Milder conditions may be treated with a suitable analgesic, a diet to prevent the animal getting fat and stressing its joints, and moderate exercise to maintain muscle tone.

In 2003, The Kennel Club announced plans to use gene technology to eradicate genetic defects caused by more than a century of inbreeding (Leake, 2003). Under the plan, owners of hundreds of pedigree dogs will be asked to have the animals DNA tested. Those found to have defective genes will be prevented from reproducing. Breeds potentially affected are bulldogs (heart problems), retrievers and springer spaniels (blindness).

Allergies

Types of allergies

Atopic reactions　　Atopic skin disease is associated with hypersensitivity to environmental allergens. Dogs, particularly small terriers, often suffer from a pruritis resulting from forays into the undergrowth on parkland. Scratching may exacerbate the condition. An important element of treating allergic reactions is removal of the allergen, but this is not always possible. Interdigital dermatitis may be precipitated by an allergic reaction to grass, and this causes the dog to continually lick between the toes. The licking and the allergic response allows bacteria to multiply between the claws. Antibiotics may be necessary; gentian violet is used topically.

Contact allergy　　Skin conditions may also be caused by using perfumed toilet soap to wash the animal or as a result of contact with material on the ground or floor, polish, etc.

Flea allergy dermatitis　　Infestation of dogs with the cat flea, *Ctenocephalides felis*, may result in hypersensitivity to flea saliva. A primary eruption with papules may be seen and pruritis is often present. Secondary infections and exacerbation due to the animal scratching also occur. Extensive measures are required to identify and destroy the source of infection (see above: Fleas).

Food allergies   Food allergies are difficult to identify and usually are found by selectively stopping and then reintroducing suspected food items. Signs include pruritis, particularly on the face, and gastrointestinal symptoms.

Treatment for allergies   Veterinary surgeons often prescribe glucocorticoids as the drug of choice to deal with allergic symptoms. Oral preparations with a short duration of action are preferred because therapy can be discontinued quickly if any adverse reactions (polyuria, polydipsia and polyphagia) occur. Typically, veterinary surgeons prescribe oral prednisolone for dogs at a dose of 500 μg/kg or methylprednisolone at 400 μg/kg daily, the amount being tapered to achieve the minimum effective alternate-day dose. In cases where glucocorticoids are considered inappropriate because of unacceptable adverse reactions, antihistamines may be used. Their effect may not be seen for 10–14 days and they are more effective as a prophylactic rather than as treatment. Oral antihistamines reported as being effective are generic chlorphenamine and diphenhydramine, clemastine (Tavegil, Novartis), and the prescription-only medicines hydroxyzine (Atarax, Pfizer and Ucerax, UBC Pharma) and alimemazine tartrate (trimeprazine tartrate) (Vallergan, Castlemead).

Combining glucosteroid and antihistamine treatment with dietary supplementation with essential fatty acids (EFA) appears to enhance the glucosteroid effect and allow a reduction in dose in some dogs, but published results vary widely. There are numerous EFA preparations available on the UK market, formulated as capsules (e.g. EfaVet, Schering-Plough) and oral liquids (e.g. Complederm, Virbac).

Hypersensitisation, involving the administration of allergens to atopic dogs to reduce clinical reactions when exposed to an allergic challenge, is reported to have been successful in 50–80% of atopic dogs.

For flea-associated allergies, 10% imidacloprid spot-on (Advantage for Dogs, Bayer) may help to reduce the incidence of flea allergy dermatitis. The condition may also be treated orally with the prescription-only medicine lufenuron, available in tablets of varying strengths (Program, Novartis).

Anal sac problems

Two anal sacs or glands are situated below and to each side of the anus in the dog. They provide a fluid that acts as a lubricant to aid defecation. Each gland has a duct opening into the anus and these may become blocked by foreign bodies, so that the secretions cannot escape. The gland may also become infected. Anal sac problems present as a 'scotting' action, when they drag their posterior along the ground – hopefully out on the grass but sometimes on a convenient carpet in the house. Tail-chasing and yelping when sitting down may also occur. In cats the condition is accompanied by excessive licking. Management is usually by gentle evacuation and irrigation; application of antibiotic or steroid cream may be necessary.

Conjunctivitis

Conjunctivitis is only one of a large number of eye problems reported in dogs but is included here because advice on this condition is frequently sought from pharmacists. It occurs commonly and has to be differentiated from other causes of pink eyes. Irritation, a bloodshot appearance and discharge are signs of conjunctival inflammation.

The causes include:

- Irritation resulting from lesions on the eyelid, eyelash obstruction or presence of a foreign body.
- Trauma from a blow or other injury.
- Bacterial or viral infection.
- Allergic response.

A superficial conjunctival congestion would suggest trauma, entry of a foreign body, allergy or bacterial infection, while deep congestion accompanied by redness around the eye is likely to be far more serious. The West Highland white terrier is particularly prone to lachrymal dysfunction, leading to dry eyes and conjunctivitis.

Conjunctivitis provides the community pharmacist with one of the most difficult veterinary situations. As far as the owner is concerned, there are perfectly good products on our shelves for human use that will surely do a similar job in animals. This may well be so, but none are licensed for veterinary use. Having been made aware of the difficulties of selling over-the-counter products for veterinary use, the well-intentioned owner may either return later for another attempt, this time without revealing for whom the product is intended, or resort to such long-standing home remedies as bathing the eyes with boric acid solution or cold tea. Clients should be referred to a veterinarian colleague. Bacterial eye infections may be treated with drops or eye ointment chosen according to the infective organism. Gentamicin (Tiacil, Virbac) and framycetin (Soframycin, Florizel) have broad-spectrum activity; chloramphenicol has similar properties and is lipid-soluble so is particularly useful for intraocular infections.

Dental disease

Dental problems are the main causes of halitosis. Although there are products for bad breath in dogs on the market, owners should be advised to have the cause identified and treated by a veterinary surgeon.

The main dental difficulties arise from several sources:

- Plaque. Dental plaque builds up as a result of feeding modern soft diets.
- Gingivitis. This is an inflammation of the gums and is generally caused by toxins liberated by the bacteria in the plaque.
- Periodontal disease. This is caused by serious escalation of gingivitis, with loss of the natural congruence of the gingival margins, dental abscesses and mobility of the teeth.

There are measures that can be taken by pet owners to prevent build-up of plaque, such as the choice of diet and various dental aids. Regular close inspection is an appropriate action.

Foot problems

- Dogs' feet often come into contact with broken glass, sharp objects, gravel, acids and other harmful materials, resulting in cut pads or webbing. First-aid measures, including gentle cleaning with water or a mild antiseptic and bandaging to stop the bleeding, are appropriate, but suturing may be required if the injury is deep.
- Foreign bodies may become lodged between the toes, leading to the formation of abscesses.
- Interdigital cysts are swellings that may occur between the toes and are caused by blockage of the sweat glands in the feet. Bathing in salt water (approximately 15 g/L) three or four times daily will help the lesion resolve.

Conditions causing diarrhoea and vomiting

Diarrhoea and vomiting are not diseases in themselves; they are common symptoms of a wide range of conditions, some serious and some more trivial. A number of causes of these symptoms are given. All treatments may be accompanied by oral replacement therapy if necessary (see chapter 3).

Diarrhoea, the frequent passage of liquid or ill-formed stools, can result from a number of aetiological factors.

- Acute diarrhoea may be caused by infection, such as *Campylobacter*, distemper, Parvo or *Salmonella*.
- Chronic diarrhoea may be caused by one or more of the following:
  - Dietary problems – intolerance of food, excess food, scavenging, poor digestion and/or absorption of food in the gastrointestinal tract (treated with dietary management and/or drugs).
  - Allergies (treated with drugs).
  - Endoparasitic infestation with helminths and protozoa (treated with parasiticides).
  - Mechanical – intestinal obstructions, including foreign bodies swallowed by the animal (may require surgical intervention).

The above factors result in one or more of the following actions that lead directly to diarrhoea:

- An increase in the fluid content of the stool, often caused by poor digestion or poor absorption in the colon.
- Hypersecretion in the small intestine due to mucosal inflammation or irritation by toxins.
- Irregular intestinal motility.

Treatment of diarrhoea   Animals with diarrhoea should be starved for 24 hours and a light balanced diet reintroduced thereafter. In most cases diarrhoea will be not be indicative of a serious condition, but owners should be vigilant if the condition persists; if there is blood in the stools they should consult a veterinary surgeon. Oral replacement therapy may be required to restore electrolyte balance.

There are four main classes of antidiarrhoeal drugs.

Adsorbents

- Given orally, these preparations reduce gastric mucosal irritation by adsorbing toxins. Examples include bismuth salts (e.g. Pepto-Bismol, Procter and Gamble), bismuth salts and charcoal (e.g. BCK, Fort Dodge) and several multi-ingredient products.
- The popular OTC product Bob Martin Diarrhoea Tablets contains bismuth carbonate, catechu powder, prepared chalk and rhubarb powder.

Drugs that reduce mobility

- Generic loperamide is used in the treatment of non-specific acute and chronic diarrhoea. It is normally restricted to prescription, but if authorised by a veterinary surgeon and labelled 'For veterinary use' it may be supplied in a pharmacy. Imodium, Arret Diocalm Ultra, etc are only authorised for human use. If labelled 'For treatment of acute diarrhoea' then, as pharmacy only (P) medicines, with prior direction by a veterinarian, they may be supplied by a pharmacist. A record should be kept.

- Other drugs that reduce motility are codeine phosphate and diphenoxylate and atropine (Lomotil, Searle). Both are prescription-only medicines.

Drugs used in chronic diarrhoea

- 500 mg sulfasalazine tablets or suspension (Salazopyrin, Pharmacia & Upjohn) are prescribed in the treatment of canine intestinal inflammation in doses of 15–30 mg/kg three times daily. The drug is degraded by intestinal bacteria into 5-aminosalicylate (which exerts an anti-inflammatory effect on the mucosal wall) and sulfapyridine. Mesalazine (Asacol, Beecham & Salofalk, Cortecs) and olsalazine (Dipentum, Pharmacia & Upjohn) are given at slightly lower doses but have the same active ingredient as sulfasalazine. All these drugs are authorised human medicines that veterinarians may supply.
- Corticosteroids, including prednisolone and dexamethasone are also used. They may be used concurrently with azathioprine (see below) to enable reduction in dosage.
- Non-steroidal anti-inflammatory drugs, such as flunixin, normally administered to dogs as a subcutaneous injection (e.g. Finadyne, Schering-Plough), may offer an alternative approach.
- The antibacterials oxytetracycline and metronidazole may help to control an imbalance of intestinal flora. Treatment may extend over several weeks.
- Severe inflammatory bowel disease can be treated with generic azathioprine (or Imuran, GlaxoWellcome), 1–2 mg/kg being given orally daily.

Parasiticides   See Endoparasitic infection in cats and dogs, above.

Vomiting and regurgitation   It is important to be aware of the differences between vomiting and regurgitation. Vomiting in the dog is a very active process, while regurgitation is a passive process. Vomiting is a complex act in which the abdominal muscles, the diaphragm and chest muscles, the larynx and the lower part of the neck all play a part. With regurgitation there is no gagging or retching and muscular effort is absent. The dog simply opens his mouth and allows partially digested food to exit. Regurgitation is used by wild dogs to provide food for young pups after a kill and may also be used by domestic animals to allow the further processing of an earlier meal. A rare condition known as megaoesophagus may also cause regurgitation.

Causes of vomiting   The causes of vomiting are varied. Diagnosis is important and in all but the simplest cases, treating without veterinary advice is inappropriate:

- Accident. The shock of an accident may involve vomiting even if no injury has been sustained to the stomach itself. Head injuries may also initiate vomiting and should be referred to a veterinary surgeon without delay.

- Disease. The symptom of vomiting is common to many diseases; e.g. infective canine hepatitis, leptospirosis, meningitis, nephritis and rabies.
- Indigestion. When the stomach is unable to process a quantity of foodstuff, it mixes it with quantities of frothy mucus and water and expels it as vomit. The material brought up is recognisable as food; it may be stained a brownish colour with bile and has a sour smell. Both the cat and the dog vomit with ease, and as soon as the episode is over the animals return to normal activity.
- Foreign bodies. Dogs may swallow all manner of small objects that can cause vomiting. In some cases the offending object may be expelled naturally in vomit or feces; in other cases surgical removal may be necessary.
- Gastritis. The stomach walls are inflamed and thickened and the mucous membrane is swollen and painful. Whenever food or liquid enters the stomach, vomiting begins immediately. The vomit has an offensive odour and comprises pieces of undigested food coated with frothy mucus. Blood may also be present.
- Motion sickness.
- Many poisonous substances (e.g. pesticides, paint, disinfectants, etc), plants and fungi will cause a dog to vomit. The overall mortality from such events is relatively modest. Vomiting should be induced with an emetic – at home by giving mustard or concentrated salt solution or, if the dog will allow, by placing one's finger at the back of the dog's throat. Milk may help in providing a demulcent effect. Immediate veterinary help should be sought.
- Stress. In dogs, stress may result from being left tied up for long periods, from ill treatment, from the use of fireworks, or moving house. Dog fights may also cause stress. Being taken to a show with hundreds of other animals may cause stress. Excessive drinking, vomiting and diarrhoea may result. The situation may be resolved by gentle support measures.

Treatment of vomiting Anti-emetics to treat vomiting fall into two main groups – broad-spectrum anti-emetics used to treat non-specific vomiting and drugs used in the prevention of motion sickness.

Broad-spectrum drugs for non-specific vomiting

- In vomiting with uncertain aetiology, broad-spectrum α_2-adrenergic antagonists in tablet or injectable form, such as veterinary acepromazine (ACP Vericore VP), and the approved human generic drugs chlorpromazine and prochlorperazine, are often used initially. They act both at the chemoreceptor sites and at the vomiting centre. Hypotension and sedation may occur as a side-effect.
- Metoclopramide is prescribed in vomiting due to gastritis and oesophageal reflux. It is a dopamine D_2 and 5-HT_3 receptor antagonist that acts at both the chemoreceptor trigger zone and gastrointestinal smooth muscle.
- Cisapride (Propulsid, Janssen-Cilag), an approved human drug, can be used when vomiting is thought to be associated with impaired gastric emptying. Erythromycin in subantibacterial dose levels is also used in this context.

Drugs used in prevention of motion sickness   Some dogs and also cats may be particularly susceptible to motion sickness.

- Diphenhydramine and cyclizine (Valoid, GlaxoWellcome) are approved human drugs. They have antihistamine activity and act directly on the vestibular apparatus, the stimulation of which is associated with activation of the vomiting centre.
- Veterinary acepromazine (ACP Vericore VP), and the approved human generic drugs chlorpromazine and prochlorperazine may be prescribed. They have sedative properties that may be useful in reducing stress associated with travelling. The canine dose for acepromazine is up to 1 mg/kg given about 30 minutes before a light meal.
- Other remedies. Pharmacists may be asked if it is safe to give pets over-the-counter travel sickness tablets. The answer is 'Yes, it probably would be'; however, these human medicines are not authorised for veterinary consumption and, as with the eye drops for conjunctivitis mentioned above, require veterinary intervention. The situation is less clear for homeopathic travel remedies like Cocculus and Tabacum and Bach Rescue Remedy. The use of ginger (a simple ginger biscuit may be sufficient) is said to be effective for travel sickness. Pet owners should ensure that the vehicle is adequately ventilated and make periodic stops for exercise.

Infectious canine hepatitis

Causative organism   Dogs of all ages may be infected with a canine adenovirus, some without showing clear clinical symptoms before sudden death.

Signs and symptoms   In acute stages of the disease the dog may have diarrhoea and vomiting, elevated temperature, jaundice and convulsions. Puppies may show signs of severe internal haemorrhaging. Keratitis (blue eye) may be seen 1–2 weeks after the start of the disease and may be the only visible sign of the disease.

Treatment/prophylaxis   An antiserum can be administered as treatment, together with glucose and vitamin K. A preparation of combined antisera is available to provide passive immunity to dogs against parvovirus, distemper and infectious canine hepatitis (Maxagloban P, Intervet).

Kennel cough (infectious tracheobronchitis)

Causative organisms   There are a number of possible causes of kennel cough, including canine parainfluenza virus, canine herpes virus and a mycoplasma, but most cases are caused by infection with the bacterium *Bordetella bronchiseptica*.

Signs and symptoms   A dry hacking cough is the most common sign of this disease. In some cases, pneumonia may occur as a complication of this disease. All of the organisms that cause this disease are contagious, so it is not unusual for all the dogs in a household or boarding kennels to rapidly become infected unless they have been vaccinated. For this reason, boarding kennels and shows usually insist on seeing a vaccination certificate before accepting animals.

Treatment/prophylaxis   Symptomatic treatment of the cough may be given with suitable antibiotics. The *Bordetella* vaccine (Intrac, Schering-Plough) is supplied as a powder for reconstitution and is administered intranasally to dogs over 2 weeks of age. Thoughts on revaccination vary widely amongst veterinary surgeons, but the consensus seems to be to revaccinate every 5–8 months depending how often the animal is likely to be kennelled. Vaccination against parainfluenza virus (Kavak, Fort Dodge) involves two subcutaneous injections, normally given from age 8–10 weeks at intervals of 2–4 weeks.

Otitis externa

Causative organisms   Inflammation of the ear canal, or otitis externa, can be caused by a number of factors, such as infection, parasites, foreign bodies, tumours and underlying dermatological (skin) disease.

Bacteria such as staphylococci, streptococci, *E. coli* and *Pseudomonas* spp. are the main causative organisms, but yeasts may also be present.

Dogs with long, pendulous ears, such as cocker spaniels, Labrador retrievers, Basset hounds and Irish setters, are certainly more predisposed to ear problems than breeds with short, erect ears. As the ear folds, it covers the ear canal and prohibits air from entering and drying the canal. The result is a moist, warm ear canal that is a perfect environment for organisms to grow, for example the yeast *Malassezia pachydermatis* and, less frequently, *Candida* spp.

The ear mite (*Otodectes cynoptis*) is a parasite that often causes a condition known as otodectic mange. This can be found on other parts of the animal's body as well as in the ear, necessitating more extensive treatment.

Signs and symptoms   Owners will notice the dog shaking its head or scratching its ears. A good sniff near the ears usually verifies a problem, as most infectious otitis ears have a pungent odour. If the infection persists, the ear canal will become inflamed and often discharge a purulent exudate, a pussy substance. Otitis externa can progress to otitis media. Signs associated with this condition are anorexia, pyrexia, depression and pain on opening the jaw.

Treatment of otitis externa and media   Topical antimicrobials are used widely in the treatment of otitis externa. Many are aimed at more than one type of organism and are combined with other active ingredients, including corticosteroids and local anaesthetic agents (e.g. benzocaine and tetracaine).

Appropriate systemic antibacterial treatment is required for otitis media.

Topical anti-infective agents

- Prescription-only ear drops containing neomycin in combination with other constituents (Auroto, Arnolds and Oterna, Schering-Plough) and polymixin B with other constituents (Surolan, Janssen) and the approved human drug fusidic acid (Fucidin, Leo) as an ointment.
- Nystatin (Canaural, Leo) and miconazole are available for fungal infections.
- Pyrethrins, monosulfiram and tiabendazole are used to treat infection with mites; the latter is included in Auroto drops (Arnolds) mentioned above. Selamectin (Stronghold, Pfizer) is effective in cats. Drops containing pyrethrin (e.g. Ruby Veterinary Ear Drops, Spencer and Secto Ear Drops, Sinclair) and dichlorophen (Vetzyme Veterinary Ear Drops, Seven Seas) are classified as GSL and may be sold in pharmacies and pet shops.

Corticosteroids   Corticosteroids are often present as a constituent in veterinary ear drops and ointments (e.g. Vetsovate Eye/Ear drops and ointment, Schering-Plough), but if the infection is extensive systemic treatment may be necessary.

Cleansing procedures   Dogs with a history of ear disease require routine cleaning of the canals to prevent recurring infection. It is not wise to use cotton buds in the ear canal, as this can be quite painful to the dog. All hair growing in the canal should be gently plucked using a pair of tweezers and the ear flushed out with an ear-cleaning product. An example of a product available to facilitate such action has propylene glycol, benzoic acid and salicylic acid (Dermisol, Pfizer). Various other formulae exist.

Parvovirus

Causative organism Parvovirus, a close relative and possible mutant of feline panleukopenia virus, appeared as the cause of a new disease in 1978–1979 in America, Australia and Europe. Until natural immunity had been established through exposure and a vaccination programme in the 1980s, dogs fell victim to the disease in large numbers and there were many deaths. The virus is extremely hardy and survives for long periods outside its host. It is transmitted by oral ingestion of virally contaminated feces.

Signs and symptoms Upon ingestion by the new host, it infects local lymph nodes, multiplies quickly and then, via the blood, moves to the small intestine, where its action interferes with the normal balance of digestive enzyme secretion and nutrient absorption. Severe haemorrhagic gastroenteritis ensues, with fluid loss from both vomiting and diarrhoea. The onslaught of bacteria and toxins in the blood will ultimately cause death. Certain breeds seem to be more sensitive to the disease, possibly related to differences in the immune system. They include Rottweilers, Doberman pinschers, and possibly black Labrador retrievers.

Treatment/prophylaxis Treatment for the disease is primarily supportive. Immunisation is usually carried out with a canine parvovirus vaccine, of which there are at least four variants on the UK market. Annual booster doses are recommended. The virus is very resistant and therefore adequate environmental disinfection is very important.

Problems with the level of immunity after vaccination with canine parvovaccine are often experienced owing to an interaction between the vaccine and maternally acquired antibodies that reduces the overall ability to resist a substantial environmental challenge. This acquired immunity can vary in both extent and the time of protection. It is recommended that the puppies' titre should be assessed before vaccination so that the optimum age for vaccination can be determined.

Poisoning

Potential poisoning episodes may arise from a number of different sources. On several occasions I have been telephoned by a distraught owner whose animal has turned a pot of paint or creosote over itself, or has consumed something that could be poisonous. Unable to contact their veterinary surgeon the owner has turned to the pharmacist. Immediate removal of the toxic agent from the animal's vicinity is vital; any unconsumed material or the container or packaging should be retained if possible for future inspection by the veterinary surgeon.

Possible agents of poisoning include the following:

- Household products, including cleaning fluids, paint products, disinfectants and bleaches, and smoke from bonfires.
- Human and veterinary medicines.
- Pesticides; e.g. organophosphates.
- Assorted chemicals; e.g. lead.
- Infested and adulterated foodstuffs caused by inappropriate compounding.
- Poisonous plants. For example, several species of daffodils and narcissus contain a mixture of alkaloids.
- Stings or secretions from other animals. For example, wasp or bee stings may need to be treated with antihistamines or corticosteroids; the toad (*Bufo vulgaris*) secretes a venom from skin glands that can be transferred to cats and dogs, causing profuse salivation. Treatment is with sodium bicarbonate mouthwashes.
- Although cats and dogs in urban areas are rarely bitten by snakes, this can be a problem in country areas. Snakebites appear as two small punctures of the skin, with swelling, pain and shortness of breath.

Below are listed some steps that can be taken to treat poisoning.

Topical contamination

- The animal should be washed with copious amounts of running water.
- Oily materials should be wiped off and the area cleaned with olive oil or a similar cooking oil.
- Vinegar may be used with alkalis.
- A weak sodium bicarbonate solution may be used for acids.
- Any affected hair or fur should be cut away.
- Veterinary advice should be sought promptly as to whether further treatment is necessary.

Ingested material

First aid   Although not generally recommended in an absolute emergency, salt and mustard deposited at the back of the throat can be used by the owner to initiate emesis.

Veterinarian action   This may involve:

- The administration of Paediatric Ipecacuanha Mixture BP (1–2 mL/kg body weight) and the approved human intravenous injection of apomorphine (Britaject, Britannia) as better alternatives.
- Gastric lavage with water, saline or a slurry of activated charcoal (BCK, Fort Dodge or the pharmacy-only human-approved product Carbomix, Penn) may be appropriate.
- Laxatives may also be prescribed to assist the removal of toxic material.
- Administration of an antidote. Antidotes may react with the toxic chemical to form something less dangerous, they may neutralise the toxin entirely or interfere with the metabolism of the toxin. See *The Veterinary Formulary*, Treatment of Poisoning section pp. 125–133, for further information.

Snakebite

Action should be taken to slow down the passage of venom round the body by keeping the animal calm and bandaging the affected limb firmly before seeking veterinary advice.

Minor cuts and abrasions

Major wound management is dealt with at length in part 5. There are a number of commercially available topical preparations that may be used to deal with minor abrasions or prevent infection of a wound after surgery. Appropriate advice should be given on cleansing and/or keeping the wound clean. Active ingredients include benzalkonium chloride, cetrimide chlorocresol and chloroxylenol in ointment, powder, lotion and spray formulations.

Antiseptic preparations containing benzoic acid, cresol or phenols should not be used on cats.

Actions necessary to keep cats and dogs healthy

Feeding cats and dogs

Nutrients

Like all animals and humans, cats and dogs require a balanced diet to grow normally and maintain health once they mature. The diet is made up of dietary components with specific functions in the body and contributing to growth, the maintenance of body tissue and optimal health. These components include water, carbohydrates, proteins, fats, minerals and vitamins and are known as 'nutrients'. There are two types of nutrients:

- Essential nutrients. These are dietary components that cannot be synthesised by the body at all, or cannot be synthesised in the quantities (or at the rate of supply) required by the body. They must therefore be provided in the diet. Essential fatty acids and most vitamins fall into this group.
- Non-essential nutrients. These are dietary components that can be synthesised by the body if they are not supplied in sufficient quantities in the diet (e.g. vitamin C can be synthesised from glucose if necessary).

Energy

A vital requirement for life is a plentiful and constant supply of energy obtained from carbohydrates, fats and proteins. Approximately 65% of the dry matter in the diet of a cat or dog is used to provide energy. Animals are capable of regulating their energy intake to meet their daily caloric requirements accurately. When allowed access to a moderately palatable balanced diet, most cats and dogs will consume only enough food to meet their energy needs. If the potential energy content of the food is low, the animal will respond by eating more. In fact, the animal's natural ability to regulate its energy intake is often modified by environmental factors. A highly palatable and energy-rich pet food leads to overconsumption. Accompanied by a lack of exercise and a sedentary, housebound lifestyle, with the consequent onset of obesity, medical problems can arise. With this in mind, it is unlikely that owners can rely on their pets controlling their energy intake, judging by the speed with which the average pet scoffs all its food. Constant overfeeding of growing dogs with high-energy food may eventually result in skeletal disorders, such as osteochondrosis and hip dysplasia. Further, excess energy is stored primarily as fat, resulting in weight gain, obesity and a change in body composition in adulthood.

The energy content of food is measured in units of calories or kilocalories. Animals cannot use all of a food's energy because losses occur during digestion and assimilation. The term 'metabolisable energy' (ME) is used to describe the amount of energy ultimately available for use by the body tissues. ME is the measure most often used to express the energy content of pet food constituents. Its value depends on both nutrient composition and the animal that is consuming it.

Food requirements

The main nutritional requirements of cat and dog food are as follows:

- Carbohydrates are the preferred source of energy, leaving proteins for tissue repair and growth, and should be available in adequate quantities in food.
- Fat provides the most concentrated source of energy. It is a source of essential fatty acids and allows the absorption of fat-soluble vitamins. It also provides texture to the food formulation and enhances palatability.
- Proteins are the main structural building blocks of the body. A regular intake of protein is necessary to maintain metabolic processes. Proteins also enhance the palatability of pet food.
- Vitamins. Most vitamins cannot be synthesised and must be administered. They are included in pet foods.
- Minerals. Necessary mineral supplementation is provided.
- Electrolytes. These aid digestion.
- Water. For an animal to survive, water is the single most important nutrient. Water is obtained from metabolic sources, drinking and food, from which it is absorbed in the large intestine. If the water content of the food is decreased (e.g. by giving dry meals) the animal will usually compensate by drinking more. A plentiful supply of fresh drinking water in addition to food is therefore very important.

Digestion and absorption

Digestion commences in the mouth with the mastication of food and the addition of saliva. Compared with the many ruminant and herbivorous species that thoroughly masticate their food (see chapter 9), cats and dogs often swallow large boluses of food with little or no chewing. Domestic cats and dogs both have six incisor and two canine teeth in their upper and lower jaws, but dogs have more premolars and molars than cats. These teeth facilitate an increased capacity to chew and crush food, actions associated with an omnivorous diet. The dentition of cats is more typical of a carnivore diet. A lack of meat can lead to vitamin A deficiency. Although both cats and dogs are meat-eating animals, dogs have evolved with greater ability to consume plant material. Digestion continues throughout the gastrointestinal tract. Waste products and undigested food are excreted in the feces.

The feeding process

Within the first 24 hours of life, cats and dogs are reliant on colostrum to provide immunoglobulins that protect against infectious disease.

Instructions for the feeding of kittens and puppies should be sought from the breeder or veterinary surgeon.

The exact feeding regime followed for older cats and dogs depends on a number of factors, including the age of animal, convenience for the owner and the number of animals being fed. Requirements for energy and certain nutrients may vary significantly during the lifetime of a pet. As with humans, greater requirements are likely during growth, reproduction and while performing physical activity or work. Decreased requirements occur during adulthood and old age, although this may depend on the breed and associated levels of activity. Weaned puppies and kittens may need up to four meals a day; for elderly animals one meal may suffice, with occasional days missed altogether.

In contrast to dogs, most cats eat slowly. If allowed uncontrolled access to food they will eat small amounts at various times during the day. Dogs eat rapidly, particularly if another animal is beside them, and this can lead to choking and overconsumption. Feeding dogs separately with controlled portions is to be preferred.

The practice of giving treats and feeding pets from the table is not to be condoned. It is much better to offer a small dog-biscuit to Fido! If treats are to be given, for example during training, specially formulated pet products are available.

Commercial pet foods

History   It was not until James Spratt, an American living in London, produced a dog-biscuit that pet food became commercially available. Before this date, owners fed their animals on home-made recipes or dinner-table scraps. After a successful launch in England, Spratt began selling his products in the USA, and was followed by a number of other competitors in the early 1900s. Commercial production in the UK began in the 1930s, when the Chappel brothers began canning a meat and cereal food for dogs. During the Second World War, a shortage of the tins in which pet foods had been packaged led to the emergence of dried food, but after the war most owners returned to familiar canned products. In the 1950s a process known as 'extrusion' was perfected, and this led to a significant breakthrough for producers of dry foods. Extrusion involves first mixing all the ingredients and then rapidly cooking the mixture and forcing it through a specialised pressure cooker (known as an 'extruder'). This process causes rapid expansion of the bite-sized food particles, resulting in increased digestibility and palatability. After drying, the pieces are coated with a palatability enhancer. Because little was known about the dietary requirements of cats and dogs, the same formula was used for both species – only the labels were different! Now, a wide range of different formulae are available to accommodate the various dietary requirements of cats and dogs.

Adult animals can still be fed on home-prepared food, but for the less experienced owner commercially prepared pet food is the best option. The foods are expertly formulated and, provided the instructions on the label are followed with respect to quantity, they ensure that pets receive a balanced diet.

Types of pet food   Commercial pet foods are available in a variety of forms, depending on the ingredients included and the manufacturing process. Foods may also be classified in terms of their nutrient content, the purpose for which they have been formulated and the quality of the ingredients. From a marketing perspective, pet foods may be categorised by outlet: e.g. grocery store, pet store or veterinary surgeon.

Dry pet food   Dry pet foods contain between 6 and 10% moisture and 90% or more dry matter. Ingredients include meat, poultry or fish, cereal grains, some milk products, vitamins and mineral supplements. The energy content is generally sufficient for most animals, except perhaps working dogs or other animals with high energy requirements. This type of food is preferred by many owners, who find it more hygienic and easier to use and keep after opening the packet. In the past, this food has been less palatable than other forms, but recent market entrants have rectified this and also increased the energy content, allowing a reduction in the total quantity needed by the animal. This in turn has reduced the production of feces. A range of products is available for different stages of a pet's life (see Figure 13.11).

Canned pet food   Canned foods contain blends of ingredients such as meats, poultry or fish, cereal grains, vegetable protein, vitamins and minerals. They are made by first blending the meat and fat ingredients with water, then adding the dry ingredients and heating. A canning and sterilisation process follows. Finally, the cans are labelled and packed.

Canned foods are highly palatable and have a good energy content. They may predispose animals to obesity if they have modest energy requirements and are constantly fed on them. The cans are easy to store and have a good shelf life, although once opened they must be

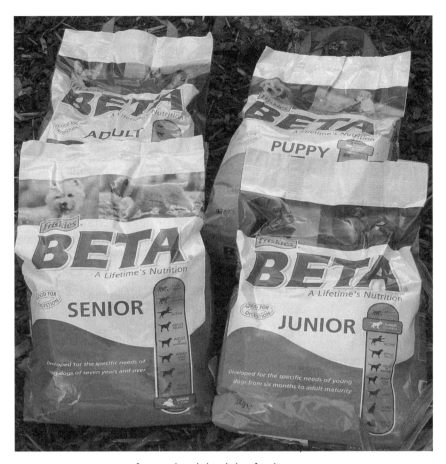

Figure 13.11 Range of age-related dried dog foods.

used within a short period of time. The higher water content partly satisfies the animals' water requirement, reducing the need for drinking.

Semi-moist pet food Semi-moist foods include fresh or frozen animal tissues, cereal grains, fats and sugar. They are highly palatable but have a lower energy content than canned foods. Owners find them agreeable because they tend to have less odour than canned foods. The idea of using fresh produce also appeals to owners.

Treats Most pet owners buy treats for emotional reasons! They are more concerned with palatability and appearance than with nutritional value, and marketing strategies take account of this. That said, some do provide nutrient supplementation, but this is not the main aim. Treats may be of the biscuit, rawhide or semi-moist type.

Probiotics and prebiotics

Pets' digestion problems are among the most common reasons for visits to the veterinary surgeon. In fact, recent studies show that 92% of pet owners rank their pet's digestive health as a major area of concern. In recent years there has been significant interest in the use of dietary procedures targeted towards improved gastrointestinal health. For humans, both probiotics and prebiotics are widely used to fortify species of bacteria seen as beneficial.

Probiotics are viable bacterial cell preparations or foods containing viable bacterial cultures or components of bacterial cells that have beneficial effects on the health of the host. The term thus includes fermented foods and specially isolated and cultured bacteria, and mixtures of bacteria with adjuvants. Most of the common probiotics are lactic-acid-producing bacteria, including species of *Bifidobacterium*, *Lactobacillus*, *Enterococcus* and *Streptococcus*. They are useful in the treatment of disturbed microflora and increased gut permeability, conditions that are characteristic of many intestinal disorders. Historically, probiotics have been more widely used in farm animals, where live microbial feed additions are used to increase weight or yield. More recently, there has been a move towards the use of probiotics in the pet food market, where animal wellbeing is a major concern. This may be driven by the fact that one of the most useful aspects of probiotic use is improved resistance to transmitted infections. To date, all probiotics for pet food use are strains isolated from humans or farm animals.

Less well known but just as effective are the prebiotics. One example of a prebiotic is chicory root, known to aid digestion in humans. It has been shown to stimulate the growth of both *Lactobacillus* and *Bifidobacterium* in the digestive system of dogs. After consuming a diet with chicory for 30 days, the number of bifidobacteria in the average dog's system can increase by 100 times.

Legislation

The manufacture and sale of pet food is comprehensively regulated in two main ways:

- All foods for animals are governed by the same legislation. As pet food is manufactured and distributed in the same way as human food, some legislation governing human food is equally applicable to pet food.
- Additionally, pet food is governed by the law that was designed to safeguard raw materials destined for the human food chain, from which the pet food

industry also sources its raw materials. Examples of this include the laws restricting the residue levels of veterinary substances in meat and those of pesticides in cereal products. In addition, there is specific legislation governing pet food.

The Feeding Stuffs Regulations 2000   Much of the EU legislation governing farm feeds and pet foods is implemented nationally through the Feeding Stuff Regulations 2000 (as amended). These regulations include provisions on labelling, additives and contaminants (see chapter 3).

Weights and measures   Prepacked pet foods are governed by the Packaging Goods Regulations made under the Weights and Measures Act. These regulations require the net weight of the product to be shown on every package and lay down rules on the size and form which the quantity declaration must take. Net weight is also an obligatory declaration under the Feeding Stuffs Regulations 1995.

The Animal By-Products Order   The use of meat as a raw material for human foods is governed largely by the Red Meat Directive, whereas that destined for use in pet food manufacture is governed by the Animal Waste Directive, which is currently being revised, and the Balai Directive, among others.

In the UK, the Animal Waste Directive is implemented by the Animal By-Products Order (ABPO). Companies have to be registered under the ABPO, which defines the ingredients and materials permitted for use by pet food manufacturers and the processing of these products.

The Balai Directive   The Balai Directive, which is currently being revised, ensures the controls in the Animal Waste Directive by harmonising requirements throughout the EU, governing the collection, handling, movement, storage and processing of raw material. These controls also cover raw materials and finished products imported from outside the EU.

Animal By-Products (Identification) Order   These regulations apply to all animal by-products not intended for human consumption. The regulations govern the movement, storage, documentation and processing of the raw animal materials not intended for human consumption. Among other measures, the regulations require that any material which is not destined for licensed or registered premises (under the ABPO) must be stained or sterilised.

Exercise for cats and dogs

A house dog should receive exercise of some type every day. A miniature breed can get exercise by chasing a ball up and down the hall, playing tug-of-war or running up and down the stairs. A larger dog should be allowed to run in a fenced garden or be taken for a walk every day. A dog that receives insufficient exercise is likely to become obese and develop physical defects. Cats normally take exercise on their own.

Routine ectoparasite and endoparasite control

Routine parasitic control is important for the animal's general state of health and will serve to minimise the chance of zoonotic infection. The necessary procedures are outlined under the relevant sections earlier in this chapter (see Figures 13.1 to 13.4).

Vaccination programmes

The theory of vaccination is covered in detail in chapter 4. In this section, examples of common cat and dog vaccines are mentioned with some indication as to when they should be administered. A Working Group was set up in 1999 by the UK Veterinary Products Committee (itself established in 1970 under Section 4 of the Medicines Act 1968) in response to concern in both the public domain and the scientific community about possible health risks related to the routine vaccination of cats and dogs. The Working Group concluded that vaccination plays a very valuable role in the prevention and control of major infectious diseases in cats and dogs. Although adverse reactions to vaccination, including lack of efficacy, occur occasionally, the Working Group concluded that the overall risk/benefit analysis strongly supports their continued use.

Cat

All cats should be vaccinated against panleukopenia virus and the two cat influenza viruses (herpesvirus and calicivirus). This is because these viruses are very common and disease can be severe.

Vaccination against enteritis (panleukopenia virus) is highly successful and the vaccine is one of the best available. Unvaccinated cats are at considerable risk of infection and the virus is widespread in the environment. When disease does occur it can be rapidly fatal and/or severely debilitating.

The two cat influenza viruses are to be found everywhere and infection with these viruses is extremely common, particularly in young cats. Vaccination against these viruses is not completely protective as the vaccines currently available do not cover some strains of calicivirus, and some cats will become infected despite vaccination. However, the use of the vaccine does normally at least prevent severe disease developing and in many cases may prevent disease entirely.

The other two vaccines currently available in the UK are for *Chlamydia* and FeLV. Not all cats necessarily need to be vaccinated against these organisms as the lifestyle or environment in which some cats are kept will mean they are highly unlikely to encounter these diseases. For example, FeLV is usually transmitted by prolonged close contact between cats, and it does not survive in the environment. *Chlamydia* also is only transmitted by direct or close contact between cats. Thus, a cat confined indoors, or confined to an enclosed run outside, may never run the risk of being exposed to these organisms.

Initially, kittens acquire antibodies from their mother's milk in the first few days of life. These antibodies protect young kittens against disease but also prevent vaccines working in the very young. Most vaccines are therefore first given to kittens at around 9 weeks of age, with a second dose at 12 weeks of age. The second dose is very important in ensuring adequate protection. Additional earlier vaccines may be appropriate if there is a particular risk of infection.

With most vaccines, further booster injections are usually required to maintain good protection. Cats should receive their first booster injection a year after the kitten vaccines are given. Subsequent annual booster injections are usually advised for at least some diseases, and currently most manufacturers can only prove that their vaccines are effective for a year.

However, some vaccines appear to induce protection that lasts much longer than a year. Some veterinary surgeons therefore advise less frequent booster vaccinations, often every 3 years subsequently, at least for panleukopenia virus and the cat influenza viruses (unless there is a particular risk of infection).

Cats can act as a reservoir of rabies virus, but they are seldom vaccinated by owners unless they are being taken abroad. Examples of cat vaccination programmes are summarised in Table 13.6.

Dog

For dogs, vaccinations are commonly given against distemper, parvovirus, hepatitis, parainfluenza, leptospirosis and now rabies (pet

Table 13.6 Examples of feline vaccination programmes

Disease	Dose regime	Booster	Example
Chlamydiosis	Vaccinated from 9 weeks, second dose 3–4 weeks later	Annually	Katavac (Fort Dodge)
Feline leukaemia	Vaccinated from 9 weeks, second dose 2–4 weeks later	Annually	Inactivated Leucogen (Virbac) Nobivac FelV (Intervet)
Feline infective enteritis	One dose at 12 weeks, further dose at 16 weeks		Live vaccine: Feliniffa P (Merial) Inactivated: Nobivac FPL (Intervet)
Feline influenza and infective enteritis (combined vaccine)	One dose at 9 weeks; another at 12 weeks in kittens, start any time in cats.	Annually	Live vaccine Nobivac Tricat (Intervet)
Feline influenza, infective enteritis and feline leukaemia (also chlamydiosis)	One dose at 9 weeks; another at 12 weeks in kittens, start any time in cats.	Annually	Inactivated Fevaxyn Pentofel (Fort Dodge)
Rabies vaccine	See canine vaccine		

Note: Immunity in kittens achieved approximately 2 weeks after vaccination

quarantine exemption scheme). Although none of these diseases is common, they are still seen and are all potentially devastating, so vaccination is an important part of the preventative healthcare of pets.

A puppy vaccination programme usually consists of two injections 2–4 weeks apart, and can now be completed by 10–12 weeks of age, depending on the vaccines used. On each occasion, the dog should be thoroughly examined and advice given on any other health concerns that may arise.

Manufacturers and most veterinary surgeons will recommend annual booster vaccinations, but there is now some controversy about the ideal interval between vaccinations. Veterinary surgeons will advise owners on the best programme to follow, depending on the local disease situation and the state of a particular dog's health. Examples of dog vaccination programmes are summarised in Table 13.7.

Table 13.7 Examples of canine vaccination programmes

Disease	Dose regime	Booster	Example
CPV + ICH	Vaccination at 9–12 weeks or if risk high at 6–8 weeks, repeated at 12 weeks	At one year then repeat vaccination at 1–2 years, thereafter according to titre	Living Nobivac DH (Intervet)
CPV + PI	As above	Annual	Living Nobivac PPi (Intervet)
CPV + CDV + ICH + PI + LPS	Vaccination at 9–12 weeks	According to titre	Inactivated Quantum Dog 7 (Schering-Plough) Intrac
KC	Owners should have their dogs protected prior to sending them into a kennel		Intranasal Solution (Schering-Plough)
Rabies	Only for dogs (and cats) being exported. 4 weeks then repeat at 12 weeks; adult animals only one dose	Every 1–2 years	Inactivated Nobivac Rabies (Intervet)

CDV, canine distemper virus; CPV, canine parvovirus; ICH, infective canine hepatitis; KC, kennel cough (tracheobronchitis); LPS, leptospirosis; PI, parainfluenza

Grooming

The objects of grooming are as follows:

- To promote cleanliness in the household environment.
- To prevent dermatological infection.
- To stimulate the circulation.
- To remove any waste products.

One should begin by combing against the lie of the hair in order to remove any particles of dirt that may have accumulated, before brushing in the direction of the hair. In spring and autumn, when the coat is changing, more careful grooming is required because quantities of dead and loose hair need to be removed to make way for the new coat. Cats, particularly long-haired varieties, benefit from regular grooming. Bathing is possible if animals are particularly dirty, and there are shampoos available for cats and dogs (see Figure 13.12). Owners should be wary of using products formulated for human use as they can cause allergic reactions, especially in small terriers such as Cairn terriers. The animals should be thoroughly dried.

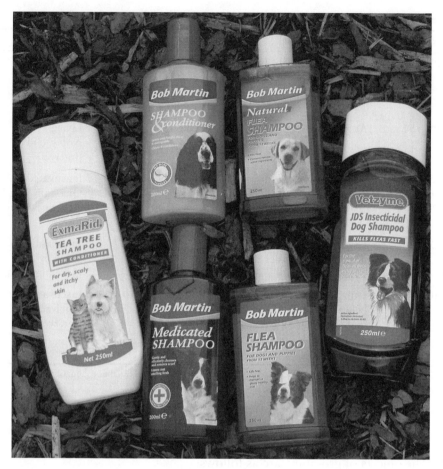

Figure 13.12 Cat and dog shampoos.

Pets are not groomed merely to make them look attractive, but to safeguard both their own and their owners' health. There are opportunities for pharmacies to keep a range of grooming products, given these health implications (see chapter 7).

Travelling abroad with cats and dogs

The Pets Travel Scheme (PETS for short) allows owners to take a cat or dog to a total of 37 countries and to return to the UK without putting the animal into quarantine, subject to compliance with a number of regulations regarding the countries of destination, the route of travel and the carrier, together with chip identification and vaccination requirements.

Preparations should ideally start not less than 6 months before the intended date of travel. When an owner has chosen his or her destination, it is advisable to visit the government website (http://www.maff.gov.uk/animalh/quarantine) or telephone the PETS helpline (+44 (0)870 2411 710) to check the following points:

- Is the country accepted into the scheme?
- Are there any additional requirements for this country?
- Which routes of travel are authorised?

The necessary actions are shown in Table 13.8.

The following countries are accepted for the scheme at the time of writing: Andorra, Austria, Belgium, Canada, Denmark, Finland, France, Germany, Gibraltar, Greece, Iceland, Italy, Liechtenstein, Luxembourg, Monaco, the Netherlands, Norway, Portugal, San Marino, Spain, Sweden, Switzerland, The Vatican, Ascension Islands,

Table 13.8 The PETS scheme – timetable for obtaining immunity from quarantine

Timetable	Action
6 months before departure	Arrange appointment with vet for insertion of microchip (ISO Standard 11784 or 11785) and then for administration of rabies vaccine.
5 months before departure	Visit vet for blood sample to ensure immunity. If no immunity, animal must be revaccinated and tested again. Once the pet has been successfully blood tested, it will be able to re-enter the UK *no less than 6 months after the date the blood sample was taken.* Following successful vaccination, they must have a health certificate signed by a veterinary surgeon.
3 months before departure	Confirm pet's travel on approved route and with approved carrier.
24–48 hours prior to return to UK	Arrange consultation with approved vet at destination for treatment for tapeworm and ticks and obtain certificate to confirm treatment completed.
Day of return travel	Ensure that pet is fit and well and that all necessary documentation is available for inspection at the port of re-entry to UK.

Australia, Barbados, Bermuda, Cyprus, Falkland Islands, Hawaii, Japan, Malta, Montserrat, New Caledonia, New Zealand, St Helena, Singapore, USA, Vanatu.

In July 2003, the UK government announced that the pet passport scheme in Europe was being extended to small mammals, including rabbits, gerbils, hamsters, guinea pigs, mice and ferrets.

Problems arising from the scheme

The availability of appropriate medicines for the treatment of exotic diseases of companion animals after the increased international movement under PETS has given cause for concern. Specifically, there have been several confirmed cases of babesiosis and leishmaniosis in travelled animals. Appropriate antiprotozoal therapies (imidocarb dipropionate and meglumine antimoniate) can be used under the cascade; however these products are not universally available outside endemic areas. Imidocarb dipropionate is available in Australia (Imizol, Coopers) and in Eire and the USA (Imizol, Schering-Plough). Meglumine antimonite can be acquired from France (Glucantime, Merial) after the granting of a Special Treatment Authorisation. The latter allows the import of a medicine licensed in another country for a specific case if it is currently unavailable in the UK, but obtaining the authorisation is a slow process. Babesiosis is an acute disease that requires rapid initiation of therapy, while leishmaniosis has potential zoonotic implications that are magnified by any delay in initiating treatment. At the time of writing, arrangements were in progress to hold stocks of such products at the Veterinary Medicines Directorate (VMD) to speed up the process of Special Treatment Authorisation and ensure that treatment can be carried out in a more timely manner.

Another problem with the scheme is the post-dating of veterinary certificates by some foreign veterinary surgeons trying to be helpful to visitors. This has happened when a road journey in excess of the 2-day second vaccination period is necessary to reach the final UK destination, and it contravenes the rules.

References

Baker K P, Mulcahy R (1986). Fleas on hedgehogs and dogs in Dublin area. *Vet Rec* 119: 161–167.

Bell J C, Palmer S R, Payne J M (1981). *The Zoonoses*. London: Edward Arnold, 1988.

Beresford-Jones W P (1981). Prevalence of fleas on dogs and cats in an area of central London. *J Zoon* 22: 272–279.

Borg C A, Woodruff A W (1974). Prevalence of infected ova of *Toxocara* species in public places. *Br Med J* 289: 424–426.

Cockrum E L (1997). *Rabies, Lyme Disease, Hanta Virus*.Tucson: Fisher Books.

Francis H, Fletcher G, Anthony C, *et al.* (2003). Clinical effects of air filters in homes of asthmatic adults sensitised and exposed to pet allergens. *Clin Exp Allergy* 33: 101–105.

Gavgani A S, Mohite H, Edrissian G H, *et al.* (2002). Domestic dog ownership in Iran is a risk factor for human infection with *Leishmania infantum*. *Am J Trop Med Hyg* 67: 511–515.

Goddard J (1997). Ticks and Lyme Disease. *Infect Med* 1997 14: 698–700, 702.

Guzman R F (1984). A survey of cats and dogs for fleas with particular reference to their role as intermediate hosts of *Dipylidium caninum*. *NZ Vet J* 32: 71–73.

Henry Ford Health System Study (2002). *Living with a dog or cat may reduce pet - allergies.* Detroit: The Henry Ford Health System (http://www.henryford.com/body.cfm?id=33666&action=detail&ref=359 last accessed 05/01/04).

Krebs J W, Noll H R, Rupprecht C E, Childs J E (2002). Rabies surveillance in the United States during 2001. *J Am Vet Med Assoc* 221: 1690–1701.

Leake J (2003). Inbred pedigree dog breeds to be 'gene cleansed'. *The Sunday Times, London*, 25 May.

Miles A (1994). A rare event letter. *Chemist Druggist* 249: 592.

Naimer S A, Cohen A D, Mumcuoglu K Y (2002). Household papular urticaria. *Isr Med Assoc J* 4 (Suppl): 911–913.

Paul A J (1988). Environmental contamination by eggs of *Toxocara* spp. *Vet Parasitol* 26: 339–342.

Pet Food Manufacturers Association (1999) *Profile*. London: Pet Food Association.

Williamson B (1995). Eradicating fleas (Letter). *Br Med J* 310: 672.

Further reading

Bishop Y, ed. (2001). *The Veterinary Formulary*, 5th edn. London: Pharmaceutical Press.

Boden E, ed. (2001). *Black's Veterinary Dictionary*, 20th edn. London: A & C Black.

Coren S (1994). *The Intelligence of Dogs. Canine Consciousness and Capabilities.* New York: Free Press.

Dunn J, ed. (1999). *Textbook of Small Animal Medicine*. London: W B Saunders.

Roach P (1995). *The Complete Book of Pet Care*. Sydney: Landsdowne Publishing.

Useful addresses

Children in Hospital and Animal Therapy Association (CHATA)
87 Longland Drive, London N20 8HD, UK
Tel. +44 (0)20 8445 7883

The Pet Bereavement Support Service
c/o Blue Cross, Shilton Road, Burford, Oxfordshire OX18 4 PF, UK
Tel. +44 (0)800 0966606

14

Other small pets

Steven B Kayne

Small mammals

A wide range of prescription drugs have market authorisations for administration to small mammals. However, not all are universally appropriate for all the species. For example, amongst antibiotics enrofloxacin (Baytril, Bayer) may be used in all species while the coccidiosidal robenidine (Cycostat 66G, Roche) is only authorised for use in rabbits. Tetracycline and tylosin are not authorised for use in guinea pigs. Full details of the applications of drugs may be found in *The Veterinary Formulary*.

Rabbits

History

Originally the European rabbit (*Oryctolagus cuniculus*) was found in the regions of Spain, Portugal and North West Africa. *Oryct* is Greek for digger, *lag* is Greek for hare and *cunniculus* is Latin for burrowing. Rabbits were introduced to England in the 11th century and used for sport, meat and, in some cases, fur (such as the angora rabbits whose fur was spun for wool). Subsequently, they were kept in hutches for breeding and meat production. By the 19th century rabbits had become pets. There are estimated to be around 4.5 million pet rabbits in the UK at the time of writing; a further 38–40 million wild rabbits roam the countryside.

Breeds

There are over 50 breeds of rabbit (ranging from the Alaska to the Vienna) and over 500 varieties. They vary greatly in size, colour and coat and are split into three main groups: fancy, fur and rex.

The fancy group includes the breeds that are kept for exhibition purposes. The first true 'fancy' breed was the English lop (whose ears sweep the ground); this was followed by the English (spotted) and the angora. They are bred for their appearance, including body shape or type and size.

Fur are shown for the colour and pattern or coat markings and rex for their particular velvety texture. Both fur and fancy rabbit breeds are included in the group called commercial rabbits, which are raised for their meat.

Animal charities have reported that domestic rabbits are one of the most neglected and ill-treated pets in the UK, because they spend most of their lives in solitude, imprisoned in their hutches at the bottom of the garden.

Housing and nutrition

Rabbits need good, secure, roomy housing with plenty of space to exercise. It should always be high enough that the rabbit can sit upright, with his ears pricked, without touching the top of the hutch. In cold weather there must be adequate protection from draughts, wind and rain. A warm, dry, comfortable bed is of the utmost importance to animals that have to spend a good deal of their time in a hutch. The sleeping compartment needs a layer of peat moss, cat litter or wood shavings about 5 cm deep with a deep layer of straw or shredded paper to provide warmth, insulation and an opportunity for burrowing. A run should be provided that allows the animal plenty of room to exercise. Rabbits like company, so a pair of the same sex will happily co-exist in a hutch outside, even in harsh conditions. Hutches should be cleaned out on a regular basis.

In their natural habitat rabbits eat a range of grasses, weeds, leaves, shoots and twigs, as well as the bark of shrubs, bushes and trees. They will also eat crops, roots, fruit and vegetables. Rabbits are herbivores and their digestive system has evolved to be extremely efficient, with the ability to eliminate indigestible fibre rapidly and ferment those fibres that are digestible. Owners often feed rabbits with fresh plants to vary the diet. Some plants can cause toxic reactions and, possibly, death. These include buttercups, clematis, elder, foxglove, holly, iris, ivy and woody nightshade.

Common conditions

Rabbits suffer from numerous conditions and illnesses and it is important to detect signs of these at an early stage. Some of the most common diseases are considered below.

Dental problems   Rabbits' teeth continue to grow throughout their life, at a rate of 2–3 mm per week. Overgrown molars and incisors can cause problems. Rabbits require a high-fibre diet to ensure the teeth are evenly worn and to prevent overgrowth. If the teeth are not worn down they grow incorrectly. Maladjusted teeth can lead to discomfort, abscesses and anorexia. The latter is a particularly serious condition for rabbits (see Gastrointestinal disorders below). Indications of dental problems include saliva around the mouth or on the chest or front paws, an inability to eat and teeth grinding. Teeth may require 'burring' or clipping by the vet to correct the problem.

Diarrhoea   Chronic diarrhoea is quite common in rabbits. Over a period of time it can make the animal unthrifty and thin in appearance; death, however, is rare. The main problem with this syndrome is an increased vulnerability to flystrike (see below). Tyzzer's disease may affect rabbits as well as rodents (see below) and generally responds to tetracyclines. Coccidiosis (caused by *Eimeria* spp.) is also a possible cause of diarrhoea, particularly in cases of overcrowding or where cleanliness has been compromised. This may be treated with clopidol (Zootechnical Feed Additives) available as a premix for addition to feedingstuff (Coyden Pure, Merial).

A major factor in rabbit diarrhoea may be the animal's diet, it should be put on a commercial dry rabbit diet, water and good quality hay, but no greens. Persistent diarrhoea cases should have samples taken for bacteriological investigation and an attempt should be made to find the cause of the disease.

Iatrogenic diarrhoea can be caused by a proliferation of clostridia in the gut following administration of certain antibiotics. Enrofloxacin (Baytril, Bayer) is a suitable alternative. It is important to maintain fluid balance. Hartmann's solution containing 3 g sodium chloride, 2 g potassium chloride, 0.147 g calcium chloride and 1.625 g sodium lactate in 500 mL sterile water may be administered by infusion for this purpose.

Eye problems   Conjunctivitis occurs in the rabbit on a regular basis. Sometimes the cause is simple, for example, following hay getting into the animal's eye. This will respond to a topical eye antibiotic such as chloramphenicol. Pasturella infections are very resistant to treatment. Cloxacillin and gentamicin ophthalmic ointments offer possibilities here.

Flystrike   Flies are attracted to rabbit droppings, either in the hutch or around the rabbit's anus. Fly eggs will hatch into maggots and initially feed on the droppings, they will then burrow into the rabbit, causing discomfort, pain and possibly death. Flystrike may be avoided by removing droppings regularly from the hutch, grooming the rabbit frequently and ensuring good ventilation. The hutch and bedding should be sprayed with an appropriate agent to deter flies and eliminate maggots and bacteria.

Gastrointestinal disorders   The ingestion of large amounts of shedding hair while grooming can result in intestinal stasis. The hair either mixes with the food and slows down its passage or it may form a hairball and entirely block the intestine. Rabbits tend to become uncomfortable with the stasis and may stop eating and drinking altogether, which may lead to more serious conditions.

Treatment involves giving intravenous fluid (in the more severe cases) or subcutaneous fluid in combination with oral fluid. Pineapple or papaya juice diluted 50 : 50 with water to reduce sugar content may be recommended. These fruits contain an enzyme known as papain that is reputed to digest hair. The juice should always be fresh or frozen, as the enzyme is not active in canned products. Other forms of treatment include laxatives, oils to help lubricate the system, and intestinal stimulants, such as the approved human drugs metoclopramide, or cisapride, to increase regular intestinal muscle contraction and motility. Owners should remove shedding hair from the rabbit regularly to prevent ingestion. Any hair not physically removed will probably be ingested when the animal grooms itself. Shedding hair can also be removed by brushing, plucking or using sticky lint rollers.

Myxomatosis   Myxomatosis is a viral disease which wiped out 99% of the wild rabbit population when it arrived in Britain in 1954. The disease was introduced and spread intentionally in a bid to reduce the population of 100 million rabbits that were causing widespread damage to crops. The sight of stricken rabbits was so unpleasant that the Pests' Act was amended to make the practice illegal.

The number and severity of outbreaks varies over time; the myxomatosis virus is notorious for its ability to mutate from year to year, and the background immunity in the wild rabbit population also varies. Southern England suffered a severe outbreak of myxomatosis in autumn 2000, which was thought to have been caused by a more virulent strain than had occurred in recent years. A handful of reports of vaccinated rabbits developing myxomatosis in these areas led to a suspicion that vaccination may not be fully effective against this possible new strain of myxomatosis and served as a reminder to all rabbit owners that vaccination is just one of a series of measures that have to be taken to protect pet rabbits from this deadly disease.

The disease starts with runny eyes and swollen genitalia. If full-blown myxomatosis then develops, the rabbit will be a pitiful sight. Severe conjunctivitis causes blindness and is accompanied by swelling of the head and genital region, plus lumps on the body. The rabbit can take a fortnight to die. There are also two atypical forms of myxomatosis: one causes pneumonia and a snuffles-like illness; the other ('nodular myxomatosis') mainly affects skin and carries a better prognosis.

Domestic rabbits do not have any genetically based immunity against myxomatosis. If an unvaccinated pet rabbit catches myxomatosis, it will almost certainly die. Pet rabbits at greatest risk are those that live outside, in contact with wild rabbits or hares, or affected by rabbit fleas – so rabbit owners who also have a dog or cat that hunts wild rabbits must be particularly careful. House rabbits are at less risk than outdoor rabbits, but can and do get myxomatosis too.

Animals can be protected with a vaccine. The myxomatosis vaccine used in Britain (Nobivac Myxo, Intervet) is made from a harmless virus called *Shope fibroma*. Antibodies made in response to *Shope fibroma* also protect against myxomatosis – this is called cross immunity. Different vaccines (including live attenuated myxomatosis virus) are used elsewhere in Europe, but tend to have more side-effects and there are concerns that they are not safe enough for use in pet rabbits.

Six-monthly boosters are recommended by the vaccine manufacturers for rabbits in high-risk areas and 12-monthly boosters are recommended for everyone else! Because myxomatosis tends to break out in autumn, the optimal time for once-yearly vaccination is late spring/early summer. Most vaccines are given entirely subcutaneously, but the myxomatosis vaccine is different. About a tenth of the dose must be given intradermally for adequate immunity to be achieved.

Parasitic infestation Rabbits are prone to a number of internal and external parasites, including fleas, fur mites, a pox virus, worms and coccidiosis, the latter often being responsible for diarrhoea. Signs of parasites are numerous, from loss of overall condition, to serious skin disease and diarrhoea, depending upon the type and place of the infection.

Ectoparasites In warm weather rabbits kept outdoors may become infested with fleas, identified by their black feces ('coal dust') when the hair is parted. Treatment is by application of insecticidal sprays or powders suitable for cats and environmental cleansing (see chapter 13).

Cheyletiella parasitovorax The fur mite can be detected by brushing the animal over a sheet of black paper, if the paper is then warmed the mites can be seen moving – from whence came the trivial name of 'creeping dandruff'. In the rabbit the mites cause an inflamed area on the animal's back. The rabbit will scratch the infected area until large raw patches appear.

Owners have reported being bitten by the mite on their arms during grooming their pet rabbits.

Ear mites (Psoroptes cuniculi) These cause reactions ranging from a mild inflammation to severe crusting that may need softening before gentle removal. A dog ear cleanser may be appropriate for this.

Ringworm is an uncommon disease of domestic rabbits and is associated with poor husbandry. Griseofulvin (25 mg/kg body weight) may be given once weekly for 4 weeks.

A zoonotic risk should be noted.

Endoparasites The two most common parasites causing neurological disease in the rabbit are *Encephalitozoon cuniculi* (also known as *Nosema cuniculi*) and *Baylisascaris procyonis*. There is continuing controversy as to the presence of the former, as most rabbits affected with this parasite remain completely normal throughout their lives. Coccidiosis (see under Diarrhoea) can also be a problem.

Parasiticides for rabbits Pet rabbits should be kept free of all parasites to keep them in optimum health and the hutch should be cleaned thoroughly if animals are affected. Unfortunately, few veterinary medicinal products for the treatment of endoparasites and ectoparasites currently have UK marketing authorisations for the treatment of rabbits. The following have been recommended:

- Ivermectin for endoparasites and ectoparasites – 200–400 µg/kg body weight by subcutaneous injection or 400 µg by mouth.
- Piperazine for endoparasites – 500 µg/kg body weight by mouth, repeated after 10 days.
- Permethrin for ectoparasites (e.g. *Cheytiella*) – used as an external dusting powder.

Pasteurellosis *Pasteurella* ('snuffles') is a common cause of respiratory disease in rabbits caused by the bacterium *Pasteurella multocida*. Most rabbits are exposed to it and harbour the organism that causes it. It can become a chronic problem that is difficult to control. Some infected rabbits will only show symptoms when under stress. The carriers can spread the problem to other rabbits without having any symptoms of their own. This can make control difficult. *Pasteurella* is spread by mating, through general contact (especially respiratory), or through wounds from fighting. The disease can be brought on by stress resulting from a number of sources, e.g. poor environmental conditions or pregnancy.

The animal will develop cold-like symptoms, with a runny nose, breathing difficulties and discharge from the eyes. Snuffles can lead to more serious problems such a pneumonia, head tilt and abscesses in the mouth and under the skin and death. The commonest cause of death in rabbits is septicaemia caused by *P. multocida* infection. Most cases are treated with antibiotics e.g. enrofloxacin (Baytril, Bayer). They sometimes need to be given for weeks or months. The majority of cases brought for treatment are chronic in nature. In these situations the bacteria has had time to become well entrenched, and there is no guarantee that antibiotics will work. If they do work the problem can recur when the antibiotics are stopped. This emphasises the need for routine general veterinary examinations every 6–12 months and a specific physical examination any time the above symptoms are noted. Minimising stress, proper diet, a clean well-ventilated environment, and fresh drinking water at all times, can help in minimising the chance of this infection. The hutch should be dry and kept at a fairly constant temperature (around 16 °C). Any damp bedding should be removed promptly.

Viral haemorrhagic disease (VHD) VHD is caused by a calcivirus, which precipitates an acute infection. This may become fatal even before the characteristic foaming at the mouth, haemorrhagic nasal discharge and convulsions become apparent. Animals that appear to survive the disease may then develop jaundice and die later. A vaccine is available (Cylap, Fort Dodge), administered by subcutaneous injection.

Rodents

Tyzzer's disease

Tyzzer's disease is a serious condition that may be zoonotic. It affects rats, mice, gerbils, guinea pigs and hamsters. Dogs, cats and horses may also be subject to infection. It was first described in 1913 and is caused by various strains of the Gram-negative bacterium *Clostridium piliforme*. The strains are usually species-specific, but an exception is the gerbil which is susceptible to infection from a wide range of strains.

Some species, e.g. mice and rats, particularly in the wild, often carry the disease without any apparent symptoms. Stress, caused by overcrowding, a change in environmental conditions, or infection may cause the disease to break out.

Animals of any age may be affected but the young seem to be the most susceptible. The disease attacks the intestines and the colon and then spreads to the liver. The organism produces a toxin that causes widespread necrosis and can cause failure of almost any organ of the body. Damage to the heart and neurological symptoms, such as loss of coordination or paralysis, are often seen. Signs of acute disease include rough coat, weakness, lethargy, watery to pasty diarrhoea and death. In gerbils a mortality rate of 80% or more of animals showing symptoms is common, death usually occurring within 48 hours of onset. Fatality rates for other species are generally lower.

C. piliforme produces spores which can live for up to 2 years in infected bedding. Spores spread though the feces of the infected animals, and infected animals can continue to produce spores in their feces for up to 2 weeks if they survive the infection. Ingestion of spores probably occurs as animals clean themselves after coming into contact with contaminated bedding.

In research facilities, spontaneous outbreaks of clinical Tyzzer's disease are most commonly seen in gerbils, hamsters, guinea pigs and rabbits. Infections in rats and mice are least likely to show symptoms. A high-protein diet has been shown to predispose animals to Tyzzer's disease.

Antibiotic treatment of infected animals has yielded variable results. Tetracycline, oxytetracycline, and penicillin were the most effective antibiotics for alleviation of clinical signs due to *C. piliforme* infection. Supporting the animal with heat and injected fluids may help.

Some authorities recommend elimination of colonies infected with Tyzzer's disease as the only sure way of stopping the infection from spreading. It is not appropriate to simply treat or remove infected animals because spores will already be spread. Infected bedding, etc. should be destroyed. Anything that may have been in contact with spores needs to be sterilised. Spores are persistent and need to be kept at 80 °C for 30 minutes to kill them. Contaminated surfaces can be effectively disinfected by treatment with bleach for 5 minutes.

Gerbils (sand rat)

Breeds As well as the Mongolian gerbil (*Meriones unguiculatus*), the breed that is normally kept as a pet, there are about 90 other breeds of gerbils and jirds that live in the dry grasslands and desert fringes from South and West Africa to Far Eastern Asia. The survival of gerbils is due to their burrowing instincts.

The gerbil species has evolved to require only limited food and water. In the wild their long hind legs allow them to cover large distances in a harsh habitat in order to collect food. Their bodies require little water as they do not sweat and they re-absorb their liquid intake producing highly concentrated urine and dry feces. Gerbils are generally very healthy robust little creatures and are not prone to frequent disease. There are 'several hundred thousand' gerbils in the UK.

Housing and nutrition   In the wild gerbils live in burrows and spend the majority of time foraging for food. They require sufficient room to eat, sleep and exercise. Ideally they should be kept in pairs or groups with sufficient room to prevent overcrowding. They need to be kept indoors.

Gerbils have traditionally been fed on hamster mixes. However, this is not ideal, as their requirements are different. Commercially available complete foods for gerbils are available.

Common diseases

Dental problems   Dental problems can occur in gerbils that have lost one of the front incisor teeth or in older gerbils which don't tend to chew as much as their younger counterparts. It is usually first identified when the gerbil begins to lose weight. To prevent the problem the gerbil's teeth should be regularly inspected and trimmed by a vet as necessary.

Diarrhoea   Diarrhoea can be a sign of Tyzzer's disease. If gerbils show signs of listlessness and diarrhoea they and any contacts should be isolated immediately. The whole colony of gerbils – infected and healthy – should be treated with antibiotics promptly.

 There is a possibility of a zoonotic risk, so owners should take appropriate precautions when handling sick animals.

Ear problems   Ear cysts, commonly caused by a cholesteatoma result in the gerbil's head being inclined to one side. The gerbil loses balance and often moves around in circles. These cysts are common in older gerbils and are untreatable, although a secondary bacterial infection of the cyst may respond to antibiotics.

Gerbils can injure their ears by excessive cleaning with the long claws of their back feet. Mites can be treated with commercial dusting powder or spray. Cages should be thoroughly washed with boiling water to prevent a return of the infection.

Epilepsy   Between 20 and 40% of young gerbils are prone to epileptic seizures, usually precipitated by stressful events, e.g. being in strange surroundings or excessive handling. The animal begins to twitch, its ears go back and it may drool at the mouth. If this should happen the gerbil should be returned to its cage and placed in a quiet area until it recovers.

Eye problems   One of the causes of sore eyes is sawdust which can get into the membranes of the eye and cause irritation. The gerbil will produce copious quantities of mucus. Treatment is in the form of antibiotic drops. To prevent further recurrence, wood shavings should be used in bedding rather than sawdust.

Nasal problems   Gerbils are easily irritated by the aromatic oils contained in some wood shavings used as bedding, and an allergic response may result on the nose and face. An antibiotic ointment is used to treat sore noses infected with staphylococcus bacilli. Gerbils chew constantly at the bars of their cage and will very often get sore noses from this rubbing action.

Respiratory infections   The gerbil develops a dull staring coat and breathing is very obviously laboured and may be accompanied by clicking sounds. Antibiotic treatment (enrofloxacin or chlortetracycline) is effective.

Ringworm   Ringworm is recognised by circular hair loss which may scab over. It can be transmitted via wood shavings and hay. Treatment is in the form of antifungal lotions. An antibiotic may be administered concurrently if the infection is particularly severe. To prevent recurrence it is essential that any infected animals are isolated and that the cage is thoroughly washed and disinfected.

There is a zoonotic risk associated with ringworm in gerbils.

Tail loss   Gerbils' tails are quite fragile and rough handling can cause the tuft to come away. Very often the bone will be left behind. Whilst it does not look very pleasant, the bone will dry out and then auto-amputate after a few days after which the end will heal over naturally.

Tumours Scent gland tumours are usually more common in older gerbils, particularly males, who tend to mark their territory more than females do. It begins as a small hard lump growing until the gerbil finds it irritating and begins chewing at it. The tumours may be removed by a vet.

Guinea pigs

History The guinea pig suffers from a crisis of identity – it has no connection with Guinea nor is it a pig! It does however make pig-like grunting noises. The guinea pig or cavie *(Cavia porcellus)* originates from South America where the Incas used to breed them for food and sacrifice. People in Ecuador, Peru and Bolivia still keep guinea pigs (known as 'Agouti'), like chicken, for food. The Spanish introduced guinea pigs to Europe in the 16th century after they conquered the Incas. Wild populations of guinea pigs still exist in South America in a range of habitats, including grassland, swamps, forest and rocky areas. Their use in medical research has led to the expression 'being a guinea pig' being adopted to describe the first individuals in which an innovative process or procedure is tested.

Breeds There are three main varieties of domestic guinea pigs:

- English are short-haired and come in one, two or three colours. They are the most common.
- Abyssinians have short to medium length hair with little rosettes and a wide range of colours
- Peruvian are long-haired guinea pigs; when their hair is it's full length (2 cm), it is sometimes difficult to tell which is the front and which the rear! This variety is the least common.

Patterns may vary. For example, tortoiseshell are usually white with another colour in patches while agouti have a 'marbled' appearance.

In all breeds, alertness is their first line of defence. Guinea pigs will spend the majority of the day looking out for predators and dangers. Guinea pigs are very vocal and exhibit interesting body language. They rely heavily on smell and constantly sniff the air looking for an indication of impending danger.

Housing and nutrition Guinea pigs live quite happily in a secure roomy hutch outdoors where they can enjoy plenty of fresh air, and in the UK, occasional sunshine! The hutch should be placed in a position that is sheltered because high temperatures can cause stress which may result in discomfort or illness. Hutches should be cleaned out on a regular basis. This is especially important in warmer weather in order to prevent flies being attracted to the hutch, leading to an infestation of maggots. In the wetter months, bedding can become damp and mouldy from extreme weather.

Guinea pigs need feeding twice a day. They require fresh vegetables and hay together with a source of protein in their diet to keep them healthy. They also need vitamin C daily as they can't produce their own and will fall ill without it.

Owners often feed guinea pigs with fresh plants to vary the diet. Some plants can cause toxic reactions and, possibly, death. These include buttercups, clematis, elder, foxglove, holly, iris, ivy and woody nightshade.

Common diseases

Abscesses   Guinea pigs are prone to suffer from abscesses in the neck and jaw area, but providing these are monitored and, at the appropriate time, lanced and drained, they are seldom, if ever, life-threatening. Abscesses can be caused during knocks or fights, or even by food that is sharp and has scratched the guinea pig.

Bumble foot   Bumble foot manifests as swelling in the foot and slight redness. It is not contagious and is treatable with antibiotics.

Dental problems   As with all rodents guinea pigs' teeth grow throughout their life so they need the opportunity to eat fibrous material to help wear down their teeth. Overgrown teeth can cause a number of problems, including abscesses and an inability to eat, and, in extreme cases, can grow back into the guinea pig's face. Regular clipping of the teeth may be necessary.

Eye injuries   Sometimes guinea pigs can be poked in the eye by stalks of hay or grass and this may cause the eye to go opaque. This will normally clear without treatment but if it persists veterinary assistance should be sought.

Flystrike   Flies are attracted to guinea pig droppings. Fly eggs laid on the animals' fur will hatch into maggots within 12 hours of being laid and will immediately start to burrow deeper into the skin or anus, nostrils, mouth and ears. If they are not immediately eliminated using antiparasitic drugs or dips, the animal will die within 24–48 hours.

Flystrike may be avoided by removing droppings regularly, grooming the guinea pig frequently and ensuring good ventilation to the hutch. A suitable spray should be used on the hutch, and on bedding, to deter flies and eliminate bacteria. Conventional fly killers or repellents in spray form should be avoided, as they can be very hazardous to guinea pigs. A mixture of citronella, lemon balm, lavender and geranium is one possibility.

Mouth scabs   Guinea pigs can cut their lips and mouths on sharp food and the resulting lesion may become infected. The condition may need treatment if ongoing.

Parasitic infestation   Guinea pigs are prone to parasitic and fungal dermatological problems, the most common of which is mange, caused by a mite that burrows into the skin surface. The resulting irritation may develop scabs with bald patches. One treatment involves massage with a combination of essential oil containing tea tree, lemon grass, patchouli, and lavender at a 9 : 1 ratio with a carrier oil. After massaging into the skin and leaving for 24 hours the oils are shampooed off. The procedure may need to be repeated after 3 days. After the first shampoo, it is important to tease out as much of the hair as possible. Other more conventional treatments are as for rabbits, with slightly higher doses; ectoparasites respond to ivermectin, while endoparasites respond to ivermectin and piperazine.

Hamsters

History   The name 'hamster' is derived from the German word 'hamstern' which means 'to hoard'. Around 1930 Professor I Aharoni of the Department of Zoology of Hebrew University, Jerusalem, captured an adult female and her litter of 12 babies near Aleppo, Syria. He gave one male and two females to the university and Dr Ben-Menahem bred them. Some of their babies were sent to England in 1931 and found to make engaging pets. Almost all pet and laboratory hamsters in the world are descended from this one family.

Breeds   The most common pet hamster is the Syrian (also known as golden) hamster *(Mesocricetus auratus)*. They prefer to follow a solitary existence and indeed will fight to the death if another hamster is introduced. Russian and Chinese hamsters (often known as dwarf hamsters) prefer to live in pairs, but the species should not be mixed. Russian hamsters are mainly white, grey and brown in colour, the Chinese hamster will have natural, dominant spots or white coats with a longer tail than the other breeds.

Wild hamsters live in hot areas of Central Asia. To avoid the heat of the day hamsters live in burrows and are nocturnal. In the cool of the evening and during the night hamsters will search for food and can travel up to 8 miles in one night. They collect food in their cheek pouches and return to their burrows and empty the cheek pouches into their food store. They are able to carry up to half their body weight in their pouches

Housing and nutrition   Hamsters should be housed indoors in a wire cage with a plastic base, a plastic hamster home or an adapted aquarium (vivarium) with a well-ventilated cover. Wooden cages should not be used as hamsters can chew their way out. Hamsters need feeding every day. As they are nocturnal animals an evening feed is better for them. They will normally wake at feeding time. The animals are omnivorous and specialist foods are available. These may be supplemented with green plant food subject to caution with the species listed under Guinea pigs above.

Hamsters do not really make good pets for young children. Their hours of activity do not fit in with patterns of a young child and it is unfair to expect hamsters (or children!) to change their natural behaviour. Hamsters are also very small and fragile and children can often be a little rough, resulting in the hamster being fearful of being handled.

Hibernation   Sudden drops in temperature may cause hamsters to go into hibernation. Hamsters may appear to be dead, but on closer inspection their whiskers may twitch; however, vital signs are often undetectable. They must be woken up so they do not get dehydrated or starve. The hamster may shiver as it wakes up, but it will stop as it becomes fully awake. They should be fully conscious in 2–3 hours. Food and water should be freely available.

Common diseases

Colds   Hamsters can catch colds from humans, so, if owners have a cold, handling of the hamster should be kept to a minimum. Symptoms are a runny nose and sneeze. When suffering from a cold, hamsters should be kept in a warm room.

Constipation If there is a lack of droppings in the cage housing the hamster, and the animal is walking with a hunched appearance, suspect constipation. Feeding with a small amount of green vegetables may relieve the discomfort.

Dental problems Special wood gnaws can be purchased from pet shops to encourage gnawing. Crunchy biscuits, dog biscuits or hamster treats will all encourage gnawing and the prevention of overgrown teeth. Regular clipping of the teeth may be necessary.

Diarrhoea Overfeeding with green food is the most common cause of diarrhoea. Animals should be fed only on specialised mix until recovery is complete.

Wet tail Wet tail is often confused with diarrhoea, but it is a bacterial infection that can cause extreme diarrhoea, with a distinctive smell. The anus and tail area of the hamster appears wet and sticky. The hamster may walk hunched up as it is in pain. The condition (that is potentially fatal) can be brought on by stress, such as weaning or separation from siblings. Hamsters with wet tail should be isolated from other hamsters as it is highly infectious. Owners should observe hygiene measures carefully. Treatment is with an antibacterial and/or antidiarrhoeal.

Mice and rats

History Both the European house mouse (*Mus musculus*) and the brown Norway rat (*Rattus norvegicus*) have been domesticated for at least 300 years. The brown rat was domesticated into what we recognise as 'fancy' or pet rats. This animal began steadily colonising Europe, and particularly England, in the early 18th century. The brown rat was quick to drive out the indigenous black rats. Because it was larger and more adaptable, the brown rat was able to thrive in environments that were not suitable for the black rats. Thus England was somewhat overrun with rats. With so many wild rats in England it was necessary to find some form of control. This led to a new career for some people, that of rat catcher. One of these men, the Royal Rat Catcher – Jack Black – can be credited as the originator of the first true domestic rats. In the course of his work, when he came upon strangely coloured animals, he kept and bred them. In the early 1800s coloured mice began to find their way into Europe and became popular, particularly in the UK. In 1895 the National Mouse Club was founded in England. They set standards for the different varieties and held shows. In the early years of the 20th century Mendel's theories on genetics were rediscovered by the scientific community. Fancy mice proved to be excellent models to use for further research. Rats were not used much for studying genetics; however, being small, easy to house, inexpensive to maintain and quick to reproduce, they became favourites for other types of research.

Breeds (varieties)   Mice and rats are both members of the animal family Muridae. A distinction in size is not always easy to identify for there are very large mice and very small rats! The animals differ principally in the structure of their tails; mice have a maximum of 180 rows of scales on their tails while rats have 210 or more.

There are now over 40 varieties of mice and they may be found in a number of exotic colours, including blue, cinnamon, pearl, sable and silver, although pet shop varieties are usually white, piebald, or 'brown'. Rats too may be found in a variety of different colours. There are substantial differences between the behaviour and susceptibility to disease of different strains of rat.

Housing and nutrition   Female mice (does) make the best pets, because their urine is less pungent than that of the male and if kept in pairs will provide company for each other. Two males will fight and a male and a female will keep reproducing. Pet mice should be kept in a wooden box or cage, with adequate ventilation to prevent condensation. They need sawdust for the cage bottom, and hay or paper to nest in. Cages should be cleaned out at least once a week. Mice should be lifted and restrained with firm pressure on the root of the tail and transferred to the hand.

Mice are basically omnivorous. They should be fed on a basic diet of whole or rolled oats, with a little hamster food and budgerigar seed given very occasionally for variety. Wholemeal bread, soaked in water and squeezed out, may be given daily. Dog biscuits are beneficial for the teeth. Carrots and boiled rice are also acceptable. Water should be available.

The tendency to become overweight is more often a problem of pet rats than mice. Overindulgent pet owners and the feeding of diets rich in seeds and nuts are most often responsible for this condition. Pet rats should not be fed chips, crisps, sweet biscuits and cake. Commercial diets specifically designed for rats are always preferred and can be supplemented with hay, whole-wheat breads, dry cereal, pasta, fruits, vegetables and non-fat yoghurt.

Mice can live for up to 2 years. They are ready for breeding when about 8 weeks old, and they can deliver a litter of up to 12 'pups' in 3 weeks.

In rats, pregnancy lasts an average of 3 weeks. Litter sizes average 6–12 pups or kittens.

Common conditions

Abscesses   Wounds (from fighting and other forms of trauma) are commonly infected with bacteria that already exist within the living quarters. Abscesses commonly result from wounds when they have gone unnoticed and untreated. Successful treatment of certain wounds (especially long and deep cuts) and abscesses require veterinary intervention. Abscesses usually need to be surgically opened because the relatively solid nature of rodent pus precludes lancing and draining.

Chronic murine pneumonia (CMP)

Causative organism   CMP or murine mycoplasmosis is the most significant and serious bacterial infection of mice and rats. It is caused by the highly contagious bacterium, *Mycoplasma pulmonis*. It may be transmitted between mother and offspring in the womb during embryonic life and by direct contact after birth. Transmission among infected and uninfected older rodents results from exchange of respiratory aerosols and sexual activity. Rabbits, guinea pigs and other rodents may also carry the causative agent but do not manifest signs of disease. The organism is relatively difficult to isolate because it cannot be grown in the laboratory using ordinary culture methods. This makes diagnosis of CMP more difficult except for the fact that the disease is so very common and well recognised.

Signs and symptoms   CMP is usually diagnosed by signs of illness (sniffling, sneezing, squinting, rough hair coat and laboured respiration) rather than isolation of the causative bacterium. If the inner ear becomes involved, a severe, often incapacitating, head tilt usually develops.

Treatment/prophylaxis   Because this disease tends to have a very chronic course, afflicted individuals should receive antibiotic treatment as soon as the first signs are recognised. Antibacterials can be added to the drinking water for long periods although some authorities claim that the drug does not reach therapeutic levels by this route and may make the water unpalatable. Tylosin may be given by intramuscular injection. Individuals exhibiting serious, life-threatening signs must be treated aggressively with injectable antibiotics if there is to be any hope of helping them. Frequently, other harmful bacteria complicate CMP. This often necessitates the use of multiple antibiotics. Elimination of the *M. pulmonis* organism from infected individuals is regarded by most experts as a practical impossibility. However, early treatment reduces the severity of the disease in affected rodents.

Complications In many mouse colonies, Sendai virus infection often complicates chronic murine pneumonia, increasing the death rate. This virus is very unlikely to infect pet mice unless they were acquired from a colony with this infection already established within its members. There is no specific treatment for this disease.

Dental problems Hereditary abnormalities of the jaw bones and/or teeth, abscessation of the incisor teeth, or injury to the jaw, may result in improper meeting of the upper and lower incisors. This in turn causes overgrowth of one or more of the incisors, with subsequent injury to the mouth. Mice and rats with this problem must have their overgrown incisors trimmed periodically by a veterinarian.

Dermatological diseases
  Barbering There are many causes of skin disease in pet mice and rats. Cage mates may be responsible for hair loss ('barbering') and/or wounds to the skin. Allergies are also a suspected cause of skin disease in pet rodents. In these cases it is wise to replace the bedding being used with plain white, unscented paper towelling.
  Ringtail Ringtail is a condition involving annular lesions of the tail in young rats. The condition is seen in rats kept in conditions of low humidity and it may become necrotic and require amputation.

Diarrhoea Tyzzer's disease (see above) most often infects gerbils and mice, though rats are also susceptible.

Eye problems
  Chromodacryorrhoea Chromodacryorrhoea (red–brown tears of rats) is a staining of the eyelids, nose and sometimes the front paws of rats which is often mistaken by the animal's owners for blood. In fact this is a normal secretion from a large gland (the harderian gland) behind the eyes. Red–brown tears are noted most often in response to stressful situations (restraint, fright, illness, etc.). It often accompanies CMP or infection with Sialodacryoadenitis virus (SDAV).
  Sialodacryoadenitis SDAV causes a highly contagious disease of rats and recently weaned mice. It is usually only acquired from a colony with this infection already established within its members. Initial signs include squinting, blinking and rubbing of the eyes. Later, sneezing and swelling in the neck region are noted. As the disease progresses, swellings below or around one or both eyes,

bulging of the eyes, red–brown tears and self-trauma to the eyes are noted. Respiratory signs may also occur. There is no specific treatment for this viral disease.

Parasitic infestations

   Ectoparasites Pet mice and rats may be infested with a variety of external parasites. Signs of mite infestation range from mild to severe scratching, with hair loss and ulceration of the skin resulting in numerous tiny scabs, most often noted around the neck and shoulders. Treatment may include injectable ivermectin. Lice may also infest the haircoats of pet mice and rats, most often on the neck and body. Louse infestations may also cause scratching, hair loss and skin wounds. Permethrin dusting powder may be used.

   Endoparasites Tapeworms and pinworms are the most common intestinal parasites of pet mice and rats. They often go undetected unless present in large numbers. Signs of infection may include weight loss, inactivity, constipation, and excessive licking and chewing of the rectal area and base of the tail. Endoparasites in mice and rats are treated with ivermectin administered subcutaneously or with piperazine added to the drinking water. Transmission of these parasites to people is possible but unlikely. Therefore, great care should be taken when handling and disposing of rodent feces. Furthermore, contact between young children and pet mice/rats and their feces should be limited and always supervised by adults.

Tumours Both mice and rats are very susceptible to formation of tumours. Rats over 2 years of age are reported to have an 87% chance of developing one or more types of tumours. Mice frequently develop tumours in a wide variety of tissue types. Leukaemia is quite common in mice as well. Both male and female rats develop benign mammary tumours, and females develop benign tumours of the uterine and vaginal linings. Because rats have mammary tissue in locations beneath the skin, other than along the underside of the belly, it is not uncommon to find lumps and bumps representing mammary tumours over the shoulders, flanks and base of the tail. These tumours are relatively easy to remove surgically under general anaesthesia.

Reptiles

The most common reptiles kept as pets are known as Chelonia and include tortoises, terrapins, lizards and snakes. These terrestrial creatures are all ectothermic, relying on external heat sources to maintain their preferred body temperature. When unwell they seek to increase their body temperature and this in turn will affect the speed with which drugs are metabolised. It is important that any disturbance in the normal fluid balance is corrected for the chelonians are prone to the deposition of insoluble urate crystals in the body cavity, joints and organs.

Tortoises

History

The inhumane importation of Mediterranean spur-thighed tortoises (*Testudo graeca*) from North Africa began in the 1890s and by the early 1950s stocks were seriously depleted. During the next 30 years collectors turned their attention to other species. In 1984 the European Economic Community, agreed to prohibit the commercial trade in tortoise species and declared them a protected species. Most tortoises in the UK are now bred in captivity and sold under licence from the Department for Environment, Food, and Rural Affairs.

Breeds

European species, such as the Hermann's tortoise (*Testudo hermanni*) and the marginated tortoise (*T. marginata*), Horsfield's tortoise (*T. horsfieldi*) from Asia and the Egyptian tortoise (*T. kleinmanni*) from North Africa, are all kept as pets.

Housing and nutrition

Walled gardens are ideal for tortoises to roam about in. Owners should allow at least 10 square metres per tortoise and ensure that the animal can neither climb over nor burrow under the surround. Garden ponds should be adequately covered to prevent the risk of drowning.

A well-ventilated waterproof house with access to a clover lawn and a paved sunbathing area is ideal for tortoises, as in both spring and autumn the animals will be able to heat up sufficiently to feed well, thereby extending their year and shortening their hibernation period. The floor should be lined with thick newspaper or dried leaves.

In a colony, male and female tortoises should normally be kept apart as the males often engage in female shell butting and leg biting as part of their courtship behaviour. Females constantly exposed to this treatment and unable to escape will feed less, produce eggs less frequently and eventually suffer from extensive shell and leg damage with an increased likelihood of infections.

Contrary to popular belief tortoises do drink, especially on waking from hibernation, when a warm bath is usually appreciated. A shallow dish about 10 cm deep, should be sunk into the ground to allow the animals to submerge their heads into the water.

Tortoises need a diet that is high in dietary fibre, vitamins and minerals, but low in fat and proteins. They feed mainly on green leaves. They will forage quite successfully in the garden on clover, dandelion, groundsel, and the leaves of various plants and bushes. The following foods can be offered: beans (leaves and pods), broccoli, green sprouts, cabbage, cauliflower, cucumber, endive, lettuce, kale, spring greens, watercress. Beetroot, carrots, cauliflower and parsnips may be grated or offered cooked. A whole range of fruits are also acceptable, including apples, blackberries, plums and strawberries.

Hibernation

The hibernation process   During autumn, as the days grow shorter, the light intensity decreases, the temperature begins to fall and tortoises prepare for hibernation. Feeding declines; it takes 4–6 weeks for their gut to empty for winter, and before they start this process in early September the tortoises need a check over. There should be no signs of wounds, abscesses, infections internally or externally, the mouth should be clean and pink, and the eyes should be alert and bright. Any fecal matter adhering to the shell or tail should be cleaned away. Weights and measurements should correspond with the Jackson chart (see The Jackson ratio below).

Any tortoise which is underweight or suffering from an ailment should not be allowed to hibernate, but should be overwintered in a vivarium. This should have a heat source and full-spectrum light for 13–14 hours to prevent hibernation. The temperatures should be around 26 °C by day and 18–22 °C at night. Fresh food and water should be provided. A simple vivarium can be provided with the light source on one end and a shelter on the other. The temperature must not go below 15 °C.

Hibernation quarters   A large, wooden, rodent-proof tea chest or box with small air holes in the sides is ideal for hibernation quarters. Both the top and the holes should be covered in wire mesh to prevent vermin entering. The base and the sides of the box should be lined with thick pads of polystyrene or newspaper. The tortoise is placed in an inner box (with air holes) and filled one- to three-quarters full with polystyrene chips, dry leaves or shredded newspaper. The smaller box is then placed inside the larger one, ensuring access is available for check-ups. The tortoise should be hibernated in a frost-free environment at temperatures of 4–10 °C.

The tortoise can be weighed individually or complete with inner box on a weekly or twice monthly basis. An adult tortoise loses about 1% of its prehibernation weight monthly. A drastic weight loss indicates that something is wrong and the animal should be brought out of hibernation immediately.

Emergence from hibernation When the animal starts moving (check regularly) it should be taken out of its hibernation quarters and the following actions taken:

- Check for discharges from the nose, eyes and tail end.
- Bathe the face and eyes and wash the mouth. Give the animal a warm bath for at least half an hour. It is important that the tortoise empties its bladder to get rid of the toxic waste accumulated during hibernation and that it replenishes its water supply by drinking. Keep the animal warm during the day and indoors overnight until the nights get warmer.
- Once out of hibernation and eating, keep it active (as for overwintering) if the weather becomes cold again.

Problems associated with hibernation Refusal to eat is natural in the month before hibernation, in cold weather, and can also be related to stress and disease, including stomatitis (mouth rot), ear abscesses, severe systemic disease (liver or kidney) and a heavy burden of ascarid worms. There should be a thorough health check and evaluation of husbandry. Blindness or disorientation after hibernation can be caused by frost damage. Refusal to eat occasionally occurs after hibernation and the possible causes are varied. Long-term rehydration therapy is necessary.

The Jackson ratio

In 1976, Oliphant Jackson, a veterinarian recorded the weights and measurements of a large number of healthy and sick Mediterranean tortoises. He observed that in healthy tortoises there is an optimum body weight which can be used as one of the criteria to assess the state of health of these species and their suitability for hibernation. If the figures for the average weights are plotted on a graph they provide very useful upper and lower guidelines. The data can also be calculated as a weight/length ratio, now known as the 'Jackson ratio' (Figure 14.1). This circumvents the problems of assessing tortoises' health because of the shell.

The carapace is measured in a straight line, which can be achieved by pressing the front of the shell against a vertical surface to push the head right in, and pressing another vertical surface against the tail end. Measure the distance between these two points in millimetres. The weight (in grams) can be measured using an accurate pair of kitchen scales, or for smaller specimens a balance or electronic scales.

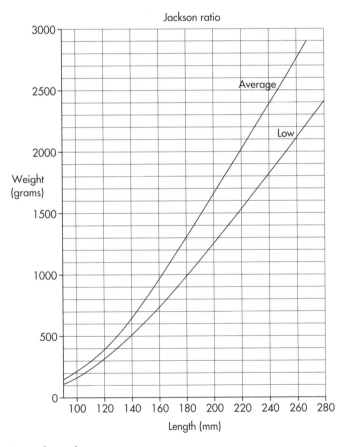

Figure 14.1 The Jackson ratio.

Common conditions

Tortoises are susceptible to a variety of illnesses for which the advice of a veterinary surgeon is required. Some of the most common are described below.

Abscesses Abscesses are common and may need surgical intervention because pus is often thick and viscous; the pus becomes encapsulated in thick fibrous material which makes access difficult.

Diarrhoea Diarrhoea is a sign of ill-health, husbandry problems, a dietary imbalance or parasite infestation. A check should be made for undigested food, mucus or worms in the feces.

Dystocia (egg binding) A female tortoise with non-specific signs of ill-health may be suffering from dystocia, pre- or post-ovulatory egg binding.

Parasitic infestation Ectoparasites (ticks, leeches) may be removed after they have been relaxed with a drop of alcohol or oil. Endoparasites (usually the roundworms *Sulcascaris* and *Augusticaecum)* may lead to unthriftiness and intestinal blockages. Protozoal infestation can also cause gastrointestinal problems.

Runny nose syndrome Discharge from the nostrils and watery eyes can be due to rhinitis, sinusitis or runny nose syndrome. The symptoms may progress from upper respiratory tract disease to pneumonia in the lungs.

Shell problems Osteodystrophy (soft shell) can result from a combination of calcium deficiency, incorrect lighting and excessive protein in the diet.

Shell breaks and injuries Depending on the severity of the injury, taping, flushing with antibiotic and removal of fragmented shell pieces will be necessary. Reconstruction may be an option.

Stomatitis (mouth rot or canker) This condition is often seen posthibernation. In the mouth it appears as a general inflammation with caseous (cheesy) material attached to the tongue, mouth and throat.

Drugs for tortoises

There are few drugs authorised for tortoises. Drugs authorised for use in other species or in humans may be administered by veterinarians for animals under their care. Examples of drugs used are:

- Antimicrobials, including ampicillin, ceftiofur and enrofloxacin.
- Ectoparasiticides include dichlorvos strip in housing control and ivermectin as a spray or in drinking water.
- Endoparasiticides include trimethoprim sulfa (coccidia) fenbendazole and tiabendazole (roundworms) and praziquantel (tapeworms and flukes).

Medication for internal use may be administered orally in drinking water or by injection.

If prescribed by a vet for an animal under his or her care fenbendazole paste designed for endoparasitic use in horses (Panacur, Intervet) may be smeared on food and is said to be well tolerated by tortoises.

Snakes

Stress

Stress and poor husbandry may be the initial cause of a number of common conditions found in snakes, including bacterial infection and parasites. For example, lesions may appear on the ventral scales. This is usually associated with a damp environment. Treatment is with povidone-iodine with an appropriate antibiotic (e.g. enrofloxacin gentamicin or tobramycin).

Burns

Snakes may find their way on to warm surfaces to maintain their body temperature and receive a nasty shock when the area heats up unexpectedly. Reports of snakes sustaining bad burns from hotplates or behind central heating radiators may be found in the literature. Topical treatment with povidone-iodine and possibly with antimicrobials to prevent secondary infection is indicated.

Parasitic infestation

Snakes can be hosts to a large number of parasites that can cause many problems including the following:

- Protozoa can cause serious diseases of the digestive, respiratory, reproductive and vascular systems (e.g. amoebiasis).
- Flukes cause illness in the respiratory and urinary systems.
- Tapeworms parasitise the digestive system.
- Roundworms and related parasites inhabit the digestive tract.

- Large numbers of mites and ticks parasitise the skin and scales of snakes, and create disease by feeding on the host's blood.

Signs of parasitism depend on the parasite and body tissue involved. External parasites may be observed by visual inspection of the skin and scales, with or without a magnifying lens, though immature stages of mites may lie dormant under scales or just inside the eye cavity. Internal parasite problems require examination of various specimens, most often blood, feces, urinary tract products, and washings from the windpipe and lungs. Special laboratory procedures are necessary to process these specimens.

The best way to avoid parasites is by adoption of good quarantine practices with new arrivals and infected specimens and maintaining hygienic cages. Systemic treatment procedures involve the use of ivermectin, fenbendazole and metronidazole. A number of specialised topical preparations are available.

Aviary and cage birds

Pigeons are covered in chapter 16. In this section 'exotic birds' are discussed. These include members of the order Psittaciformes known as psittacines (budgerigars, macaws, parrots, etc), canaries and finches. Most birds will thrive in captivity given an appropriate diet, clean housing and freedom from stress. However, like fish (see chapter 17), changes in environmental surroundings or variations in diet can precipitate disease. There are a number of ways by which the chance of disease can be minimised:

- Observance of highest standards of hygiene; bird owners should wash their hands after touching their stock for both their own and their birds' benefit.
- Prevention of contamination of outdoor aviaries with a waterproof cover to prevent entry of wild bird droppings or rodent feces that might contain transmittable sources of disease. Attention to food and water dispensers is particularly important.
- Quarantining of sick birds for at least 2 weeks to prevent the spread of disease and to allow a return to full strength before return to the colony.
- Monitoring of new birds to ensure no evidence of illness. Exotic birds imported from overseas should have been subject to a period of quarantine before delivery, but nevertheless vigilance is a sensible precaution.

Common conditions

Stress

Stress in birds often leads to eating disorders and increased susceptibility to disease. Common sources of stress are:

- Cats, rodents and squirrels, seen as natural predators, are all potential causes of stress for cage birds. A cat walking across the top of an aviary will cause panic, particularly amongst breeding birds. A recent innovation involves a device that emits high-energy pulses of ultrasonic sound. It appears to deter rodents and cats effectively.
- Within the cage or aviary one individual bird may become uncharacteristically aggressive during breeding and upset the harmony that normally exists.
- Changing housing arrangements may cause stress.
- Crowded and poorly ventilated housing.

Affected birds should be removed to a 'hospital cage' or well-ventilated cardboard box and kept warm at around 30 °C. A dark environment aids relaxation and sleep. Because the bird is not feeding, its metabolic rate and body temperature drop and death from hypothermia is a risk. As the bird recovers, the temperature should be slowly returned to normal.

Respiratory conditions

Aspergillosis   Fungal infection affecting parrots and raptors (birds of prey). Causes breathing difficulties that are unresponsive to antibiotics.

Avian tuberculosis   Symptoms include lethargy and progressive weight loss.

Avian tuberculosis can be zoonotic.

Pasteurella   A serious bacterial infection affecting young birds which causes breathing difficulties and some diarrhoea. Prompt administration of antibiotics is required.

Chlamydiosis (ornithosis, psittacosis)   Chlamydiosis, ornithosis or psittacosis are conditions resulting from infection with *Chlamydia psittaci* which is associated with cold-like symptoms, dripping nostrils, enteritis and exhaustion. Plumage is ruffled. Many species of wild and captive birds carry the bacterium and there are several serovars showing different degrees of virulence. Treatment is with antibiotics.

This condition is zoonotic. Cage and aviary dust is a source of inhaled infection for humans. The most serious infections have resulted from contact with parrots and ducks in Europe and turkeys in the USA. A less virulent form may be caught from pigeons (see chapter 16).

Digestive tract

Fowl pest (Newcastle disease)   This is a viral condition spread by wild birds and causes bloody diarrhoea and paralysis of the legs. Affects psittacines and poultry. There is no known treatment for this condition.

Going light syndrome   Going light syndrome is characterised by loss of weight, lethargy and fluffed up plumage. The condition may be helped by feeding probiotics.

Salmonella poisoning   Salmonella poisoning results from ingestion of contaminated food, poor hygiene and contact with rodent feces. Signs and symptoms include stained feathers around the cloacal vent and lethargy. Treated with antibiotics.

   There is a zoonotic risk.

Eye problems

Eye infections often result from minor injuries and rubbing. They may be treated with ophthalmic ointments or drops. The latter tend to be washed away by secretions so ointment is better. Perches should be disinfected to prevent reinfection when the bird scratches its eye.

Miscellaneous problems

A number of feather, feet and bill problems may also be seen by bird owners, including some of bacterial, viral and protozoal origin. Regular clipping of overgrown claws or malformed bills should be carried out.

Parasite infestations

Ectoparasites   Ectoparasites include red mites, biting, sucking and feather lice, fleas and ticks. Red mites can carry the protozoan *Lankesterella*; this is usually fatal. The most conspicuous parasites found on birds are scaly-face mites (*Knemidocoptes pilae*) found most frequently on budgerigars. One form of treatment is to rub the affected area with petroleum jelly which interferes with the mite's respiration.

Endoparasites   Roundworms, tapeworms and protozoans (*Coccidia*, *Leucoctozoa* (see above) and *Leukesterella*) cause a number of problems in birds.

Reproductive system

Egg binding   A distressing condition found in young female birds that is generally caused by mineral imbalance and calcium deficiency. The ovum becomes blocked in the reproductive tract. It may be possible to ease the egg out with gentle pressure using a lubricant and tweezers.

Drugs for birds

Avian drugs may be administered by a variety of routes: oral, in the drinking water, by addition to feed, by injection, by topical application and by nebulisation. The armamentarium includes antimicrobials, parasiticides, anaesthetics, sedatives and non-steroidal anti-inflammatory drugs as well as drugs from several other therapeutic groups. Few of these drugs have marketing authorisations for bird species in the UK (see chapter 3).

Amongst the large number of antibiotics used in avian medicine, the following are recommended in *The Veterinary Formulary*:

- Dermatological problems: amoxicillin with clavulanic acid (co-amoxiclav) available as Synulox (Pfizer) or sulfadiazine with trimethoprim (Delvoprim, Intervet, or Duphatrim, Fort Dodge).
- Gastrointestinal and urinary tract infections: aminoglycosides (e.g. streptomycin, gentamicin and tobramycin) with sulfadiazine and trimethoprim.
- Respiratory tract infections: amoxicillin with clavulanic acid (co-amoxiclav).

Other antimicrobials used by veterinarians include ketoconazole, metronidazole, nystatin, oxytetracycline and tylosin.

Drugs such as pyrethrins, fipronil and carbaril (and in other countries some organophosphates) are used to control mites and lice in birds. Environmental control is achieved with a dichlorvos-impregnated strip (Vapona, Sara Lee).

Fenbendazole or levamisole orally or in the drinking water may be used 4–6 monthly for endoparasitic prophylaxis but should be changed periodically to reduce the risk of resistance. Ivermectin may be applied to the skin as a spot-on preparation; it may also be administered by injection, but not to budgerigars and finches.

Commercial birds

A market exists for the supply of parasiticides for a variety of commercially farmed birds including ostriches, poultry and game as well as for raptors used to hunt. These opportunities are obviously limited and pharmacists wishing to become involved should seek specialist training before embarking on what is a fascinating area of practice.

Further reading

Bartlet R D, Bartlett P P (1996). *Turtles and Tortoises*. Hauppauge: Baron's Educational Services.

Bishop Y, ed. (2001). *The Veterinary Formulary*, 5th edn. London: Pharmaceutical Press.

Hart-Davis D (2002). *Fauna Britannica*. London: Weidenfield and Nicolson.

Roach P (1995). *Complete book of pet care*. Sydney: Lansdowne Publishing PTY.

Taylor D T (2002). *Small pet handbook*. London: Harper–Collins.

Tilford T (2001). *The Cage and Aviary Bird Handbook*. London: New Holland.

15

Health and nutrition of horses

Michael H Jepson

It is estimated that there are over 850 000 horses and ponies in the UK at the present time, most of which are kept for riding. Figures from the relevant ministries in England, Scotland and Wales only give information about horses and ponies grazed on agricultural land, with no indication of the numbers of equines being kept on domestic premises, and therefore do not give an accurate picture of the equine population. The only subdivision on the census form is between animals owned and not owned by the occupier of the agricultural holding. There are approximately 2000 horses in the Greater London area – police horses, dray horses, animals belonging to riding establishments, and so on.

Horses and ponies, together with donkeys, are the most common species of the genus *Equus* that are kept domestically. The transition from being a major contributor to commercial haulage in the past to their present predominant role for riding for pleasure has resulted in equines being often considered today as 'companion animals' or even pets. However, it is worthy of note that, for some years and currently, there is considerable interest in reviving the use of heavy-breed draught horses in the UK, though this has been largely limited to show competitions and use by some breweries for promotional purposes and for local deliveries in a traditional way.

It needs to be recorded that in some European Union (EU) member states horse meat is still used for human consumption, that horses are raised as food-producing animals and that horses may be exported between countries to provide meat for human consumption. Where this is the case, the restrictions that apply to the use of certain drugs or maximum residue limits will apply, and will be referred to later in this chapter. Broadly speaking, this is not an issue in the UK, and it is potentially relevant for any community pharmacist to consider whether there is a place for those animal medicines that can contribute to equine health, especially in the locality of a community pharmacy. Medication for routine treatment of conditions that do not require diagnosis by a veterinarian, such as infection with gastrointestinal tract worms, can be appropriately supplied together with general advice about the choice of drugs available, frequency of treatment and the way in which, for example, the potential for resistance may be minimised by changing the chemical nature of the active ingredient used. A large proportion of horses and ponies are kept at livery stables and riding schools. Shared grazing is the norm, so it is imperative to worm horses regularly in order to maintain good health.

Sources of detailed or more specific information are reasonably and readily available to any pharmacist and details of some of these are included at the end of this chapter.

In the UK, Ireland and some other countries, horses may also be bred for specialist performance and leisure activities and are completely disassociated from human consumption. EU legislation requires that horses intended for breeding and production are accompanied by a passport, confirming whether or not the horse is intended for human consumption and, importantly, the passport includes a section that records all medicines administered to the animal. This legislation is important to the veterinarian in particular, as it enables the use of medicines, on appropriate occasions, that do not have an established maximum residue level.

Nutrition

Horses are herbivores, though their digestive system appears less specialised than that of the ruminant (see chapter 9). The equine stomach is simple but the intestine is considerably modified, with an enlarged colon, in order to digest the large quantities of roughage required. Microbial synthesis in ruminants and in horses makes these animals unlikely to experience thiamine deficiency. However, symptoms have been reported in horses that have consumed quantities of bracken (*Pteridium aquiline*), which contains thiaminase, a thiamine antagonist. The horse grazes one or two mouthfuls at a time by using its very strong and mobile lips to draw grass between its pairs of incisor teeth. The grass is ground briefly between the molars and swallowed. Horses avoid grass soiled by their feces. Domesticated horses are routinely fed concentrates, but this may cause a problem if they contain too much grain. While the horse's teeth are suitably modified to crush grass into small pieces, they seem less able to crush grain efficiently. Food boluses normally pass quite rapidly through the stomach into the intestine, but if too much uncrushed grain is present this may swell in the stomach, causing distension and pain or colic.

Management

Awareness and understanding of equine management has greatly increased in recent years, and many former losses due to disease and injury are now avoided. The two major rules of management are to avoid overcrowding and to establish and maintain cleanliness. These fundamental needs, with so many parallels in health terms elsewhere, apply irrespective of the number of horses or of the size of the establishment. Unfortunately, pressures that favour economics often result in unsatisfactory compromise. It is important for all those concerned to recognise that the prevention of disease and injury is optimised by good nutritional management, housing and hygiene, vaccination programmes and internal and external parasite control. It is poor practice to rely on veterinarian service, only when an acute situation presents. The prophylactic control of many conditions and diseases should be the rule, and this is where pharmacists have a role to play alongside veterinarians. Animal health and welfare require team cooperation with the animal owner.

It should be emphasised that product literature for medicinal products with marketing authorisation for use in animals will give precise details about the animal species and indication(s) to which the licence applies. It is illegal, for other than a veterinarian under the 'cascade' arrangement, to direct the use of a product outwith the licence (see chapter 3). Certain cough remedies have frequently been purchased by horse owners for administration to their animals. Pharmacists should be alert to this situation, which on occasion may raise issues of short-term animal welfare, but such products are invariably licensed only for human use and may legally be supplied only on the authorisation of a veterinarian if intended for animal use.

One of the commonest causes of horses being 'out of action' is lameness. In part this is associated with the considerable demands put on horses in racing, jumping and other related athletic activities. However, poorly fitting shoes, damaged ligaments or broken bones can also be responsible. The appropriate treatment may include the use of non-steroidal anti-inflammatory drugs, which requires accurate veterinary diagnosis. Other problems may arise from ill-fitting equipment (e.g. saddles).

Endoparasite control

Horses harbour a wider variety of nematodes than any other domesticated animal and a worm control programme is essential, the more so since many horses in suburbia are limited to shared grazing. It is not surprising that established livery stables and riding schools usually already have suppliers of horse wormers and are only likely to change if dissatisfied. However, for those horse and pony owners whose animals are not stabled at livery, there is the option of obtaining supplies of pharmacy and merchant supply (PML) wormers from a pharmacy or from a veterinarian if the animal(s) are under his or her care, or from a merchant. A limited number of products may also be obtained from a registered saddler. Merchants and registered saddlers may also supply PML products to non-commercial users. As in other situations, pharmacy opening hours and the convenience of location, together with informed advice about dosage and frequency, are potentially significantly advantageous factors for pharmacists to demonstrate.

Nematodes or roundworms are the most common group of equine parasites, and horses and ponies can be host to the worms at certain stages of their life cycle (see Figure 15.1).

The principal parasitic worms infecting horses are detailed below and are frequently referred to in veterinary data sheets or summaries of product characteristics on anthelmintic products. There is also an admirable summary in the Royal Pharmaceutical Society of Great Britain's (RPSGB) Veterinary Pharmacists' Group leaflet, available for quick reference and for customers (see Further reading).

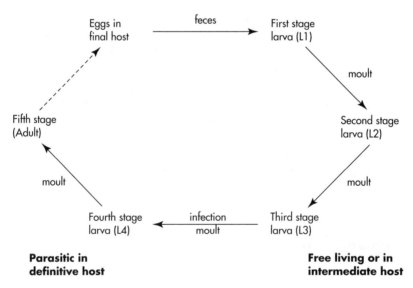

Figure 15.1 Typical nematode (roundworm) life cycle.

Endoparasite statistics are daunting, but a properly planned and conscientiously recorded worm control programme can provide comprehensive regular treatment of these endoparasites.

Worms in foals

Foals are young horses of either sex, up to 1 year old. Usually, they start to eat grass between 3 and 4 weeks of age and are weaned when 4–6 months old. Large roundworms, known as ascarids, and threadworms are the most important endoparasites. Worms and their treatment are important because a heavy worm infestation, or 'burden', can affect the performance, growth and general health or 'thrift' of horses and ponies. A severe infection can even be fatal. Worm infestation may also put an animal under considerable stress, thereby increasing its vulnerability to other diseases. Diarrhoea and colic can occur, though these may be due to other causes requiring veterinary advice.

Large roundworms (Parascaris equorum)

These can be over 30 cm long. One female parasite can lay up to 200 000 eggs a day. The eggs are resistant to disinfectants and are capable of surviving for several years outside the horse. The sticky outer coating of the eggs enables them to stick to most surfaces, including feeding bowls and stable walls. Foals can carry over 1000 adult round-worms, which can cause severe ill-thrift.

Threadworms (Strongyloides westeri)

These only cause disease in very young foals. Infective larvae can be transmitted via the mare's milk, causing diarrhoea in the very young foal. Diarrhoea, which is common in foals, may be due to other causes, including bacterial or viral infections, and requires veterinary advice. Threadworms can also infect foals via the skin in unhygienic conditions.

Control

Fenbendazole, ivermectin and oxibendazole are suitable drugs for worm control in foals.

Worms in adult horses

Large and small redworms, pinworms and lungworms are the most important endoparasites affecting adult horses.

Redworms

Large redworms (*Strongylus vulgaris*) cause the most serious worm infection in older horses. They are a very common cause of recurring bouts of spasmodic colic, which is a debilitating condition capable of killing an apparently healthy horse. As many as 30 million eggs a day can be passed in feces by an unwormed horse, thereby severely contaminating the pasture. The infective larvae develop on the grass and are subsequently ingested by other grazing horses. The larvae then penetrate the gut wall and migrate to the cranial mesenteric artery, causing damage and the formation of blood clots. If these clots should break off and obstruct a major artery to the gut, irreversible damage may ensue and the horse may die. The mature larvae return to the gut to develop into egg-producing adults, from 1 to 5 cm in length, which complete the parasitic life cycle by attaching themselves to the gut lining, where they cause blood loss.

Small redworms (*Cyathostoma* spp.) have a life cycle that differs from that of large redworms. The ingested infective larvae pass to the large intestine, forming modules in the gut wall. Here, the time taken to develop into adults varies greatly, from less than 3 months to much longer. Significant infection results in ill-thrift, anaemia and the possibility of diarrhoea, which may alternate with constipation.

Both small and large redworms are controlled by routine anthelmintic dosing. Over 80% of larvae may be removed by the use of either increased dosage in accordance with product information leaflet or data sheet guidance, or by use of routine dosing for 5 consecutive days within an overall control programme.

Pinworms or seatworms (Oxyuris equi)

In their adult stage these worms live in the large intestine. The female lays cream-coloured eggs on the skin around the anus. This results in intense itching that causes the animal to rub the tail area. These parasites are controlled by routine worming, and are not usually considered to be a serious problem.

Lungworms (Dictyocaulus arnfieldi)

These can be up to 6 cm long. The larvae migrate to the lungs, where they mature. Infections in the horse frequently cause coughing, but coughs may also be caused by bacterial or viral infections and require veterinary advice. It is estimated that up to 90% of donkeys may be infected, but few show likely symptoms or any ill-effects. It is considered good management practice to graze horses and donkeys separately where possible.

Formulations containing ivermectin or mebendazole are licensed for the control of lungworms.

Bots (Gasterophilus equi *and* G. nasalis)

These are not worms but larvae of the fly *Gasterophilus*, and are an important internal parasite of horses. Gadflies are airborne in the UK between June and October and lay eggs on the horse's hair, especially around the legs and belly. The horse licks the area, causing the eggs to hatch, and taking the larvae into the mouth. The larvae develop in the stomach, where they remain for 8–10 months before being expelled in the feces in spring. After pupating, adult flies develop and lay eggs and the cycle continues.

Bots cause pain, gastritis and can result in mechanical obstruction of the gut.

Control can be achieved by using products containing ivermectin or moxidectin. Haloxon was used formerly but is no longer authorised for use in the UK. Regular grooming is important for the removal of eggs.

Liver fluke (Fasciola hepatica)

Liver fluke or fascioliasis is uncommon in horses, which are fairly resistant to infection by *Fasciola hepatica*. Symptoms include loss of weight, lethargy and poor performance. There is a possibility of anaemia, jaundice and diarrhoea. Diagnosis is from the identification of eggs in feces and the elimination of other possibilities. Patent liver fluke infection occurs in donkeys and treatment with triclabendazole has proved effective, though the product Fasinex (Novartis) does not have an authorised indication for use in equines.

Worming treatment and programmes

The wide variety of nematodes that horses can harbour commonly cause ill-thrift, diarrhoea and sometimes colic, while migrating *Strongylus vulgaris* larvae damage the cranial mesenteric artery. Gastrointestinal nematodes may be controlled by treating newly acquired animals with a broad-spectrum anthelmintic, examples of which are included in Table 15.1. This should be concurrent with regular dosing of all ponies, horses and donkeys at 6–8 weekly intervals throughout the grazing season (see Figure 15.2).

During the winter, the frequency may be reduced to 3 monthly, but the advice given in the product literature should be taken into account. Risk factors are variable and include the stocking rate of the grazing land. As previously stated, one unwormed horse can pass out an incredible 30 million large redworm eggs in one day, which represents a severe threat to other horses. Avermectins may give a longer period of protection than other chemical groups, but reliance on anthelmintics can be reduced by the frequent removal of feces from paddocks and grazing land, preferably twice a week. Early winter is the optimum time to treat migrating large redworms with a five-day course of fenbendazole or ivermectin.

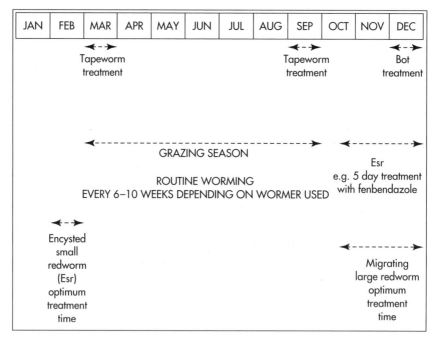

Figure 15.2 Example of an optimal worm-control programme for horses. (Modified from Hoechst 'Panacur' data sheet.)

It is of increasing importance to rotate the wormers used in the grazing season on an annual basis to minimise any risk of drug resistance. Once again, the pharmacist's knowledge of chemistry can be applied to ensure that the annual rotation is based on the use of different chemical groups and not just of a product name.

Pyrantel is the drug of choice for routine tapeworm treatment, advisably twice a year and at twice the dose rate for strongyles.

Figure 15.2 shows a typical worming programme.

Table 15.1 summarises the chemical groups of licensed parasiticides with their mode of action.

Good practice and practical summary

- It is important that groups of horses living together should all be treated with anthelmintics at the same time.
- Repeated treatment at regular intervals is essential, as not all worms are killed and animals are constantly subject to reinfection from pasture or stable.
- Overgrazing of pasture should be avoided and the level of pasture contamination reduced by removal of dung. Where possible, grazing areas should be rotated.
- The dosage of anthelmintics should be related to the weight of an animal. The RPSGB Veterinary Pharmacists' Group leaflet provides a table relating approximate weight in kilograms to the height of a horse, which is tradition-

Table 15.1 Distinctive chemical groupings of endoparasiticides

Chemical grouping with symbols used on some labels	Endoparasiticides	Mode of action
Benzimidazoles '1 – BZ'	Fenbendazole Mebendazole Oxibendazole	Disrupt parasite energy metabolism by binding to a protein required for nutrient uptake etc.
Tetrahydropyrimidines '2 – LM'	Pyrantel	Interferes with parasitic nerve transmission, leading to neuromuscular paralysis.
Avermectins '3 – AV'	Ivermectin Moxidectin	Interferes with parasite nerve transmission by opening chloride channels in the postsynaptic membrane.
Organophosphates 'OP'	Haloxon	Inhibits cholinesterase, thus interfering with neuromuscular transmission in parasite.

ally measured in 'hands'. A hand is four inches (10 cm), measurement being made at the withers (the ridge between the shoulder bones of a horse). The metric equivalent of 12 hands is 122 cm.

- data sheets/summary of product characteristics for anthelmintic products and product information leaflets detail dosage in relation to animal weight and in some instances to breed of horse or pony. Dosage by oral syringe or dosing gun is preferable to in-feed dosing as this ensures that the full dose is received by the horse.
- It is of particular importance for the horse owner to keep a worming record sheet and to keep it up to date. The leaflet referred to above incorporates a simple record sheet. Many product manufacturers also supply record sheets. Distributors, such as the nearest Vetchem pharmacy (see chapter 7) can advise about availability and supply.

Ectoparasite control

Flies, midges and lice

Fly repellents are products frequently associated with horse-wormers, as they can help control the intermediate host of bots, the gadfly. They will also control stable and nuisance flies such as *Musca* and *Hydrotaea* and, dependent upon the licence indications, lice.

Formulations may include citronella oil, diethyltoluamide or dimethyl phthalate in gels, liquids, creams and/or aerosol sprays.

Licensed products include those listed in Table 15.2.

Cooper's Fly Repellent Plus for Horses (Schering-Plough) is applied by sponge. Deosan Deosect (Fort Dodge) is applied, after dilution, by sprayer or sponge.

Sweet itch

Sweet itch is a common recurring dermatitis that results from hypersensitivity to saliva from the bites of midges, especially *Culicoides* spp. and flies, during the summer months. Susceptible horses should be housed overnight or earlier, during the midge season. Benzyl benzoate lotion is licensed for use on horses other than those intended for human consumption. Carr & Day & Martin Killitch (Quay Equestrian) emulsion is a benzyl benzoate 25% emulsion for application to the mane and tail. Day Son & Hewitt Sweet Itch Lotion (Quay Equestrian) contains piperonyl butoxide 0.5% and pyrethrum extract 0.4%.

Table 15.2 Fly repellent products

Active ingredient	Product name	Indications
Permethrin 1.05% Citronellol 2%	Fly Repellent Plus for Horses, Coopers (Schering-Plough) (GSL)	Biting and other flies; Biting louse; midge – *Culicoides pulicaris*.
Diethyltoluamide 10% Dimethyl phthalate 10% Citronella 3%	Extra Tail (Kalium)	
[a]Cypermethrin 5%	Barricade 5% EC (Sorex) (PML)	By spray after dilution, control of flies and lice.
[a]Cypermethrin 5%	Deosan Deosect (Fort Dodge) (PML)	Residual insecticide for control of flies and lice.
[a]Permethrin 4%	Day Son & Hewitt Switch (Quay Equestrian) (GSL)	Pour-on, which aids control of sweet itch.
[a]Permethrin 1.05% Citronellol 2%	Lincoln Fly Repellent Plus (Battle Hayward & Bower) (GSL)[b]	Repel and kill biting flies.

[a]Not to be used on horses intended for human consumption; [b]the same active ingredients are in emulsion products labelled 'Lincoln Sweet Itch Control' and 'Lincoln Lice Control Plus'. GSL, general sale list; PML, pharmacy and merchant suppy.

Other conditions affecting horses

Most of the other conditions to which horses are subject are best dealt with by a veterinarian. Cough treatments and liniments to ease muscle strain and rheumatism are available over the counter but delay in appropriate treatment can be costly. Most horses are relatively expensive companion animals to maintain and the responsible owner will recognise, for example, that antibiotics may be necessary to treat a respiratory disorder after proper diagnosis.

Consequently, only brief reference will be made to the following conditions as they are largely intended to be understood as background information.

Gastrointestinal tract

Colic is a vague term that is applied to symptoms of abdominal pain, especially in horses. A large number of conditions can produce abdominal pain and include the following:

- Acute indigestion, often a consequence of feeding unsuitable food, and flatulent colic from the build-up of gas.
- A heavy parasitic worm and bot burden.
- A severe organic disorder, such as a rupture of the stomach, enteritis, peritonitis, impaction of food materials or obstruction of the colon or strangulation of the bowel.
- The approach of parturition in a pregnant mare.
- Grass disease.
- Anthrax, a common symptom of which is abdominal pain.

Most cases of colic result from the disruption of normal gut motility, are benign, not life-threatening, and respond to veterinary therapy. As there may be little to differentiate benign from more serious cases, veterinary attention is indicated in all but very mild, self-limiting cases.

Treatment   The main aim of treatment is to relieve pain and correct the underlying cause after diagnosis. Medication may include spasmolytics, analgesics, sedatives, non-steroidal anti-inflammatory products, lubricants, endoparasiticides and fluid electrolytes.

Diarrhoea

Diarrhoea must be considered separately in relation to foals and adult horses.

Foals   Foals commonly experience diarrhoea of small intestine origin which is unlike that in the adult horse. Foal heat diarrhoea or foal heat scour is of short duration, is seen as a normal physiological event, lasting 2–4 days during the second week of life after birth, is self-limiting, and treatment is rarely necessary.

Other causes of diarrhoea in the foal may include bacterial infection, rotavirus infection and parasitic damage.

Treatment   Treatment in all cases is to minimise dehydration by administering oral fluids and electrolyte preparations. Intravenous fluids may be required in severe cases. Protectants and adsorbents may be beneficial in the foal, as may probiotic preparations containing freeze-dried lactobacillus and *Streptococcus faecalis*. Antibiotics have limited use and may exacerbate the condition. (See also the section Diseases controlled by vaccines below.)

Adult horses   Adult horses may contract diarrhoea from a variety of sources, which can include bacterial, viral and parasitic infections, nutritional imbalance, stress, toxicities and drug side-effects. This can include the use of antibiotics, especially broad-spectrum therapy with drugs like the tetracyclines. These acute forms of diarrhoea are most commonly associated with inflammation of the caecum and large colon. Because of the extensive surface area of the mucosal surfaces involved, such inflammation can produce massive exudation of fluid and rapid dehydration, with huge electrolyte and acid–base imbalance. Prompt veterinary attention is required, as is the use of large volumes of intravenous fluids.

The commonest bacterial cause of acute diarrhoea is salmonellosis, which is a potential zoonosis.

Chronic diarrhoea in the adult horse is commonly associated with parasitic infection, most notably with the migration of small redworm larvae (*Cyathostoma*) through the mucosa of the caecum and large colon. This is known as 'larval cyathostomiasis'. Chronic diarrhoea may also be caused by such conditions as inflammatory bowel disease, idiopathic colitis and neoplasm. As specific diagnosis may be extremely difficult, treatment may be limited to being symptomatic.

Treatment   Medication may include endoparasiticides, fluid electrolytes, antibacterials, probiotics and injectable corticosteroids, though the latter should not be given to horses with early enterocolitis.

Respiratory conditions

Cough

As in other animal species, including humans, cough and coughing can be of varying aetiology. Equine influenza, other virus infections, laryngitis and bronchitis are common causes. In addition, an allergic or asthmatic cough is frequently audible in the autumn. Cough is also associated with 'strangles', which is an acute contagious fever of horses, donkeys and mules caused by *Streptococcus equi* and requires prompt veterinary attention. If coughing occurs when the horse's temperature is normal (37.7 $\pm$ 0.5 °C), the cause may be due to lungworm infestation. The outdated terms 'broken wind' and 'heaves' may still be used to refer to a long-standing, dry, short and hollow persistent cough, perhaps with audible wheezing and some nasal discharge. There may be several different causes, not all of which are chronic or irreversible, and they all require reliable diagnosis by a veterinarian.

Treatment Mucolytic agents, which reduce mucus viscosity in the tracheobronchial tree, may be prescribed for chronic coughing in horses. Reduction in viscosity facilitates removal by ciliary action and expectoration. Two drugs are currently licensed in the UK, bromhexine (Bisolvon oral powder) and dembrexine (Sputolosin oral powder), both of which are prescription-only products.

Expectorants increase the volume of secretions in the respiratory tract, thereby aiding their removal by ciliary action and coughing. Traditionally ipecacuanha, squill, guaiacol and ammonium salts have been included in expectorant formulations, though their efficacy is unproven. At present there is no product licensed containing any of these expectorants for such use in horses in the UK.

Chronic obstructive pulmonary disease

This is most commonly caused by fungal spores, such as *Aspergillus fumigatus*, in hay and straw and is an allergic response to inhalation of allergens. Viral infections may also predispose to allergic bronchitis. Stabled horses, especially from 6 to 10 years old, are particularly susceptible. The condition is exacerbated by dust, by hay or straw that contains moulds, and possibly by food mites. Prevention is better than cure. The avoidance of adverse conditions, by keeping horses at pasture or boxed in clean stables with shavings, peat or shredded paper and dampening hay as required, is to be preferred. Stables with high levels of ammonia may aggravate the condition.

Chronic obstructive pulmonary disease initially and principally affects the small airways, and breathing difficulty or dyspnoea is worse at night, as it is with human asthma. It can progress from a mild form to a moderate to severe form, and can precipitate more serious complications, which makes differential diagnosis even more important.

Viral infections

Viral infections affecting the respiratory tract are potentially of major and economic importance world-wide. Equine influenza is highly contagious and tends to occur in epidemics. Young horses in training or other groups are particularly susceptible. Vaccination is widely employed (see under Diseases controlled by vaccines below).

Skin conditions

Dermatitis

'Dermatitis' describes any inflammation of the skin and may be produced by myriad agents. These can include external irritants, allergens, trauma (including burns), or be of bacterial, viral, fungal or parasitic origin. There may be an association with concurrent systemic disease or hereditary factors. Scratching the irritating area is a common indicator, and there tends to be progression from erythema and papules to skin lesions, which may then become secondarily infected.

Treatment   Although palliative measures rarely lead to a cure and topical applications are likely to be licked or rubbed off, both topical and systemic palliative therapy may be appropriate until the underlying cause is determined. Thus, before the application of a topical product, the treatment area needs to be prepared by clipping away the hair and removing any contaminating debris with disinfectants or cleansing agents. There is a range of suitable products available containing either quaternary ammonium compounds or chlorhexidine or povidone–iodine (see chapter 3). Restraining devices, such as hobbles and Elizabethan collars to prevent licking, are best avoided as they contribute little to the comfort of the animal. However, licking may be reduced by feeding or exercising the animal, either of which acts as a distraction. As is to be expected, formulations for treating skin disorders include creams, gels, lotions, liniments, ointments, pastes, powders, collodions, sprays and shampoos. In choosing the form of formulation, the role of the vehicle in the formulation must be recognised. It may aid penetration of the active drug constituent and influence the level of hydration of the skin, be protective or have a mild anti-inflammatory effect.

A cream base or aqueous cream alone will act as an emollient in the treatment of dry, scaling lesions, while soothing and hydrating the skin. Frequent application may be necessary as well as desirable.

Lotions are particularly suitable for application to hairy areas and for lesions with minor exudation and ulceration. Lotions that contain volatile substances may sting when applied and care should be taken with nervous or excitable animals.

Ointments are more occlusive than creams and are preferred for use with chronic dry lesions; they should be avoided with exudative lesions. They are also very effective emollients.

Pastes are less occlusive than ointments as they normally contain a very high proportion of finely powdered solid constituents. They are porous and capable of absorbing exudates (see also under Sweet itch above).

Dermatophilosis or rain scald This is caused by *Dermatophilus congolensis*. It is prevalent in wet weather, and grazing horses that are subjected to persistent wetting of the coat are most susceptible to it. It appears as an exudative dermatitis, especially on the back and quarters, but also affects the lower limbs and the lines of rain water drainage. Hair matting and a 'paint-brush' appearance follows the accumulation of exudates. The disease is self-limiting in dry conditions. Shelter to enable the coat to dry out should be provided in order to ensure that the signs are not due to some other cause, such as mud fever.

Mud fever This is common when wet and muddy conditions underfoot prevail. Such conditions encourage the development of cracks or fissures in the skin, known as chapping. This allows the ingress of bacteria into the skin, especially of the lower limbs. The bacteria most implicated are *Staphylococcus aureus* and *Dermatophilus congolensis* (see under Dermatophilosis or rain scald, above).

Treatment Treatment requires adequate housing to facilitate drying, and probably the application of appropriate antibacterials, antiseptics and disinfectants after local debridement. It is important to ensure reliable confirmatory diagnosis.

 There may be a zoonotic risk from mud fever, and appropriate precautions should be taken.

Ringworm or dermatomycosis

This is found world-wide and is a very important skin disease of horses. The causative organisms are predominantly species of *Trichophyton* and *Microsporum*. The disease is most prevalent in riding and racing stables and transmission may be by direct contact or indirectly from grooming equipment, tack, clippers or a contaminated horsebox. Young horses are relatively more susceptible because of the lack of previous exposure; some resistance can develop with age but reinfection is possible. The incubation period is up to 4 weeks, most cases occurring in the autumn or winter at the time of housing.

Ringworm is a zoonosis and cases have been recorded in which initial infection was followed by subsequent transmission between children in a classroom.

Initial signs develop as raised patches of skin followed by the breaking of hairs and the development of round crusty lesions. The lesions may be inflammatory, exudative and less commonly, pruritic. They occur most commonly in the saddle, girth or neck areas, especially those rubbed by tack. Hypersensitivity may lead to oedema, suppuration and necrosis. Microscopic examination of a skin scraping or hair sample and isolation of the organism is necessary to confirm diagnosis. Infection is usually self-limiting, with spontaneous remission in 1–3 months.

Treatment Successful treatment requires medication of the animal, which will shorten the duration of the disease, and decontamination of the environment. Ideally, infected animals should be isolated. Griseofulvin is given orally for the systemic treatment of ringworm in horses, either in the form of an oral paste or granules. All the products are prescription-only and brand names include Dufulvin, Equifulvin, Grisol-V and Norofulvin.

Diseases controlled by vaccines

All diseases of horses that are controlled by vaccines are endemic in the UK, except rabies.

- Equine herpes virus 1 and 4. These may cause respiratory disease and abortion.
- Equine influenza, characterised by mild fever and persistent cough.
- Tetanus.
- Equine viral arteritis, a contagious disease world-wide.
- Rabies, for which vaccination is not routinely used in the UK.
- Enteritis.

It is considered advisable for horses to always be vaccinated against tetanus and equine influenza, and several combination vaccines are available for this purpose. All the authorised equine vaccines are classed as prescription-only medicines and an immunisation programme appropriate for individual horses will be best advised by the veterinarian responsible for the animal's care. The use to which the horse is put and the extent of contact with other horses are factors to be taken into account, as well as the rules of the Jockey Club when relevant.

Enteritis in foals may be of viral, bacterial, protozoal or environmental and management origin. However, rotavirus is the most common cause of diarrhoea in young foals. At present there is an inactivated rotavirus vaccine available under a provisional marketing authorisation, subject to the ongoing collection of data on efficacy in use. The vaccine is given to pregnant mares to provide passive transfer of rotavirus antibodies to foals.

Pharmacists may be in a position to respond to enquiries about the respective details of passive versus active immunity, live versus killed vaccines, the storage and handling of vaccines, and contraindications and side-effects (see chapter 4).

The correct storage (usually at 2–8 °C) and transport of vaccines is crucial to their efficacy, and the manufacturer's recommendations should be followed carefully. Otherwise, the preparation is in danger of becoming completely ineffective, to the detriment (including financial) of all concerned.

Aseptic procedures, so familiar to all pharmacists, cannot be presumed to be understood by all those who have occasion to handle medicines, especially injections and vaccines. Abscesses and the transmission of incidental infections can be minimised by the use of only sterile needles and syringes and the application of aseptic precautions. Animals are moving targets; the injection site should be clean and the animal may require appropriate restraint.

Foot conditions

When the enormous pressures and stresses a horse puts on its legs and feet are taken into account, it is hardly surprising that horses can suffer from a range of adverse foot conditions that justify brief reference. They range from laminitis to the result of bad shoeing, but include corns and cracked heels.

Laminitis

This is most common in ponies and in fat or unfit horses. All four feet are not necessarily affected and the inflammation may only be transitory, followed by congestion of the laminae. There are a considerable number of causes.

- The commonest cause is the ingestion of excessive amounts of soluble carbohydrate, or 'grain overload'.
- Damage to the tiny arteriovenous shunts within the highly vascular laminae of the foot.
- Damage by bacterial endotoxins and trauma.

- High-level corticosteroid administration.
- Allergic-type reaction to certain medications, including anthelmintics and hormonal drugs, has been suggested as a factor.

Laminitis can be a potentially life-threatening condition and should always be regarded as a serious disease, requiring prompt veterinary attention and appropriate nursing care, such as is associated with expert farriery. Shoeing is especially important in treating chronic cases. Awareness of some of the causes of such conditions is useful and important if the pharmacist is to encourage prompt referral to a veterinarian. Treatment may include the use of a local anaesthetic to block the digital nerves and give immediate pain relief. Associated medication may include acepromazine, phenylbutazone and corticosteroids.

A horse's hooves require regular attention. Hoof oils, together with a wide range of grooming aids, represent a large and expanding market when once established. Attention to ill-fitting saddlery may also be important, as this can be the cause of sore mouth corners from an unsuitable bit, saddle sores and other injuries.

Veterinary wound dressings

These have been slower to be developed and adopted in practice than dressings for human use, as will be discussed in more detail in chapter 18. There is increasing recognition of the value of using appropriate dressings, such as semi-permeable adhesive films (Tegaderm and Opsite) on wounds where granulation tissue is established and wound exudate is declining in order to accelerate re-epithelialisation. Adhesive hydrocolloid dressings (Granuflex, Comfeel and Tegasorb) applied to the rumps of horses have resulted in a decrease of up to 30% in healing time from injury to hair regrowth and will remain *in situ*. However, a pharmacist's knowledge of modern wound dressings can contribute not only to wound recovery but also can markedly strengthen professional relationships with both veterinarian and animal owner. The management of wounds is covered in detail in chapters 18 and 19.

As seen from earlier chapters in this book, the opportunities for many pharmacists to develop their involvement in helping to contribute to the healthcare and welfare of animals, including horses, is considerable and can be professionally very satisfying.

Further reading

Aiello S E ed. (2000). *The Merck Veterinary Manual*, 8th edn. Rahway: Merck and Co.

Bishop Y, ed. (2001). *The Veterinary Formulary*, 5th edn. London: Pharmaceutical Press.

Blood D C (2000). *Pocket Companion to Veterinary Medicine*, 9th edn. London: W B Saunders.

Boden E, ed. (2001). *Black's Veterinary Dictionary*, 20th edn. London: A & C Black.

Hayes M H (2002). *Veterinary Notes for Horse Owners*, 18th edn. London: Ebury Press.

Royal Phamaceutical Society of Great Britain Veterinary Pharmacists' Group (1999). *Has Your Horse Got Worms? Ask Your Pharmacist About Appropriate Treatment*, revised (free leaflet). London: RPSGB.

Smith B P (2002). *Large Animal Internal Medicine: Diseases of Horses, Cattle, Sheep and Goats*, 3rd edn. St Louis: Mosby.

Watson D, ed. (2002). *The Henston Large Animal and Equine Veterinary Vade Mecum*. Peterborough: Veterinary Business Development.

16

Pigeon healthcare

Michael H Jepson and Barrie Wilton

Pigeons, like domestic poultry, cats, dogs and livestock, are subject to and infected by endo- and ectoparasites as well as by the usual range of bacterial and viral infections affecting most living creatures. It is estimated that about ten million pigeons are kept by about a quarter of a million pigeon fanciers, primarily for racing and showing, including show breeds with names such as rollers, tipplers and tumblers. This is in addition to pigeons raised and intended for meat production. 'Pigeon fanciers' is the commonly used term for owners. Pigeon racing is not only a hobby; to an increasing number of fanciers it is a profitable living. Birds bred from good stock may be worth several hundred thousands of pounds.

Pigeon fanciers are usually able to diagnose the more common ailments of their birds, such as simple catarrh, which is often called 'one-eyed cold', and the two protozoan infections, coccidiosis and canker or trichomoniasis. However, relatively few medicinal products have marketing authorisation in the UK for use in pigeons, which differs from the situation in some other European countries. While pigeon fanciers may treat symptoms and use prophylactic medication as part of a disease prevention strategy, it should be emphasised that the specific diagnosis of a disease and its appropriate treatment by a veterinarian depends on the birds being under his or her care and requires specialist veterinary knowledge and experience. Treatment may be dependent upon the use of the prescribing 'cascade', which at present is only legal for veterinarians to use. In addition, not all veterinary surgeons would claim to have the appropriate specialist expertise.

Pigeon fanciers tend to be keen and acute observers of their birds, and pigeon clubs, rather like bee-keepers' associations, act as an important focus for sharing knowledge and experience.

Pigeon fanciers are more geographically scattered than is generally realised and are not confined to former mining areas of northern England, so check your Yellow Pages for local clubs. About one million

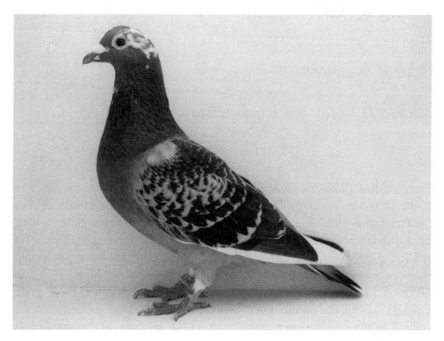

Figure 16.1 Racing pigeon. (Courtesy K Moore, 'Topcolor'.)

Box 16.1 Pigeon fancier's lung

Pigeon fancier's lung is a form of extrinsic allergic alveolitis in which the repeated inhalation of avian antigens provokes a hypersensitivity reaction in susceptible subjects. It is probably the most experienced allergy amongst pigeon fanciers, and has caused many of them to give up their pigeons.

Three main patterns of disease may be recognised:

- Acute progressive
- Acute intermittent non-progressive
- Recurrent non-acute disease.

Some patients present for the first time with established lung fibrosis without having experienced acute episodes, whereas others continue to have intermittent acute episodes for many years without progressing to permanent lung damage. Fanciers who develop the disease have often remained in a state of equilibrium with the antigen for many years before the onset of symptoms, and in some patients established disease may regress despite continued exposure to antigen.

Ideally, treatment of extrinsic allergic alveolitis consists mainly of avoiding contact with the inciting antigen, and complete cessation of exposure to pigeons is the safest

continued

Box 16.1   (continued)

advice for patients with pigeon fancier's lung. However, this may not be necessary in all cases, and fanciers are usually highly committed to their sport. Under these circumstances there are simple precautions that can be taken which will allow fanciers to continue their hobby nd minimise their symptoms. Respiratory protection masks have been shown to improve symptoms, to prevent a reaction to antigen challenge, and to reduce the level of circulating antibodies. The protection provided by masks is not complete, however, since most masks permit penetration of particles less than 1 μm in diameter, and leakage through defects in the fit of the mask to the face allows particles to bypass the filter. Sensitised fanciers should wear a loft coat and hat, that are removed on leaving the pigeon loft, to avoid continuing contact with pigeon-derived antigens carried on clothing or hair. Time spent in the loft should be kept to a minimum and, whenever possible, the fancier should avoid activities associated with high levels of antigen exposure such as 'scraping out' or cleaning the loft. Fanciers should be advised not to transport pigeons on the back seat of a car since this can result in very high levels of airborne antigen in an enclosed space. Antigen avoidance and respiratory protection should be continued at pigeon shows. When highly sensitised patients have given up pigeons completely, they will still face a risk of residual antigen exposure in their home and, more likely, continued exposure through their social circle if they remain in close contact with other pigeon fanciers. Some fanciers find it helpful to increase the level of ventilation in their loft, but resulting air turbulence may generate as many airborne particles as are eliminated to the outside by ventilation. The administration of corticosteroids may assist in controlling symptoms.

From: Bourke S, Boyd G. (1997). Pigeon fancier's lung [editorial]. *Br Med J* 315: 70–71.

birds are raced each weekend during the season from Easter to mid-September, and most of us would never know as they are mostly transported by road. Gone are the days when baskets of pigeons were a common sight on railway platforms!

The pigeon year

In order to adequately understand how best the optimum health of domesticated pigeons may be sustained, it is necessary to have a basic understanding of the 'pigeon year', which can be divided into six periods:

- Wintering.
- Pairing-up.
- Breeding.
- Training and racing old birds.

- Training and racing young birds.
- Moulting.

Wintering

This is the period from the end of the body moult until 'pairing-up' takes place for the new season. The birds moult the last of their main wing-feathers around November and so the wintering period lasts from approximately November to March in the UK. However, the actual length of this period is determined by whichever racing system, usually either 'widowhood' or 'natural', the fancier uses to race his or her pigeons.

During the wintering period, the birds need to be kept fit and given sufficient food to maintain their body temperature in very cold weather. It is important to avoid overfeeding, with its consequent obesity.

Pairing-up

In general, this period is either from late December to January or from mid-February to March, but is again determined by the system chosen by a fancier for the racing of his or her birds and by the distance of the longest race planned for the birds. Thus, between the Christmas break and the end of March fanciers will be pairing their birds and getting them settled, and the fancier will select both the mate and the nestbox for the respective pairs.

Pigeon race rules require that each bird has a ring on its leg that includes a number registered to the current owner of that pigeon. The ring also indicates the identity of the country, the year of ringing, a letter prefix and a number; an example might be 'GB 99 D 25068'. Rings have to be placed over the foot during the first 7 days of life as after that time the foot is likely to have grown too large. Rings for the current year are available from 10 January, so that a bird carrying a ring dated '03 could not have been bred earlier than 2003. In the year of a bird's 'birth', it is classed as a 'young bird'. From 1 January of the next year, the bird becomes an 'old bird'. The age of a bird classed as 'old' is usually immaterial except that some pigeon clubs will not allow birds that are less than two seasons old to enter very long races.

Breeding

The breeding period covers the time when the birds are being paired, nest-building, egg-laying, incubation, feeding the young, and the period until the young, known as 'squeakers', are weaned. This is usually up to about the end of March or April. The fancier will usually aid the nesting process by supplying some straw or special nest material, which the birds can use to line the bowl provided in their nestbox.

The hen will normally lay her second batch of eggs about a month after the first, even though the first pair of squeakers will not have been weaned.

It usually takes about 44 hours from fertilisation for the hen to produce a completed egg, and two eggs are laid a day apart. Incubation lasts 18 days from the first egg laid, and weaning usually takes place about 21 days after hatching. Laying and rearing may continue for whatever length of time the fancier chooses, and if artificial light was used in the short winter days at the beginning of the year, it may continue throughout the year. In practice, the fancier breeds for only a small part of the year, which is related to the chosen racing system. These systems are described in the following sections.

It is a characteristic of pigeons that both sexes incubate. The hen incubates from late afternoon, and overnight to about nine in the morning. The cock takes over when the hen leaves the nest, and the shifts are repeated from late afternoon. Both sexes also feed the young and both produce 'crop milk', with which they feed them during the first few days after hatching. Subsequently, the parents gradually add hard corn to the squeakers' diet. Feeding is by regurgitation.

Training and racing old birds

Birds that are paired early in the season, for example at the end of the Christmas holiday, may be trained as early as February if the weather is favourable. Birds that are paired later, perhaps around 8 March, are more likely to be trained from mid-April. The racing system chosen and the distance of races envisaged will have influenced the training schedule. The two basic systems for racing pigeons are called: 'natural' and 'widowhood'. Pigeon racers in the UK still follow imperial rather than metric measurements of distance, so for convenience all distances in this chapter are given in miles and yards rather then kilometres and metres.

The natural system

This is so called because the pairs follow the natural cycle of mating, laying, incubating and rearing before repeating the complete cycle.

This system is preferred by many fanciers when competing in long-distance races of 500, 600 or 700 miles or more. Pigeons will start to drop and then regrow their wing feathers after rearing their first squeakers of the season. Consequently, natural flyers pair up much later. Their birds have not reached an advanced stage of the moult before the date of the longest race of the season in June, which is nearest to the longest day of the year and when daylight hours are at their maximum. In order to race by this system, it is necessary to keep records of when the eggs are laid, so that, for example, on the day of the race for which the pigeon has been selected the bird has reached a stage of its nest cycle known as its 'nest condition'.

Nest cycle stages may be summarised as:

- Sitting: 7 days.
- Sitting: 10 days, which is when the crop-milk is forming.
- Due to hatch, the eggshell just chipping.
- Feeding a big youngster. This is when the next eggs are due to be fertilised and the cock bird is staying very close to the hen, and is a suitable time to send the cock to the race. This is known as 'driving', in other words driving the hen to nest again.

Different pigeons and the two sexes race better at different stages of the nest cycle, which means the fancier must produce the best nest conditions for particular birds in order to get the maximum result from an individual bird for a particular race. Thus, it is essential to keep accurate and detailed records, for each pair of birds, of the races in which they have competed. Under the natural system, most fanciers will race either the cock or the hen, or even both on the same day. However, whereas the cock can race when the hen is due to lay, it would be inappropriate to race the hen if there is a likelihood that she will lay en route to the race point. If the fancier wishes to save the eggs of a pair of birds destined to race on the same day, the eggs can be placed under other birds until the first bird returns from the race.

Fanciers use various strategies to encourage birds to achieve greater speeds, such as:

- Placing an egg from another nest that is just chipping under one of the birds to be sent to the race, so that it feels the movement of the hatching youngster, and believes that it is its own.
- Placing a recently hatched youngster from another nest under the chosen race bird to stimulate a response similar to the above, but at a later stage of the nest cycle.
- Placing under the chosen pair a bigger youngster than their own, to provoke the same stimulus.

These ploys can bring forward the timing of a pair's nest cycle by a day or two, enabling adjustment of the nest condition to one that is most appropriate for the individual bird for racing.

Widowhood

Many fanciers prefer this system of racing for short distances of up to 250 miles, known as 'sprint' races, but the system is also used for all distances. One recognised advantage of this system is that birds can be sent each week to race up to 400 or 500 miles as training flights, thereby obviating the need for the fancier to take them for training.

The system is called 'widowhood' because after the birds are paired and the hen lays her first pair of eggs, and irrespective of whether or not the pair rear their squeakers, the birds are kept in separate sex groups. Thus, the cocks are kept in their nestboxes and the hens are kept in other nestboxes out of sight of the cocks. The birds are put together again briefly, for a few minutes, before they are placed in baskets to take to the club for race marking. An essential feature of the system is that the hen is always waiting in the cock's nestbox when he returns from the race, or at the early part of the season whenever the cocks are being trained.

Some fanciers race their hens in the widowhood system instead of the cocks, in which case the references to cocks and hens above need to be reversed; it will be the cock who is waiting for the hen on her return. Similarly, other fanciers send birds of either sex to a race, leaving the opposite sex at home awaiting the arrival of their mate, or they may alternate between cocks and hens from one week to the next.

The basic aim is to provide an added incentive to race home rather than just to fly home.

Separation of the birds, as described above, for most of the race season affects the rate at which the birds moult, which is slowed down. By contrast, in the natural system of racing the moult continues faster and the birds reach the stage in the moult when they cease to be able to race much sooner, unless they are paired up later in the season.

The widowhood system and the corresponding loft design, enables the 'widowed' birds to be rested and have peace and quiet during the week between races, which mostly take place on Saturdays. Inevitably, in the natural system, there is constant movement of birds in and out of their boxes as they feed their squeakers or spend their share of time incubating their eggs.

Training and racing young birds

The main purpose of training is to reinforce the pigeon's natural homing instinct to return to the loft by the shortest route and to build and maintain athletic fitness. In young birds, it enables them to gain confidence in their reliance on their homing instinct. How pigeons achieve this is still not conclusively proven, although several theories have been postulated.

Birds are taken to increasing distances from the loft before racing commences and training may be continued after racing has started if considered necessary. If the natural system of racing is used, it may be necessary to continue training throughout the season to keep the birds in a fit condition. In the widowhood system, intensive pre-race training is more usual and there is less training, if any, once racing has started. This can enable the fancier to spend more time in the loft, ensuring heightened awareness of the birds' habits, preferences, state of health and their general wellbeing. Factors which facilitate birds being less perturbed by the fancier's presence and loft maintenance and are increasingly tame can make the difference between winning and losing.

Moulting

Moulting is a natural function for any bird when fit and healthy. Starting at hatching, a squeaker grows a set of feathers, which then moult and a new set is grown in proportion to the bird's increasing size and weight. It is most likely that this second growth takes place at a similar time to that of the old birds (old birds are birds at any time after 1 January following their year of birth). Smaller body feathers moult quickly during warm humid weather, most usually from late July to September or October, depending on the weather. Most crucial to a pigeon fancier is the moult of the flight feathers in the wing. A pigeon fancier sees the moult as the growth of new feathers in perfect condition rather than the discarding of old feathers. The replacement of sound feathers in a good moult indicates a fit pigeon and augurs well for the next year's racing. Pigeon fanciers have always to look ahead and pay careful attention to the next part of the season.

The wing moult

Moulting of wing feathers takes place in step in each wing, starting in the middle of the wing and working outwards to the long flight feathers. Each feather is longer than the previous inner one, except for the outer-most, which is slightly shorter than the one before it. Feathers are counted from the middle feather, called number 1, which is the first to moult, and there are ten 'primary flight' feathers in each wing, called primaries 1–10. From the wing-middle back towards the body of the bird are the 'secondary flights', which are secondaries 1–10. The primary flights provide the main power source for flight, which means speed. Hence the need for the fancier to control the timing of the wing moult of a particular bird so that it relates to the races for which the bird has been selected. Control is achieved by planning the time that the birds have their first nest, as this is the time from which the wing moult will be triggered. If the bird is not stressed at any stage, the wing moult will progress as described above. Unpaired birds moult much more slowly, and as widowhood birds are seemingly unpaired for much of the season the wing stays in racing shape for a much longer time.

Short-distance 'widowers' can be paired in December and then trained earlier in the new season, since they will have stopped racing earlier. Longer-distance widowers are paired a little later; pigeons under the natural system may not be paired until about the end of the first week in March. It will depend upon how many old primary flight feathers the fancier requires by the time of the longest daylight hours. The last four flight feathers, 7–10, should still be in place from last year's moult by that time, or the power of the bird's flying will be adversely affected.

Races increase in distance as the season progresses, so that birds that are sent not more than 200 or 300 miles, even though paired early, will have stopped their racing for the season before reaching the critical stage of the wing moult.

To enable young birds from the current season to develop their athletic ability and skill at homing, their moulting condition is largely ignored and, except when their heads are almost bare of feathers, they are raced weekly or fortnightly.

Race marking or 'basketing'

Races are grouped into three categories:

- Sprint or short distance: up to about 250 miles.
- Middle distance: 250–400 miles.
- Long distance: 500–700 miles.

The terms 'flying north road' and 'flying south road' are used by fanciers and indicate the direction in which the birds were transported to the race starting point. For example, if birds from the English Midlands were transported to Scotland and liberated to fly back to the Midlands, they would be called 'north road birds'. Similarly, birds taken to France to fly back to the UK would be called 'south road birds'. The east and west directions are ignored, which no doubt reflects the overall shape of Great Britain.

Before the start of a race, pigeons are taken by their owners to the club responsible for organising the race and each pigeon has an elastic, numbered ring placed over its foot onto its leg. This is the 'race rubber' and the number on it is recorded on the race entry form against the permanent ring put on the pigeon at about 6 days old. In some races, birds also have a letter and number, such as 'A4' or 'B12', applied with a rubber-inked stamp on a wing feather. This is also recorded against the pigeon's identification ring number. These measures are designed to prevent cheating and the fancier remains ignorant of these identifications until the bird arrives home. On arrival home, the elastic ring is slipped off the bird's foot and placed in a special timing device and struck so that it records the time it was 'clocked', and the time and bird's ring number are noted on a form which the fancier takes back to the club on the 'checking night'. If wing marking has been used, this would also be noted on the form. Subsequently, the previously secured timing clocks are opened by the club, the rubber rings removed and checked against the details on the recording form. The time at which the birds were liberated at the start of the race is known to the minute and the time of arrival at home to the nearest second. The distance of each loft from the liberation site is known to the nearest yard, from all of which can be calculated the ground speed of the bird. Further checks are made to confirm the integrity of the recording equipment and corrections are made where necessary. The bird having the highest velocity, in yards per minute, is recorded as the winner and each bird completing the race will have its velocity recorded too, if necessary to two decimal places.

Common conditions affecting pigeons

Watery droppings

One condition that is frequently seen in pigeon flocks is loose or watery droppings. It may be a symptom of many diseases or infections, including those caused by:

- Roundworm infestation.
- Protozoa responsible for coccidiosis and trichomoniasis (canker).
- Salmonellosis.
- Paramyxovirus.

Mixed infections are common, and stress may be an additional factor. In addition to appropriate therapy, supportive care and loft hygiene to eradicate the causative organisms are most important. The risk of spreading an infection must be addressed and minimised. Keeping stress to a minimum is also crucial, as birds suffering from stress are more prone to disease.

Paramyxovirus

Between 1981 and 1983, a disease of pigeons resembling the neurotropic form of Newcastle disease in chickens spread across Europe, and was first reported in Great Britain in the summer of 1983. The disease is mainly caused by infection with a variant avian paramyxovirus of the serotype 1 group, PMV-1, which produces a debilitating illness that is often fatal. The disease can upset breeding and training schedules in racing pigeon lofts and has been the cause of considerable financial loss. Newcastle disease in poultry, caused by a different strain of paramyxovirus, is a notifiable disease in the UK.

No disease treatment for pigeon paramyxovirus is currently available, but there are vaccines that are used to immunise pigeons and protect against infection. The virus could potentially spread to commercial poultry.

Today, under The Diseases of Poultry Order 1994 (SI 1994 No. 3141) as amended, it is obligatory for all racing pigeons entered for races or shows that take place wholly or partly in Great Britain to be vaccinated against pigeon paramyxovirus (avian type 1). The legislation includes procedures to be followed regarding the movement of birds, the disinfection of premises and vaccination to ensure continued protection of poultry from Newcastle disease.

It should be remembered that the large feral pigeon population will continue to act as a potential reservoir of infection for the racing pigeon population.

In pigeons the virus is spread in droppings or feces and from nasal secretions. Young birds are relatively more susceptible to disease, which is why vaccination should not be delayed beyond the time recommended by the vaccine manufacturers.

Clinical signs include:

- Watery, discoloured feces.
- Nervous disorders, such as paralysis, twisting of the neck and a lack of coordination.

Non-specific symptoms include ruffled feathers, increased thirst and listlessness.

There are currently two authorised inactivated vaccines, containing suitable adjuvants, available in the UK, both of which are pharmacy

(P) medicines (see Figure 7.4, page 182). The dose by subcutaneous injection is either 0.2 or 0.25 mL, and is given to young birds at any time from 3–6 weeks of age, normally in February or March. It is most important to check the vaccine's data sheet for specific conditions. The injection site is at the base of the neck. All pigeons in a loft should be vaccinated. Vaccination should be at least 2 weeks before the first race or show of the season. For sustained protection, a booster dose is required every 12 months and the months of October to November (5–6 weeks before pairing) are appropriate. The slaughter withdrawal period for these vaccines is nil.

One of the two vaccines available uses a suitable oil as adjuvant and it is appropriate to refer to the warning about accidental self-injection with oil-based vaccines. This can cause severe pain and intense swelling, which may result in ischaemic necrosis and loss of a digit. Prompt medical attention is essential and details of the product involved should be available.

Pigeon fanciers have been known to delay vaccination until the young birds are considered large enough to handle more easily, and are less likely to suffer stress. However such delay is not recommended or within the manufacturers' dosage guidance, and also leaves the young birds vulnerable to a greater risk of infection.

Pigeon pox

Pigeon pox is a disease caused by a poxvirus that is characterised by lesions of the mouth and eyes.

Birds can be vaccinated from 5 weeks of age, and all birds in the loft should be vaccinated. Old birds should be revaccinated annually outside the racing season (between 30 September and 31 December), and this can be done at the same time as paramyxovirus vaccination. The vaccine, which is a powder for reconstitution (formerly a pharmacy product, now reclassified as a pharmacy and merchant supplies medicine (PML)), is applied on the lower leg or breast after the removal of a few feathers. The vaccine is brushed in one direction into the plucked follicles. A reaction should be observable in about 4 days. If little or no reaction is produced, vaccination may be repeated after 5–7 days but birds that are already immune from previous vaccination are less likely to show a reaction. Birds remain infectious until the vaccination sites have healed, and until then they should be isolated from other stock.

Pharmacists are in a position to supply vaccination record cards, advise and provide information on the appropriate injection site and optimum age for primary vaccination. Pigeon fanciers should be advised not to put their fingers anywhere near their eyes when handling live vaccine or sick birds, in order to prevent the risk of infection by conjunctivitis.

Parasite problems

There are three parasite problems in particular for which routine prevention is necessary: gastrointestinal roundworms, coccidiosis and trichomoniasis (canker). Several pharmacy (P) only and general sale list (GSL) products are available for routine administration, as listed in Table 16.1. Further details may be found in *The Veterinary Formulary* and from manufacturers' data sheets.

A typical loft will contain 30–100 birds and individual treatment for parasite infection control may be neither practical nor appropriate. Most group medication is given in the drinking water. A typical pigeon consumes about 50 mL water per day; the amount drunk will depend, for example, on the season, the bird's clinical condition and whether nestlings are being fed.

Table 16.1   Preparations for pigeons (Adapted from *The Veterinary Formulary*)

Indication	Active ingredient	Product (manufacturer)	Legal class
Coccidiosis	Amprolium	Coxoid Liquid (Harkers[a]);	GSL
	Clazuril	Appertex Tablets (Harkers[a]);	GSL
	Sulfadimethoxine	Coxi Plus (Alpharma)	POM
Trichomoniasis (canker)	Carnidazole	Spartrix Tablets (Harkers[a]);	GSL
	Dimetridazole	Harkerkanker (Harkers[a])	GSL
GI roundworms	Fenbendazole	Panacur Capsules (Intervet UK);	GSL
	Piperazine	Biozine Powder (Harkers[a])	GSL
Immunisation against paramyxovirus disease	Pigeon paramyxovirus vaccine, by subcutaneous injection	*Colombovac PMV(Fort Dodge); Nobivac Paramyxo (Intervet)	P P
Vaccination against pigeon pox	Pigeon pox vaccine, by brushed application	Nobivac Pigeon Pox Vaccine (Living) (Intervet); Colombovac PMV/Pox (Fort Dodge); Combination pack, vaccines in 2 vials	PML P

(*continued*)

Table 16.1 *Continued*

Indication	Active ingredient	Product (manufacturer)	Legal class
Lice and mites	Malathion	Duramitex (Harkers[a])	GSL
	Pyrethrins	Anti-Mite & Insect Spray (Johnson's)	GSL
		Anti-Pest Insect Spray (Johnson's)	GSL
		Caperns Mite Powder (Bob Martin)	GSL
		Kil-Pest (Johnson's)	GSL
		Pigeon Insect Preparation (Johnson's)	GSL
		Rid-Mite (Johnson's)	GSL
Dietary supplements	Compound multivitamins and mineral preparations	Collivet (Harkers[a])	
		Pigeon Minerals (Harkers[a])	
		Omni-Vit (Harkers[a])	
		Vetreplex (Vetrepharm)	
		Vitamix (Oropharma)	
		Harkervet Plus (Harkers[a])	
	Oral fluids	DextroTonic (Oropharma)	
		Electrovet (Vetafarm)	
		Fortalyt (Oropharma)	
		Spark (Vetafarm)	
		Vitalyte (Vetrepharm)	

[a] Harkers, now part of Petlife International Ltd, Bury St Edmunds, Suffolk, UK
*See Figure 7.4, page 182

Pharmacists can advise about such things as the careful measurement of an oral powder to be added to drinking water; the unsuitability of galvanised drinkers (drinking water dispensers) for preparations containing substances such as citric acid and copper sulfate; and the fact that unused medicated water must not contaminate water courses, ditches or drains.

The Veterinary Formulary provides informative details on drug administration and parasiticide therapy that complements data sheet information.

Worms

Gastrointestinal roundworms   The roundworms found in pigeons include pigeon ascarids (*Ascaridia*), which are about 20–90 mm long and 1 mm in diameter, and hairworms (*Capillaria*), which are usually up to 25 mm long and very fine, as their common name implies. Adult ascarids are found in the intestine and a very heavy worm burden (infestation) can lead to blockage of the intestines. A severe hair-worm infection may lead to diarrhoea (possibly blood-tinged) and weight loss.

The life cycle of roundworms is direct. Adult worms in the intestine shed eggs that are passed through into the droppings, where the eggs mature and become infectious after about 1–2 weeks, depending on the prevailing climatic conditions. Eggs that are ingested by a pigeon will hatch and develop into adult worms. The adult worms will subsequently lay eggs, thereby completing the life cycle and enabling the whole process to start again.

Effective drugs for the treatment and control of gastrointestinal roundworms invariably have some side-effects. Oral levamisole can cause vomiting and has a bitter taste in drinking water. It is usually found necessary to withhold drinking water for a limited time before providing medicated water. In severely infected birds, levamisole may have to be given by injection. As benzimidazoles may cause feather abnormalities during feather development in young birds and during moulting, it should be avoided at these times.

Product information leaflets, data sheets and summary of characteristics product (SPC) all include full details of dosage and frequency. *The Veterinary Formulary* includes a summary table of parasiticidal doses of drugs for pigeons in its section on guidance on the prescribing and dosage of antimicrobial drugs.

Tapeworms   Tapeworms or tapeworm segments may be identifiable in the droppings but can be confused with starch grains. Infestation with tapeworms is much less common than with roundworms and is likely to occur only in birds that have access to fields and gardens.

The life cycle of the tapeworm, in contrast to that of the round-worm, is indirect. Eggs shed by adult worms in the intestine are passed through into the droppings but then ingested by an intermediate host, such as a beetle. Birds will become infected when eating an insect that contains a developing tapeworm. The life cycle is completed when the tapeworm matures to adulthood in the intestine and lays eggs.

From a basic understanding of these life cycles, it can be seen that the potential sources of infection are diverse and include pigeon lofts, baskets used for transporting pigeons, and newly acquired birds introduced to the loft, if not previously treated for worms. Free-living and free-range birds are at risk from infected insects in the soil.

Control and treatment   Good loft hygiene is of paramount importance. The level of contamination in a loft can be reduced and minimised by frequent removal of droppings to ensure that the worm eggs are eliminated before becoming infectious. Regular use of a medicated floor dressing is also advisable. As with all domesticated pets and livestock, birds can be dosed with a suitable anthelmintic at regular intervals to control worm infestations. It is not possible to kill all infecting worms as birds are constantly exposed to reinfection. Hence the need for retreatment and for the simultaneous treatment of groups of birds in lofts.

Routine treatment is strongly recommended. Praziquantel is often given twice a year, initially in March or April and then after racing, before pairing in October.

Protozoa

Coccidiosis ('going light')   Coccidiosis in pigeons is caused by the protozoa *Eimeria labbaena* and *E. columbarum*. As in many other species affected by coccidia, including game birds, calves, lambs, cats and dogs, it is the young that are most susceptible, but older birds become carriers. It is noteworthy that coccidiosis is of major economic importance and concern in the poultry industry. The oocysts or eggs are passed in the droppings and can survive in the environment for long periods. On maturing they become infectious, which can be in as short a time as 2 days after the eggs are shed in the droppings, depending on the prevailing climatic conditions. When infectious oocysts are ingested by pigeons, their life cycle is completed in the intestine. By invading the gut wall, where they multiply, they cause damage that is manifested in the clinical signs of the disease. These include diarrhoea (possibly blood-tinged), weight loss, reduced feeding, increased thirst, loss of eye colour and dull plumage.

Control and treatment   Good loft hygiene is essential. The loft floor should be kept dry, particularly around the drinking water containers. The use of regular medication with an anticoccidial will help ensure that the disease is kept under control.

Routine treatment is usually before pairing in October or November and once during the racing season.

The following anticoccidials are currently authorised for use in pigeons for prophylactic control:

- Amprolium hydrochloride oral solution.
- Clazuril tablets 2.5 mg.
- Sulfadimethoxine oral powder (see Table 16.1). These products must not be used in pigeons intended for human consumption.

Prolonged intermittent or continuous medication may be required for severe coccidiosis.

Trichomoniasis (canker)   Trichomoniasis is caused by the protozoon *Trichomonas gallinae (T. columbae)*. Infection is common but clinical signs of disease are usually only seen in young birds or debilitated adult pigeons. Young birds usually become infected from the parent bird during feeding, and if crop milk is infected any contamination in the nest can affect a hatchling's navel before it has completely closed.

Clinical signs of the disease   Initially there are yellow plaques or deposits visible in the bird's throat and also in the upper respiratory tract. Other non-specific signs, including diarrhoea, listlessness and decreased feeding, are a result of the invasion by the organism of internal organs, especially the liver.

Control and treatment   Regular medication will control the disease in flocks.

Special care should be taken when administering medicated drinking water to birds during hot weather, or to breeding birds, because an increase in water consumption may lead to drug toxicity.

Routine treatment is appropriate after egg-laying and before hatching, while the birds are sitting.

Carnidazole tablets (10 mg) are authorised for the treatment and prophylaxis of canker in pigeons (see Table 16.1). Carnidazole, like metronidazole, is thought to interact with DNA, destroying its ability to act as a template for DNA and RNA synthesis.

Ectoparasites: lice, mites and ticks

Several species of these ectoparasites are to be found on pigeons, most of which live for their whole life cycle on the bird. Eggs are laid, hatch and mature, and the parasites feed on the blood, body fluids or feathers of the pigeon. Ectoparasites that show variations of this pattern include some that lay eggs in the environment and attach themselves to the bird for feeding, and the red mite, which only invades the pigeon at night. During daylight, red mites hide in crevices and nest bowls away from light, and so are not to be seen on birds during the day. At night they can be seen on pigeons by the light of a torch.

In general, these parasites cause damage to plumage, and severe infestation causes debilitation and may lead to anaemia. Red mites leave skin blemishes that may be visible, and severe infestation in young birds can prove fatal.

Control and treatment Control requires regular treatment of the whole group of birds and any newly introduced birds at the same time. The use of an insecticide formulated for use in pigeon lofts when the birds are present can help to eradicate those parasites that do not live permanently on the pigeons. Permethrin or pyrethrins are used on birds for the control of lice and mites and pesticides containing malathion and permethrin are available for use in the loft and on fittings.

Other conditions

Other diseases of sufficient importance to mention are discussed in the following sections.

Salmonellosis and other bacterial infections

This is also referred to as paratyphoid and wing paralysis.

 The *Salmonella* group of bacteria is widely distributed in all animals and can affect humans. It is a notifiable disease.

In pigeons, as a gut infection it may cause diarrhoea, which has a characteristic green slimy consistency. If the organism spreads to other parts of the body, it may cause swelling of the joints, resulting in leg stiffness and wing droop or paralysis. If the septicaemic infection spreads to major organs, such as the liver, heart, kidneys and spleen, the result is likely to be rapid debilitation and loss of balance. Similarly, if the brain is affected, paralysis and loss of balance will follow. The consequence may be chronic diarrhoea, permanent paralysis or death. *Salmonella* is spread in excretions from infected birds and animals and through eggs. It is thus possible to be infected from birth, though infection is more likely to be oral. The disease follows ingestion of sufficient bacteria by a susceptible bird.

Although the infection may be treated with appropriate antibiotics, it is possible for up to 25% of affected birds to remain as carriers, capable of infecting new disease-free birds added to a flock. Carrier birds need to be identified and culled. At least three negative fecal culture tests are considered necessary in order to confirm that a bird is not a carrier, as the test has limited reliability because salmonellae are not secreted continuously from the gut.

Prevention relies heavily on good hygiene and good ventilation of the loft, which must include attention to preventing the access of vermin and wild birds to the loft.

Pigeons, like other birds and mammals, may contract bacterial infections from a number of other opportunistic microorganisms present in the environment. Thus, diarrhoea can be caused by *Escherichia coli* present in the gastrointestinal tract. *E. coli* may also enter the circulatory system and cause septicaemia. Other bacteria capable of multiplying in the blood and causing problems, such as abscesses, include *Staphylococcus*, *Streptococcus* and *Corynebacterium*.

Treatment with an appropriate antibiotic is likely to be necessary and to be prescribed by a veterinarian before laboratory identification and confirmation of the particular bacterium and strain.

Preventative measures again relate to the importance of loft hygiene. As these diseases are contagious and can be spread by infected birds, such birds should be isolated.

Haemophilus catarrh (owls head)

When a pigeon presents with heavy catarrh and much swelling around and especially of the eyes (hence the common name), a bacterial respiratory infection with *Haemophilus* is likely and will probably require antibiotic treatment and a veterinary prescription. As with a number of other conditions, including mycoplasmosis, adequate ventilation of the loft is an important preventative measure. It is also considered that birds are more vulnerable if under stress.

Respiratory disease

This may also be referred to as coryza, mycoplasmosis or infectious catarrh.

The performance of racing pigeons is comparable to that of any athlete, dependent as it is on respiratory function of maximum efficiency. Among other things, this implies freedom from any infection. Modest breathing difficulty may not be evident but even a slight infection may adversely affect a bird's maximum flight speed. A severe infection will have a marked adverse effect on flight. Visual signs in affected birds include watery mucus discharging from the nostrils and the mouth. Later this will become more purulent with an unpleasant smell and be associated with rasping breathing (see also the section on Ornithosis below, which causes catarrhal discharge.)

The causative organism is one of the mycoplasmas, which are distinct from bacteria and viruses. They resemble a large virus in size, and different species have been identified in humans, dogs, pigs, fowls, turkeys, rats and mice. They seem to be particularly prevalent in the lungs.

The disease is spread from bird to bird by direct contact, mainly from droplets respired or coughed out. Mycoplasmas are also excreted in feces but only survive for a short time outside the bird. It is believed that a low level of mycoplasma infection is probably universal, but is enhanced under conditions of stress and may make birds more vulnerable to other infections.

Preventative measures include good loft ventilation and the minimising of stress from overcrowding, poor-quality feed and water, parasitic infection and poor hygiene. The organism can be killed by suitable disinfectants. Travelling in baskets and even new accommodation can have adverse effects.

Ornithosis

This is common in pigeons in the UK and is caused by the microorganism *Chlamydia psittaci*. The condition is known as 'psittacosis' in the parrot family. Conjunctivitis is usually evident in affected adult birds. The disease can be lethal in young birds and it is claimed that up to 80% of young birds in a loft may die of the disease. It is also a zoonosis, and when pigeon fanciers present with flu-like symptoms at a pharmacy or a doctor's surgery they should inform their pharmacist and/or general medical practitioner that they keep pigeons.

Chlamydia are found in the droppings, nasal and beak mucus, tears and crop milk of diseased birds. Transmission is most likely by droplet infection or the inhalation or ingestion of infective particles, but may also involve wild pigeons, which are widely infected, vermin, insects and even humans.

As a respiratory disease in young birds it often appears to be latent, but it probably affects flight adversely. It may cause severe diarrhoea and wasting of body weight, and may lead to death.

The disease does respond to antibiotic treatment when properly diagnosed.

Control is again of particular importance and it is crucial to minimise stress and to maintain good standards of loft hygiene and to exclude vermin and wild birds so as to prevent the risks accruing from their droppings.

Aspergillosis

This is not a common condition in pigeons, but is a disease affecting the tissues of mammals and birds. It is caused by *Aspergillus fumigatus*, a widely distributed fungus that occurs in dust and damp food.

Infection most likely occurs through inhalation of the fungal spores or orally. Once in the bird's tissues, hyphae grow out from the spores, as with ringworm fungi, and from the branching filaments more spores are produced. Various organs and tissues can be affected and this may result in abscess formation.

Signs of the disease include breathlessness and green fungal deposits in the mouth. Externally, dandruff and fragile feathers may result. Unless treated promptly, the disease can be fatal.

Prevention is crucial because effective treatment of the established disease is uncertain. The loft and food store must be kept dry.

Medication and drug administration

As a consequence of the limited number of preparations for which marketing authorisations have been sought for use in pigeons, preparations available for use in other species, especially poultry, are frequently prescribed by veterinarians. When this is necessary and the cascade procedure is followed, it is required that the pigeon owner should be informed and his or her consent obtained for using any preparation prescribed beyond the data sheet or SPC authorised indications and recommendations.

Where the pigeons are intended for human consumption, it is of the utmost importance that the withdrawal periods, as stated by the manufacturer, are adhered to for any preparation authorised for use in pigeons. If a preparation is not authorised for use in pigeons or if no withdrawal period is given, then standard withdrawal periods must be applied.

Methods of drug administration

Medication may be given to pigeons either individually or in a group. In most situations it is usually necessary to treat all pigeons together as a group, or the whole loft. Where a few birds are clinically ill, they may best be treated individually, while also treating the rest of the group simultaneously, as most of the birds are likely to have contracted the same infection.

Individual treatment can be given by crop tubing, by mouth as tablets, capsules or liquid, or by injection. Injections, such as the paramyxovirus vaccine, should be given subcutaneously on the back at the base of the neck, pointing the needle posteriorly in the mid-line to avoid the plexus of vessels in the neck.

It is possible for some medicinal products to be applied topically either for local treatment or for percutaneous absorption and systemic effect.

Most drug medication for routine prophylactic treatment is given in the drinking water. For this purpose, drug dosage is frequently calculated on the assumption that a typical pigeon consumes about 50 mL a day. Unfortunately, this is an imprecise assumption, as the daily variation may be as great as 15–250 mL. In cold weather, during rest periods and during illness, water consumption will be low. Conversely, in hot, dry weather, when the birds are racing, when feeding nestlings, and in birds with certain clinical conditions associated with severe diarrhoea, water consumption will greatly increase. It should also be recognised that the unpalatability of certain medicines will result in reduced water intake, most noticeably on the first day of treatment. It can be helpful to withhold water for a few hours before medicated drinking water is supplied. As some individual birds seem to consistently refuse medicated water, they represent a threat to the possibility of reinfection and the apparent failure of treatment.

Pigeons normally drink mainly after feeding and so consume most of their daily intake of water over a short period after the main daily feed. As pigeons are frequently provided with water in excess of their needs and drinking containers are hygienically emptied and refilled several times daily, it is all the more essential to be able to accurately assess the amount of water actually consumed, rather than the amount offered. The required quantity of medication for the appropriate quantity of water can then be reliably determined.

Attention to the disposal of medicated water may also be necessary, and the manufacturer's product information should be followed carefully as disposal must not be into drains, ditches or watercourses.

If the medication is insoluble, it may be appropriate to incorporate it into the feed. There may, however, be a problem if the medication does not adhere to the feed grains, as pigeons can be selective feeders and are capable of avoiding items other than the feed grains. To prevent this problem, the estimated amount of food to be consumed daily is placed in a suitable container and sprinkled with a small quantity of vegetable oil. After thoroughly mixing the oil with the feed, the calculated amount of oral drug powder is added and mixed well. The medicated feed is then ready. Alternatives to vegetable oil that are often used are lemon juice and live unpasteurised yoghurt.

Because the amount of medication likely to be consumed by an individual bird is so variable, sick birds should be isolated and given medication individually. It is also important to ensure that external sources of water from garden ponds, bird baths or rainwater in general are avoided when birds are receiving mass medication from drinking water.

It has been noted in *The Veterinary Formulary* that the absorption of many drugs from the digestive tract of pigeons is believed to be relatively poor and may be adversely affected by bird grit containing calcium and magnesium salts. Consequently, the dosage, particularly of prescribed drugs, may require some adjustment.

The pharmacist's involvement

The keeping of racing and show pigeons should not be seen only as a well-established hobby mainly restricted to mining or former mining districts, but as a national activity for a very dedicated, enthusiastic, wide-ranging group of people. There is much investment of time and money and extensive expertise involved in the pigeon fancy, and pharmacists, as health professionals, are in a position to support this. Interested pharmacists who acquaint themselves with the pigeon year (see under The pigeon year, above) will recognise the opportunity and need to establish a planned programme for prophylactic medication, vaccination and the use of food supplements appropriate to the requirements of breeding birds, racing birds old and young, and moulting birds. The product range literature of the medicine manufacturers can provide useful guidance, and addresses are given in the *The Veterinary Formulary* and in the *Compendium of Data Sheets for Veterinary Products*. The RPSGB's free 12-page booklet *Pigeons – Ask your pharmacist for advice on common conditions affecting pigeons* is most informative, and the Royal Pigeon Racing Association also publishes free leaflets. Pigeon fanciers are often prepared to lavish much care and attention on their birds, especially on champion racers or breeding stock, and a single bird may be valued at several thousand pounds. The value of the medicines, equipment and feed market is estimated to be well in excess of £20 million a year.

Further reading

Bishop Y, ed. (2001). *The Veterinary Formulary*, 5th edn. London: Pharmaceutical Press.

Palmer D A (1994). *Pigeon Disease and the Vet*. Dewsbury: Twigg Printing.

The Racing Pigeons (vaccination) Order (1994). SI no. 944. London: Stationery Office. (Now applicable only to racing and show pigeons.)

Royal Pharmaceutical Society of Great Britain Veterinary Pharmacists' Group (1999) *Pigeons – Ask Your Pharmacist for Advice on Common Conditions Affecting Pigeons*, revised (free leaflet). London: RPSGB.

Schrag L (1994). *Healthy Pigeons: Recognition, Prevention and Treatment of the Major Pigeon Diseases*, 7th edn [English translation]. Hengersberg: Schober.

Useful websites

Racing Pigeon Portal: http://www.pigeonportal.co.uk
The Royal Pigeon Racing Association, Cheltenham, UK
Website: http://www.rpra.org.uk

17

Fish

Steven B Kayne

One area of veterinary health that currently receives little interest from pharmacists involved in pet care is that related to fish. This is a pity because uniquely fish are not subject to the provisions of the Veterinary Surgeons Act 1966 and there are no statutory restrictions on the diagnosis and treatment of fish diseases by non-veterinarians. However, fish are subject to the Medicines Act 1968 so prescription-only medicines (POMs) may be prescribed only for fish under the control of a vet.

Fish have certain advantages over land animals. Being cold-blooded they do not have to expend energy in maintaining body temperature, nor do they have to support their weight. They are more efficient at converting food into flesh and with relatively small amounts of inedible bones and offal their attractiveness as a source of food is obvious. The farming of fish for human food, for restocking angling waters or as bait is big business but access to this market is likely to be restricted to a few 'expert' outlets in appropriate areas of the country. It is with ornamental fish that a realistic opportunity exists for the community pharmacist, even though the majority of treatments available are unlicensed medicines.

Morphology

The external body form of a fish is a function of the environment in which it has evolved and lives. How it feeds, how active it is, whether it is a predator or potential prey, are some of the salient features. Unlike most land-dwelling animals, fish have evolved several unique traits in their outside coverings, including scales, fins and protective mucus. Fish slime, or mucus, is a vital component of the skin/water interface. When fish are moved from aquarium to aquarium, or they are in a weakened condition from transporting, their stress levels are increased and their protective slime coating may be lost. The slime has fungicidal and bactericidal action and any damage to it may contribute to infection of the skin. Most fish have seven fins, although some have six and others have eight. These fins allow fish to steer and move forward and backward. Because water is 800 times denser than air, fish require a tremendous amount of muscle strength and coordination. The powerful tail fin coupled with a large efficient muscle-filled body gives the fish the necessary strength. On the outside of the skin most fish have compact rows of protective scales.

Locomotor adaptation reflects the problems associated with moving through water, for example, drag and buoyancy.

Fish eyes are similar in structure to those of other vertebrates, the main adaptation being the almost spherical shape of the lens. The field of view is generally determined by the position of the eyes on the head; in predatory fish the eyes are positioned at the front so that the intended prey may be clearly seen, while in non-predatory fish the eyes are located at the side of the head and provide a good defence vision in a wide arc.

Sense receptors enable fish to orientate themselves in three dimensions within the aquatic environment. Fish rely heavily on the sensory perception of sound, which in water is transmitted as pressure waves. This is achieved through a system of canals and pits located below the skin that recognises low frequency sounds. An inner ear picks up sounds at the other end of the spectrum.

Chemoreceptor sites concentrated in the nasal openings, the mouth and around the head respond to chemicals diffusing through the water. They act as olfactory and taste organs.

A simple two-chambered heart, with two valves, pumps blood sluggishly through an extensive system of arteries, veins and capillaries and this forms the basis of a cardiovascular system.

The respiratory system needs to be extremely efficient because fish require oxygen for life, and their environment contains only 5% of the gas. Large volumes of water have to be moved over the surfaces of the mouth and gills to achieve absorption. The latter occurs by simple diffusion. Blood flowing into the gills has a lower oxygen concentration than the surrounding water, so oxygen moves into the blood. Most aquaria need aeration to supplement aquatic oxygen – the more crowded and warm the aquarium, the more aeration required.

Environment and disease

The aquatic environment

Since fish comprise 80% water, it is not surprising that their health is greatly influenced by any alterations in their aquatic environment. Most fish keepers rely on domestic tap water for filling an aquarium. Public water suppliers add many chemicals, such as chlorine, to kill bacteria; unfortunately, these chemicals can be harmful to fish. Appropriate products are available to neutralise toxic additives before stocking an aquarium filled with tap water. However, many fish experts use untreated tap water for their fish. When filling a fresh aquarium they will do it over a few days, but if changing only 25% they will check the temperature and pour the water straight in. Most experienced fish keepers consider that pH and hardness (see below) to be the most important things to worry about in tap water.

pH is a measure of the concentration of hydrogen ions in the water and is an indication of the balance between acid and alkali. pH 7.0 is neutral, being neither acidic nor alkaline. The lower the pH value the more acidic is the water and the higher the value the more alkaline. Since pH is measured on a logarithmic scale, then each full pH point is ten times more acidic or alkaline than the adjacent one. For instance, pH 8 is ten times as alkaline as pH 7, pH 9 is 100 times as alkaline as pH 7.

Appreciation of this feature is particularly important when the water has turned green – a common feature in fishponds particularly. The green water is caused by myriads of small green organisms, and their act of photosynthesis can make the pH shoot up to 10, which is 1000 times more alkaline than pH 7. This level of alkalinity puts the fish under stress and is the frequent cause of onset of disease. It is important therefore to monitor the pH of ponds, particularly during periods of high light intensity when the water may turn green. The best cure is to eliminate the green water.

pH levels should be adjusted to suit the fish. Most tropical fish can live happily in water with pH levels ranging from 6.8 to 7.5 whereas levels up to 8.5 are acceptable for cold-water fish. All fish are quite sensitive to rapid pH changes and some fish will only thrive in water outside the normal pH range, e.g. some South American fish need quite acid water of pH 5.5–6.0 for comfort. Commercial pH adjusters are available.

Water hardness is another factor which can be critical for some fish and plants and is caused mainly by salts of calcium and magnesium. It is commonly expressed either in mg/L of calcium carbonate or in German degrees of hardness [°DH]. 1°DH is equivalent to 17.9 mg/L of hardness expressed as calcium carbonate.

Most tap water in the UK has a hardness between 200 and 450 mg/L calcium carbonate and is suitable for most common cold-water and tropical fish.

Other chemicals that may cause problems are:

- *Ammonia.* Ammonia poisoning, the leading cause of fish loss, is most likely to occur at toxic levels in a newly established tank where the process of biological filtration has not been established ('New Tank Syndrome'), in an old aquarium where the pH has become alkaline, or in an overcrowded tank. Ammonia, which destroys the mucous membranes of fish, is secreted by fish directly through the gills as a waste product, and also produced by the bacterial breakdown of fish waste, uneaten food and plant by-products. This causes the ammonia levels in the tank to reach toxic levels, known as ammonia poisoning. Ammonia can be removed by using a liquid ammonia remover, which is placed directly in the water, or by using ammonia chips, which are put into the power-filter canister.

- *Nitrites and nitrates.* Nitrites are converted by beneficial bacteria into nitrates. High levels of nitrites indicate that the breakdown of organic materials is incomplete and that the aquarium does not have adequate biological filtration. Nitrites are less toxic than ammonia, but can still kill fish if the levels are too high. Nitrates, on the other hand, are generally harmless to freshwater fish provided excessive build-up is avoided by regular partial water changes.

- *Sodium chloride.* Although salt is associated with marine aquariums, freshwater aquariums can benefit from small doses as well. A lack of sodium (salt) in the water will break down the slime coat of fish (see below).

- *Calcium and magnesium salts.* 'Water hardness' is a measure of the amount of calcium and magnesium salts present in the water. Too much hard water causes a white crust to form on parts of the aquarium. Hard water also makes it difficult to adjust the pH. Various chemicals are available to help soften the water.

- *Pathogens.* Many potential fish pathogens are a constant and natural part of the environment and under normal circumstances do not cause disease. For example, fish often carry protozoan parasites that feed mainly off surplus tissue and are kept under control by the fish's immune system. However, if there is an alteration in one or more environmental features – temperature or pH – then this delicate balance is likely to be upset. Disease-causing organisms may be introduced into the environment on new fish stocks, plants or decorative items. These pathogens upset the immunological balance of the existing community and therefore new fish should be carefully quarantined in a separate aquarium for a minimum of 2 weeks.

Stress and disease

Stress is one of the most critical factors in fish health. 'Stressors' such as handling, overcrowding and inappropriate mix of fish types (e.g. mixing with aggressive breeds) are vital factors in fish health. Improper nutrition is also a commonly overlooked stressor of fish. Many fish can live on minimal nutrition, with old or stale flake foods, but this poor nutrition is a cause of chronic stress. A variety of well preserved dry foods as well as freeze-dried, fresh, and frozen foods specifically designed for individual species are necessary to prevent chronic nutritional stress. Disturbing the tank through banging on the glass, constantly netting fish, or rearranging décor stresses fish and should be kept to the necessary minimum. Probably the most significant stress for fish is bringing them from the wild or an aquaculture pond, through the wholesaler, into a domestic aquarium. Poor water quality is another source of stress. It may be due to excessive hardness, unsuitable pH or waste products, such as nitrites or ammonia, either already in the water or produced by the fish (see above).

Response may involve the release of adrenaline and cortisol, and the fish may take hours or even days to recover equilibrium, depending on the severity of the stress. Although the fish may successfully adapt to the new conditions, growth, breeding ability and disease immunity may all be impaired. Constant exposure to stressors causes significant extension of the adaptive phase and a reduction in the chances of survival. Minimising stress is an important part of good fish keeping. While it is impossible to eliminate all stress, we fortunately have the ability to limit or prevent many of the causes of stress. Acute stress is more obvious and needs to be addressed very quickly. Chronic stress is often not visible and may take weeks and months to develop. By looking at the prevailing conditions in the wild with respect to variables such as temperature, pH, water hardness and shade or brightness, we may be able to optimise the environment for captive fish in an attempt to avoid stress.

Preventing disease

There are a number of precautions that may be taken on a regular basis to reduce the risk of an outbreak of disease:

- The water quality and temperature should be monitored regularly with commercially available testing kits to ensure that the environment is suitable for the fish being kept. To limit the occurrence of toxicity the Ornamental Aquatic Trade Association recommends the following values: free ammonia < 0.01 mg/L, nitrite < 0.125 mg/L, nitrate < 40 mg/L, dissolved oxygen > 5.5 mg/L.
- Water temperature can greatly affect the concentration of free oxygen in the water. As the water temperature increases, the free oxygen concentration decreases. Stagnant or poor quality water also contains less oxygen.
- A filtration and aeration system should be installed.

- The water should be partially changed regularly and chemicals added as appropriate to make domestic tap water suitable for aquarium use. Customers should be advised to wash their hands thoroughly after contact with aquarium contents.
- The fish should be fed a varied and balanced diet.
- The mix of species should be carefully chosen.

Treating disease

Ornamental fish

Despite taking the precautions detailed above, disease of bacterial, fungal or protozoal origin may still strike. Prompt diagnosis and treatment will give the fish a better chance of survival. Fish should be monitored constantly for differences in appearance or behaviour that might signify disease. Unusual swimming movements (e.g. flicking or rubbing against solid objects), inability to maintain balance, or hiding behind decorative stones are often signs that all is not well.

Figure 17.1 shows the location of the most common problems; Table 17.1 details the various signs and symptoms that may be expected. Most infections are caused by similar situations. By following a few basic precautions most of these infections can be prevented.

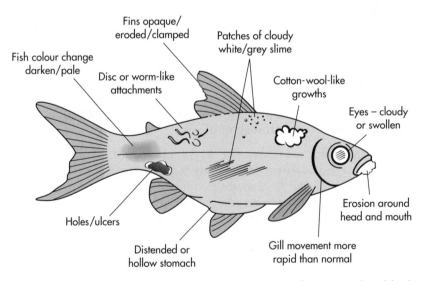

Figure 17.1 Location of the most common problems in fish. (Reproduced by kind permission of Interpet, Dorking, Surrey.)

Table 17.1   Signs and symptoms of fish diseases (Reproduced with permission of Interpet Limited, Dorking, Surrey.)

Symptom	Definite symptom of disease	Possible symptom of disease
Fish gasping; rapid gill movement; fish hanging near surface.	Bacterial gill disease. Poisoning/water quality.	White spot. Velvet. Slime disease. Higher form parasite.
Flicking & rubbing.	White Spot. Velvet. Slime disease. Higher form parasite.	Poisoning/water quality.
Peppering of gold spots.	Velvet.	
Patches of slime.	Slime disease. Poisoning/water quality.	
White spots (sugar grain).	White spot.	
Disc or wormlike attachments on body/gills.	Higher form parasite.	
Gills pale/eroded.	Higher form parasite. Bacterial gill disease.	White spot. Velvet. Slime disease.
Cloudy eyes.	Slime disease. Poisoning/water quality.	
Cotton wool growths.	Mouth rot. Fungus.	
Fins eroded/opaque.	Fin rot.	Internal bacterial infection.
Mouth/head erosion.	Mouth rot.	
Eyes swollen (pop-eye).		Internal bacterial infection.
Distended/hollow stomach.		Internal bacterial infection.
Holes/ulcers.		Internal bacterial infection.
Fish colour darkens.	Poisoning/water quality.	Internal bacterial infection.
Unexplained deaths.	Internal bacterial infection.	
Darting around.	Poisoning/water quality.	
Unable to maintain balance.	Swim bladder problems. Poisoning/water quality.	Internal bacterial infection.

Precautions include:

- Checking that the conditions in the aquarium are suitable for the species to be kept, e.g. temperature, pH, water hardness.
- Maintaining excellent water quality at all times.
- Removing any dead or diseased fish from the tank.

- Treating all diseased fish.
- Never introducing diseased or sick fish into a community tank.
- Preventing injuries from fighting or unsuitable habitats.

It is beyond the scope of this section to cover fish diseases comprehensively; however, some of the more commonly seen problems are listed below.

Bacterial gill disease

Bacterial gill disease, as the name suggests, is caused by bacteria (e.g. *Flexibacter* spp.). Bacterial erosion of the delicate gill membrane causes suffocation of the fish. Bacterial gill disease often occurs after the gills have been damaged by poor water quality. Affected gills are pale or grey/brown in colour with heavy mucus production and clear signs of erosion. Treatment with proprietary medicines plus the addition of 0.2% aquarium salt is recommended. Water conditions must be checked, as poor water contributes greatly to the onset of this disease.

Fin rot

Fin rot caused by *Aeromonas*, *Pseudomonas*, and *Flexibacter* spp. often begins with red streaks in the fins that are soon followed by abnormal lightening of the edge of the fin and then a fraying or rotting of the fin membrane and edges. This infection can lead to a complete rotting of the fin and can spread to the body and lead to death. Infection occurs from bacteria that are already in the water, but do not cause problems in healthy fish. Injury to the fins, stress, or poor water quality can all lead to an increase in these infections. Infected fish can be bathed in a salt solution (make sure your species of fish can tolerate this) or given topical treatment of the affected area with gentian violet. Treatment tanks with appropriate antibiotics added are sometimes used. There are also a number of proprietary treatments in the UK that use phenoxyethanol. One particularly effective variant is an emulsion that disperses rapidly in water.

Fungus

Fish fungus is caused by species such as *Saprolegnia*. Fungus spores are present in all freshwater aquaria. A disease outbreak is usually a secondary infection of an area of the fish's skin or gill barrier which has been damaged. The growth looks like cotton wool. It is essential to prevent the fungus spreading deep into the tissue or over the gills. An appropriate treatment (see below) will stop the fungus spreading and destroy it. The medicine remains active for several days to ensure that full healing occurs.

Internal bacteria

These diseases are caused by a variety of bacteria species, e.g. *Pseudomonas flourescens*, *Aeromonas hydrophila* and *Virio marinium*. Internal bacterial infections spread throughout the fish's tissue and internal organs. Symptoms vary, depending on the acuteness of the disease. In some cases the fish will just darken in colour, become listless, stop feeding and die. In others, severe symptoms exist (ulcers, abdominal and eye swelling and destruction of the central nervous system) and the fish goes on to die. It is essential to catch these diseases as early as possible or treat as a precaution as soon as they are suspected. Previously, the only effective treatment against internal bacteria was veterinary prescribed antibiotics. Over-the-counter medicines are available and will improve the chances of successful treatment of internal bacterial infections. Bacterial problems, such as dropsy, ulcers and septicaemia, are very difficult to cure if the disease is too far advanced, but the medicines will help to prevent further deaths.

Internal parasites

Fish are host to a wide array of internal parasites although symptoms are often not visible. Occasionally there may be difficulties arising from infestation with *Hexamita* and *Sanguinicola* spp., and intestinal tapeworms and roundworms. A number of treatments are available (see below).

Lice

The adult fish louse, *Argulus*, is a flat disc-shaped crustacean measuring up to 10 mm in diameter that attaches itself to the skin and fins of a fish by means of twin suckers. It inserts its mouthparts into the body of the fish to feed on blood and this causes intense irritation. Reddened lesions appear and these may become subject to fungal infection. These parasites principally affect garden pond fish during the summer months. Adult females leave the fish to lay batches of eggs in long gelatinous capsules. Juvenile parasites emerge within 3–4 weeks and develop into adults. Treatment with organophosphate insecticides will kill both juvenile and adult forms of *Argulus*.

Mouth fungus (mouth rot)

Mouth fungus or columnaris disease shows all the signs of being a fungus but is actually a bacterial infection usually caused by *Flexibacter columnaris*. Fish do not always show external symptoms but may die in just a few days. Diagnosis is normally only possible on a postmortem examination. This disease may be responsible for some unexplained deaths. The bacterium is commonly present in aquarium water, on dead organic material, or even on healthy fish skin, and may invade damaged or unhealthy skin and the surrounding tissues. The bacterium appears to be more pathogenic under hard-water conditions with a pH above 6. The initial lesions develop into off-white fluffy growths resembling cotton wool. The lips and inside of the mouth are the most likely places to be infected. Small, off-white to grey, marks may be seen on the head, fins and gills. Any existing injuries or diseases of the mouth, incorrect pH, high levels of nitrate, low oxygen concentrations, or even a vitamin deficiency, can increase the risk of fish developing this disease. Bath immersion using a treatment containing phenoxyethanol is normally effective. Good husbandry is important in preventing the disease.

Slime disease

Slime disease is caused by protozoa, e.g. *Chilodonella*, *Ichthyobodo* (Costia), *Trichodina* and *Brooklynella* spp., and Trematodes (flukes), e.g. *Gyrodactylus* and *Dactylogyrus* spp. These parasites spend the whole of their life cycle on the fish, although infective young parasites may be released into the water to spread to new hosts. The parasites live on the skin and gill surface, eating gill and skin tissue debris. If their numbers increase rapidly they may irritate the skin and gills, causing excessive mucus production and usually killing the fish by smothering the gills and hence causing suffocation. Treatment will quickly and effectively eradicate gill and skin parasites and remove the mucus build up, therefore aiding the fish's respiration.

Swim bladder problems

The swim bladder is a smooth, gas-filled organ found in the abdomen and helps the fish to control its buoyancy and maintain its position in the water. A fish will either add to or decrease the amount of air in the bladder to help it move up or down in the water. Swim bladder problems are caused by bacterial and viral infections or hereditary problems. Internal bacterial infections can affect the function of the swim bladder, making it difficult for fish to maintain position. Fancy goldfish with their short body form are particularly prone to this problem. Treatment for swim bladder problems involves raising the temperature to 27 °C and using a proprietary treatment. The fish should be fed sparingly.

Velvet

Velvet disease is caused in freshwater aquaria by the protozoan parasite species *Oodinium pillularis* and in marine water by *Amyloodinium* spp., both of which have a similar life cycle to white spot (see below). The symptoms of velvet usually involve the skin and lungs. Mild infections will usually only infect the gills and the fish may show minimal symptoms. As the infestation becomes more severe, the gills will become inflamed, bleed, and the lung tissue will begin to die. The fish will show signs of irritation and distress, with rapid breathing and lethargy. As the inflammation increases, the fish will lose its ability to transport oxygen across the gill membranes resulting in a fish that shows symptoms of suffocation; if treatment is not initiated death will often result.

The parasites attach themselves to a host fish where they feed and grow. As they mature the parasites fall from the fish and develop into cysts encased in a membrane on the substrate. Here the cysts divide forming 64 new cells per cyst within 4 days whereupon the membranes burst freeing the cells into the aquarium to find a new host. If the cells fail to find a host within 24 hours they die.

Velvet usually only arises when poor aquarium conditions prevail and is highly infectious. Increasing the temperature to 28 °C and application of a commercial chemical treatment containing copper is most effective. Dimming the aquarium lighting also aids recovery.

White spot

The ciliated parasite *Ichthyophthirius*, more commonly known as white spot or 'ich', is a very common fish disease capable of affecting virtually all fish species. It is also claimed to be especially prevalent in koi. Ich has a fairly complex life cycle that has a major bearing on treatment methods. The white spot parasite forms a nodule under the skin or gill epithelium. It constantly turns and moves under the skin, feeding on destroyed cells and body fluids and finally 'punches' its way out of the skin when mature. The parasite then attaches itself to a plant or some other object and forms a capsule around itself. Inside the capsule, the 'tomont', as it is now called, repeatedly divides, producing up to 1000 'tomites' that finally hatch from the capsule and swim to find a fish host. These small tomites are the infective agent. They burrow into the fish's skin and the cycle starts all over again. Clearly, with each turn of the cycle the number of parasites increases dramatically. White spot cysts, each containing an active 'trophont', appear as small white nodules on the skin, gills and fins, giving the fish the appearance of having been dusted with salt. In the early stages of the disease, fish are likely to flash and rub against objects because of the irritation. At a later, advanced, stage they will become lethargic and spend most of their time sitting on the bottom of the tank. It is only the free-swimming stage of the parasite that is susceptible to treatment; neither the trophonts under the epithelium or the tomont cysts can be killed. Prolonged immersion in 1–2 g/L salt solution was widely recommended in the past, but far better commercial treatments are now available.

Treatments for fish diseases

A variety of proprietary treatments such as those effective against fin rot, fungus, white spot and velvet are available from specialist suppliers, along with a number of broad-spectrum aquarium antibacterials and antiparasite treatments. These are preferable to extemporaneous formulae as they are often based on chemicals that may not be readily available in generic form from pharmacies. If used according to the manufacturers' instructions these products can be extremely effective.

Bacterial and fungal infections

Treatments include antiseptics (e.g. acriflavine, benzalkonium chloride), methylene blue and phenoxyethanol. In addition there are some prescribed antimicrobial drugs, e.g. ampicillin, chloramphenicol, oxytetracycline and sulfadiazine with trimethoprim (Sulfatrim, Vericore AP), that may be administered either by injection, mixing with food or by adding to the aquatic environment.

External parasites

Treatments include copper (0.3–0.5 mg/L), formalin (15–25 mg/L), malachite green (0.1–0.5 mg/L) and methylene blue (1–8 mg/L). Leteux–Meyer mixture is a stock solution containing malachite green 3.3 g/L in 35–40% formaldehyde solution. It is applied in a bath at a concentration of 25 ppm for 1 hour. Sea lice infestation may be treated with azamethiphos (Salmosan, Novartis) in a bath at a concentration of 1 ppm for 30–60 minutes.

Internal parasites

Treatments include dimetridazole, metronidazole, furazolidone, mebendazole and piperazine citrate.

Commercial fish farming

Losses in salmon farming are often due to disease. These diseases are classed as parasitic, bacterial, viral or fungal. The high stocking densities of fish in aquaculture render them particularly susceptible to disease and parasites. Moreover, most waters are populated by wild fish which may carry and be susceptible to disease agents. Measures have to be taken to minimise the likelihood of disease outbreaks in farmed stock.

Furunculosis is a major factor affecting fish management, particularly salmon. The appearance of large furuncles produces unsightly fish that cannot be sold and ultimately may prove fatal. Treatment is with a variety of antimicrobials including amoxicillin (Aquacil, Vericore and Vetremox Fish, Vetrepharm), oxytetracycline (Aquatet, Vetrepharm and Tetraplex, Vericore AP) and sulfadiazine with trimethoprim (Sulfatrim, Vericore AP).

The introduction of new and efficacious injectable vaccines to prevent furunculosis has shown encouraging signs of success and vaccines have largely superseded antibiotic treatment which was becoming less effective due to the development of resistant strains of the causal agent A. *salmonicida*. Although oral administration of vaccines is still a relatively new technique, the development of oral vaccines could improve welfare by reducing handling. Vaccines that protect against several diseases are desirable because they further reduce handling. Sea lice, which erode the skin causing tissue damage, have traditionally been controlled using dichlorvos and more recently hydrogen peroxide. However, the development of resistance by some sea lice has reduced the effectiveness of dichlorvos. Concern has also been expressed about possible effects of dichlorvos on the marine environment.

Adult trout are subject to a wide range of problems, some more serious than others. Endemic bacterial problems include enteric red mouth for which vaccines are available and bacterial kidney disease for which there is no effective treatment or vaccine. Cold-water diseases caused by *C. psychrophila* can also occur.

Acknowledgement

The author acknowledges the kind assistance received from Dr Neville Carrington, FRPharmS, in writing this chapter.

Further reading

Andrews C, Exell A, Carrington N (2002). *The Interpet Manual of Fish Health*, revised edn. Dorking: Interpet Publishing.

Carrington N (1999). *An Interpet Guide to the Healthy Aquarium*. Dorking: Interpet Publishing.

Shepherd J, Bromage N, eds. (1992). *Intensive Fish Farming*. Oxford: Blackwell Scientific Publications.

Wall A E, Wildgoose W H (2001). *Prescribing for fish*. In: Bishop Y (2001). *The Veterinary Formulary*, 5th edn. London: Pharmaceutical Press.

Part 5

Management of wounds

18

The management of animal soft tissue injuries

Sarah Cockbill

Over the last 35 years there has been extensive research into human wounds and consequent evolutionary changes in their management (Turner, 1992). The same cannot be said about the management of animal wounds over the same timescale as, although there have been dramatic changes in veterinary medicine and practice during that period, there has been little or no sustained interest shown by practising veterinary surgeons in the management of animal wounds. These wounds occur frequently and need to be assessed and treated in the same way as those of their human counterparts. Their management is more complicated than that required for human wounds as there are small (but significant) species-vital sign variations to be taken into consideration when deciding upon a suitable treatment regime. The original *passive* plug-and-conceal materials, such as gauze, Gamgee tissue and absorbent cotton, are no longer extensively used to manage human wounds. Products such as vapour-permeable films, alginates, hydrocolloids, hydrogels and foams have been developed for the management of human wounds, and all of them control the microenvironment surrounding the wound and contribute in different ways to the enhancement of the healing cascade. However, their application to the management of animal injuries is only just beginning to be evaluated. Manufacturers are moving towards the development of *bioactive* materials, which will lead to improved healing by direct stimulation of one or more of the steps in the healing cascade.

Many veterinary surgeons still consider that wounds will heal despite attention, not because of it (Cockbill and Turner, 1994, 1995). As a consequence, veterinary wound management is still in its infancy and in many instances any therapy which may be selected is done so with consideration of little but its price, which will be passed on to the animal's owner. In contrast, unlike in the management of human soft tissue injuries, the commercial value of the animal plays more than a significant part in the perceived cost-effectiveness of any new treatment. It follows that the principal areas where there will be veterinary interest in the use of modern wound management materials will be the small animal and equine areas, as most farmers will consider sending casualty cattle and sheep straight to the abattoir before spending any extra money on veterinary fees and materials. Unless an owner is convinced by his veterinary surgeon that a new, more expensive regime will prove to be cost-effective in the long term there is no incentive for him to agree to change from any existing therapy. The result is that, although veterinary surgeons may be interested in new types of wound management products developed for human application and their possible use, after modification, for the management of wounds in animals, there is no observed need by manufacturers to ensure that they understand the correct application of these materials. There can therefore only be a limited evaluation of any possible advantages in their mode of action over existing therapies (Cockbill and Turner, 1994).

There are approximately 20 000 registered veterinary surgeons in the UK (register held by the Royal College of Veterinary Surgeons), of whom approximately 75% are in practice and see, on average, 20 animals each (large and small) per day. Undoubtedly it is a very small percentage of these animals which will visit the veterinary surgeon for the treatment of wounds (of whatever aetiology), but the figures do give some idea of the potential number of patients that could present with wounds needing treatment over a selected period.

There are seasonal variations in the demand for wound management products. For example, in the UK hunting accidents occur between November and March (the hunting season), and can number as many as 1000 per week; flap injuries and stab wounds from hedges are the most common. These figures indicate the potential scale of wound management in domestic animals and illustrate the market size available to surgical dressing manufacturers. Figures have not been included for other domestic pet animals, such as rabbits, hamsters and guinea pigs, exotic animals, such as iguanas, fish and birds, all of which could need some sort of wound care during their lifetime; inclusion of these animals would therefore revise the quoted figures upwards.

Structure of the skin

In all animal species the skin is the largest organ of the body, and consists of a complex three-tiered structure. Its function is protective. It covers the other organs, plays a role in temperature regulation, allows removal of waste products, incorporates sensors for the detection of pain, external pressures and external temperature changes, absorbs sunlight (thus aiding in its conversion to vitamin D in at least humans), and acts as a waterproof barrier. The skin is composed of several layers: the outer epidermis and stratum corneum, which protect against injury and contamination; the dermis, containing the capillary network, which provides nutrients and removes waste; the sensors for detecting pain and immediate environmental changes; and the subcutis, from which the dermis and epidermis develop. The stratum corneum also acts as a barrier to the loss of water from the body and its destruction is an important contributory factor to the development of shock with severe burns. Skin also contains sebaceous glands, hair follicles and sweat glands, which arise in the dermis. The proportions of these vary between animal species according to the environment in which they live. A dog such as a husky, which comes from an inhospitable climate, has a dense layer of insulating fur close to the skin surface which traps air, thereby insulating the animal against extremes of temperature. This layer of fur is covered by another layer of thicker hair which is water-repellent, thereby protecting the animal against inclement weather. Horses which need sophisticated temperature control have a higher number of sweat glands than other animal species.

The cornified cells on the surface of the skin do not contain blood vessels or nerve endings but consist of keratin, which is continuously shed as squames. About 1 g of keratinised cells is shed each day as dandruff. Shed cells are replaced by new cells produced by the basal layer, and these continuously migrate to the surface of the skin. The thickness of the epidermal layer varies from a thin membrane at internal flexures (e.g. at the elbow) to thick, compacted layers at points which bear considerable pressure (e.g. the palms and soles).

The outer surface of the dermis (the papillary layer) is formed of ridges that project into the epidermis. The papillary layer contains blood vessels, lymphatics and nerve endings. The blood supply is distributed between outer vessels, which nourish the epidermal cells, and deeper vessels, which lie just outside the lower subcutaneous layer of fat. The elasticity of the skin and its ability to retain and lose water rapidly are the consequence of the presence of a network of collagen fibres. The dermis also contains sweat glands that are distributed unevenly over the body. Thick skin contains a high proportion of eccrine glands, which secrete sweat throughout life.

Beneath the dermis is the fat-containing subcutaneous layer, which is highly vascularised. It insulates internal structures from excessive heat and reduces heat loss in cold climates. Because of its spongy texture and flexibility, it may also dissipate the effects of physical trauma.

Classification of wounds

A wound can be defined as any process which leads to the disruption of the normal architecture of a tissue. It should always be remembered that all wounds are not identical and that there is no single wound management product suitable for all wounds at all stages of the healing process. Wounds need to be assessed at each stage of the healing process and an appropriate dressing regime devised for the wound at that time. They may be closed (contusions, bruises, ruptures and sprains) or open (abrasions, lacerations, avulsions, ballistic, penetrating, hernias and excised or surgical wounds). Open wounds are by far the most common in the domestic species.

Wounds may be classified according to the number of skin layers affected and whether tissue has been lost. Simple surgical incisions do not involve loss of tissue. Conversely, traumatic wounds and chronic wounds are frequently accompanied by varying degrees of tissue loss. Damage limited to the epithelial tissue alone is regarded as a superficial wound which will heal rapidly by regeneration of epithelial cells. A partial-thickness wound involves the deeper dermal layer and includes vessel damage, and its repair process is therefore more complex. A full-thickness wound affects the subcutaneous fat layer and beyond, and healing of this wound will require the synthesis of new connective tissue to aid wound contraction. It therefore takes the longest time to heal (Mast, 1992; Yardley, 1998).

In the management of wounds and the use of wound management products, however, subdivision into clean and non-infected wounds is essential. Contaminated wounds should never be closed without thorough removal of all the damaged tissue (debridement), and even then it may be necessary to delay closure until the risk of infection has receded.

Animal wounds may be classified by several methods, which are based on the degree of contamination within the wound, its depth, and the location on the body. The likelihood of wound healing and the treatment required to facilitate this must depend on all these factors. The most popular concept of dealing with wounds involves minimal interference. This, from a veterinary point of view, revolves around the removal of any impediment to normal wound healing rather than the use of any magical substance or technique to actively encourage it.

Wound healing

Wound healing is a complicated and precise series of events which involves cellular, physiological, biochemical and molecular processes that result ultimately in connective tissue repair and the formation of a fibrous scar (Peacock, 1984). The process follows a specific sequence of phases, which may overlap. The first phase is the inflammatory (reaction) phase; it is followed by the proliferative (repair) phase and finally by the maturation (regeneration) phase (Peacock, 1984; Leaper, 1986). The process also depends on the type of tissue that has been damaged and the nature of the tissue disruption. Deep open wounds in bone do not heal in the same way or at the same rate as superficial epithelial wounds, largely because bone tissue consists of up to 65% inorganic calcium-based matrix.

The objective of any wound management regime is to heal the wound in the shortest time possible and with minimum pain, discomfort and scarring to the patient. Success in fulfilling the objective will be assisted by an understanding of the healing process and a knowledge of the contributions that the existing range of wound management products can make to initiating and maintaining the optimal microenvironment for healing.

The process of healing is the replacement of damaged tissue by new living material, with the intended reconstruction of the original structure. Wound healing is accompanied by the formation of a permanent new structure lacking functional ability: the scar.

The following description of the mechanism of wound healing is derived from current knowledge about the process in humans. At present, very little is known about the precise mechanism of wound healing in different domestic animal species, which may differ in some aspects from that in humans, but it is known that the same cell types are involved, so there seems to be no valid reason why the same fundamental principles cannot be applied and the same outcomes expected.

Healing by primary intention

If the two apposed surfaces of a clean, incised wound (which has not been subjected to a significant degree of tissue loss) are held together through the use of sutures, wound management products or surface adhesives, healing will take place from the internal layers outwards. The process of healing by first intention is initiated by the movement of epithelial cells from the two edges of the wound towards its centre. They usually meet and commence interlocking within 4–7 days of the incision. The reappearance of normal skin follows the keratinisation and thinning of the epidermis. The pre-trauma strength of the tissue will never be completely regained.

Primary wound closure should be performed relatively soon after the wound has been inflicted. Closure should be undertaken when it is certain that healing will continue uneventfully. Additional requirements are:

- A short time lapse since injury.
- A minimal degree of contamination and tissue trauma.
- Thorough debridement and lavage to provide tissue suitable for suturing.
- Good haemostasis and the absence of tension or a dead space.

If wounds are properly evaluated, managed and closed then they should heal within 7–10 days after operation. Otherwise, haematoma, seroma and/or infection may result, with the necessity for extended wound management.

Delayed primary closure is wound closure 3–5 days after injury. During this time the wound is managed medically to improve its chances of uncomplicated suturing and healing. This type of closure is indicated in three basic wound types:

- New wounds with severe secondary contusion.
- Heavily contaminated or infected wounds.
- Relatively clean, sharp wounds several days old, which do not have devitalised tissue and no appearance of infection.

This type of closure is beneficial because it allows observation of contused, contaminated or infected tissue and progression of inflammation. It also allows staged debridement of the wound and maximum wound drainage. If closure is properly performed, healing should be complete within 7–10 days. If the procedures are improperly completed, wound infection may result and extended wound management may be needed.

Healing by secondary intention

If there has been significant loss of tissue in the formation of the wound, healing will begin by the production of granulation tissue at the base of the wound. The process of healing by second intention always involves contraction of the wound, and the degree of contraction is greatest during the first few days after the wound has been inflicted.

Secondary closure of a wound is closure 5 or more days after the time of injury, when the wound has formed healthy granulation tissue.

This type of closure is indicated when it has been necessary to manage contused or infected tissue. It is also performed when the wound, as presented to the veterinary surgeon, is already in the repair phase of wound healing and has a well-developed bed of healthy granulation tissue.

Delaying wound closure helps ensure that all infection and necrotic tissue have been removed. Closure of wounds in the presence of granulation tissue is generally more difficult because the tissue is not pliable, and therefore suturing the edges of this type of wound does not provide the cosmetically acceptable appearance of a wound closed by primary intention.

The mechanism of healing may be most usefully considered chronologically, although it must be remembered that the process is continuous and well-defined stages do not occur in practice. The process of wound healing follows a specific sequence of phases, which may overlap.

Stages in the healing process

Stage 1: the inflammatory/reaction phase

The inflammatory phase consists of the immediate reaction and a protective tissue response to an injury. This initial phase is the beginning of the healing process. It may continue in a normal wound for up to 72 hours. Inflammation is characterised by pain, heat, redness, swelling and loss of function at the site of the wound. These classic signs of inflammation can be seen almost immediately after an injury, and are also characteristic of an impending wound infection. They are outward signs of damage, and result from vasodilatation caused by the secretion of histamine and enzymes from damaged tissue, and from the passage of plasma into the affected area due to increased capillary permeability (diapedesis). The plasma transports antibodies, leucocytes (particularly polymorphs), growth factors, macrophages and fibroblasts to the site of damage, and these elements start the repair process by clearing debris and damaged tissue by phagocytosis. The purpose is to destroy, dilute or isolate the injurious agent and the injured tissues.

The drop in potential difference across the edges of the wound after injury acts as the stimulant for Hagemann factor XII, which is responsible for activation of the healing cascade (Barker, 1986). The effector systems within the cascade – the plasminogen cascade, the complement cascade, the kinin cascade and the clotting cascade – interlink to control infection and regenerate tissue. They release chemical mediators, such as complement C5a, fibrin degradation factors, platelet activity factors, and vasoconstrictors, such as histamine and serotonin (Leaper, 1986).

Initially, cessation of blood flow from the wound is achieved by vasoconstriction, lasting 5–10 minutes, which reduces blood flow and isolates the wound. This is followed by, but separate from, haemostasis, with the deposition of fibrin and the formation of a blood clot. This clot maintains haemostasis and creates a provisional matrix for the migration of cells (monocytes, fibroblasts and keratinocytes) to the wound, with the consequent release of their cytokines and mediators. When blood flow is controlled, vasoconstriction is followed by active vasodilation of all the local small vessels, which allows the influx by diapedesis of a protein-rich exudate containing antibodies and various complement fractions together with other substances essential to the healing process, such as growth factors and cytokines (Kunimoto, 1999; Haroon et al., 2000).

Immediately after injury, platelets aggregate and release coagulation factors and growth factors that are vital for haemostasis and initiation of the wound-healing process. The platelets forming the clot are activated by exposure to collagen or microfibrils and to platelet-derived growth factor (PDGF), which is produced by the erythrocytes damaged during injury. The platelets adhere to the subendothelium exposed after injury, flatten, and release a prostaglandin, which encourages aggregation, and, in combination with vasoconstrictors (histamine and serotonin from mast cells), reduce immediate blood loss before the initiation of the clotting cascade (Wahl and Wahl, 1992; Kiritsy et al., 1993). Activated platelets release several growth factors – PDGF, platelet-derived epidermal growth factor, epidermal growth factor (EGF), transforming growth factors α and β (TGF-α, TGF-β), heparin-binding EGF and insulin-like growth factor-1, which stimulate cell growth and migration at the injured site from within their alpha granules. These growth factors stimulate the orderly migration of cells (neutrophils, then macrophages, then fibroblasts) into the wound site (Haroon et al., 2000). Activated platelets also stimulate the intrinsic coagulation system, which converts fibrinogen to a fibrin mesh to produce a thrombus stabilising the platelet plug (Bennet and Schultz 1993; Kiritsy et al., 1993; Declan, 1999).

Oedema is observed together with an increase in wound temperature and pain caused by the action of histamine, kinins and prostaglandins (Schaffer and Narrey, 1996). This permeability may last for up to 1 hour. The occlusion of the local wound lymphatic channels by fibrin prevents the spread of the inflammation. During inflammation the white blood cells (neutrophils) migrate to the wound area and, together with macrophages, they ingest bacteria and cell debris by phagocytosis. The successful macrophage function normally indicates the end of the acute inflammatory reaction.

The chemoattractants released by the platelets stimulate the rapid influx, again by diapedesis, of neutrophils and monocytes from the circulation to the wound site (Peacock, 1984). Neutrophils and monocytes have a common origin (a pluripotent bone marrow stem cell) and overlapping functions. Once the monocyte becomes phagocytic, it is referred to as a macrophage. Both macrophages and neutrophils are able to kill and digest bacteria and damaged tissue and thus help prevent infection by organisms that may be introduced into the host through the wound. Neutrophils are short-lived and die once they have phagocytosed bacteria and necrotic tissue, but they continue to aid healing as they release toxins that further stimulate the inflammatory response and contribute to the activation that produces macrophages from monocytes. Macrophages also serve as an important source of growth factors that regulate the wound-healing response (Wahl and Wahl, 1992; Kiritsy *et al.*, 1993).

Growth factors and cytokines are polypeptides transiently produced by cells that exert their hormone-like function on other cells via specific cell-surface receptors. Their activities overlap and the effect of most of them depends on the group and pattern of regulatory molecules to which the cell is exposed (Harding and Scott, 1983). Growth factors are so named because of their stimulatory effect on cell proliferation. They display both stimulatory and inhibitory activities even with the same cells, depending on the state of activation and differentiation of the cells and the presence of other stimulating factors.

Macrophages are pivotal in bringing about the first stages of healing, after which they then control and direct it, before finally stopping it when the repair is complete. The cells modulate the immune response by induction of lipoxygenase products through stimulation of the arachidonic acid cascade (Bennett and Schultz, 1993). In addition to aiding debridement at the wound site, they are involved in the secretion and synthesis of the collagenases neutrophil elastase and matrix metalloproteinase 8 (MMP 8) preparatory to laying down new extracellular matrix (connective tissue). They are another source of the growth factors PDGF and TGF-β and regulate fibroblast migration and proliferation by the production of the cytokine interleukin-1β (IL-1β) (Schultz and Mast, 1998; Shah *et al.*, 1999).

Stage 2: the repair phase

Proliferation The inflammation phase overlaps the proliferation or repair phase. This begins with a period of cellular proliferation. During the transition from inflammation to proliferation the number of inflammatory cells decreases while the number of fibroblasts within the wound site increases. Fibroblasts are attached to the site and synthesise collagen, beginning on the fourth or fifth day of injury and continuing for 2–4 weeks. Capillaries are formed by endothelial budding with the production of granulation tissue and the lysis of the previously produced fibrin network. Specific chemoattractants (growth factors TGF-β and PDGF) stimulate the influx of macrophages (Schultz and Mast, 1998). At the surface of the wound epithelial cells are beginning to cover the tissue defect. The end of this phase is marked by the re-epithelialisation of the wound surface (Witte and Barbul, 1997; Frank *et al.*, 1999).

The first stage of this process is the restoration of vascular integrity (angiogenesis), which involves the migration, proliferation and organisation of endothelial cells under the influence of the following growth factors: acidic fibroblast growth factor (aFGF), tumour necrosis factor β (TNF-β), wound angiogenesis factor, vascular endothelial growth factor and EGF. The regeneration of capillaries and arterioles continues until equilibrium of arterial and venous blood pressures is obtained within the microcirculation. Endothelial cells are organised so that developing tissues are ensured a supply of oxygen and nutrients. This is achieved as capillary loops infiltrate into the wound space (Kiritsy *et al.*, 1993; Bennett and Schultz, 1993; Steinrech *et al.*, 1994).

Also during this phase, extracellular matrix (ECM) components are deposited to replace lost or damaged tissue. Fibroblasts are attached to the site and synthesise collagen, beginning on the fourth or fifth day after injury and continuing for 2–4 weeks. Capillaries are formed by endothelial budding, with the production of granulation tissue and the lysis of the previously produced fibrin network. This follows the migration of activated fibroblasts and macrophages, the proliferation of endothelial cells, the production of ECM and the secretion by fibroblasts of tropocollagen, together with the formation of collagen fibrils (Kerstein, 1997). At the surface of the wound epithelial cells are beginning to cover the tissue defect, which now approaches maturation.

The macrophages involved in granulation tissue formation produce cytokines which stimulate cells to activate fibroblasts to protein synthesis and to proliferation, to activate endothelial cells to make adhesion factors and various mediators, and to activate T and B cells

(Schultz and Mast, 1998). Macrophages also stimulate new blood vessels from the surrounding tissue to grow into the wound. Their appearance heralds the next stage of healing.

Fibroblasts also secrete a range of growth factors which play a part in this phase of the wound-healing process. These are: insulin-like growth factor 1, basic fibroblast growth factor (bFGF), TGF-β and keratinocyte growth factor (KGF). bFGF and PDGF stimulate connective tissue formation and directly enhance epithelisation. EGF and TGF-β increase the rate of epithelialisation, whilst KGF stimulates keratinocyte proliferation (Wahl *et al.*, 1987; Desmouliere *et al.*, 1993). Epithelial cells adjacent to the wound site are also an important source of these growth factors. Fibroblasts, in addition to macrophages, are a major source of MMPs which degrade the ECM at an appropriate point and also of tissue inhibitors of MMPs (TIMPs), which are proteolytic enzymes responsible for the elimination of fibres which do not contribute to the structural strength of the wound (Schultz and Mast, 1998; Madlener *et al.*, 1998; Nuomeh *et al.*, 1999; Vaalamo *et al.*, 1999).

The action of the macrophages and polymorphs continues in all damaged tissues, irrespective of their degree of vascularisation, up to the fifth day after trauma. Even if the wound is clean and the number of polymorphs is consequently reduced, the repair mechanisms will continue. However, if the number of macrophages is reduced healing will cease. This is thought to be a consequence of the directing role which macrophages undertake and of their involvement in the production of fibroblasts, which synthesise the body's principal structural protein, collagen. The presence of collagen may be detected in fresh wounds from as early as the second day.

Organisation   Depending on the severity of the wound and its site, the proliferative phase may begin as early as the third day and last until the end of the third week. This phase marks the period of regaining of order within the wound, and the production of collagen reaches a peak from about day 5 to day 7. Fibroblasts act as the source of new collagen, the greatest production occurring in a slightly acid environment.

Endothelial cells produce buds which fuse and subsequently differentiate into blood vessels (i.e. arterioles, capillaries and venules). In an adequately nourished patient, these vessels are supported within the scaffolding of collagen fibres, producing granulation tissue. The amount of granulation correlates directly with the extent of inflammation that occurred in stage 1 of the healing process. This in turn depends on how effectively dead tissue, foreign bodies and infection have been excluded from the wound site. The importance of a clean environment, a healthy immune response and a well-nourished patient cannot be overstressed. The overproduction of granulation tissue will result in an outsized and usually unsightly scar.

Degradation of collagen requires collagenases which are members of the MMP family. Collagen turnover requires a complex regulatory system and is a normal process even in intact skin, but under certain conditions, such as wound repair, the rate of synthesis and degradation is increased. In chronic wounds MMP 8 has high activity, which may be a contributor to wound chronicity.

Once repair has taken place, the wound will still undergo a continued phase of regeneration or maturation.

Stage 3: the maturation/regeneration phase

This is the longest stage of wound healing and can last from 3 weeks to 2 years after the original injury. This phase overlaps with the repair phase and consists of a series of dynamic processes in which the composition of the ECM continually reflects a balance between synthesis and degradation of the components present in the wound. As described previously, fibroblasts produce tropocollagen molecules, which combine to form collagen fibrils, filaments and fibres. There is an increase in the tensile strength of the wound, which, in cavity wounds, is accompanied by contraction caused by modified fibroblasts called myofibroblasts. As collagen is deposited the fibroblasts disappear. The wound will now be covered by epidermis and maturation will continue. Fibroblasts continue to be important as they are responsible for the deposition of matrix materials and are the source of MMPs and TIMPs, as described above (Schultz and Mast, 1998).

Collagen type III, which is synthesised during granulation, is replaced by collagen type I, which is stronger and gives the tissue greater tensile strength. As this collagen develops there is a decreased demand for oxygen and nutrients within the wound, and there is therefore a reduction in the microvasculature.

As granulation is completed the wound edges contract, thereby reducing the size of the defect. This is achieved by the transformation of fibroblasts to myofibroblasts, which contain contractile proteins. The degree of contraction varies with the depth of the wound. Vascularity is reduced and the inflammatory cells leave the healing site. The new tissue which develops is known as scar tissue, and this will only ever reach between 70 and 80% of the original tissue strength (Hunt and Hussein, 1992; Whalen and Zetter, 1992; Moulin et al., 2000).

Figure 18.1 is a diagrammatic representation of the functional interlinking of the cells and growth factors involved in the wound healing process.

In addition to the mechanisms described above, two other processes must be considered, particularly if there has been a loss of tissue in the formation of a wound.

Contraction   Wound contraction is a natural healing process which allows open wounds to heal almost as rapidly as those that have been sutured. Contraction appears to be mediated by myofibroblasts, which

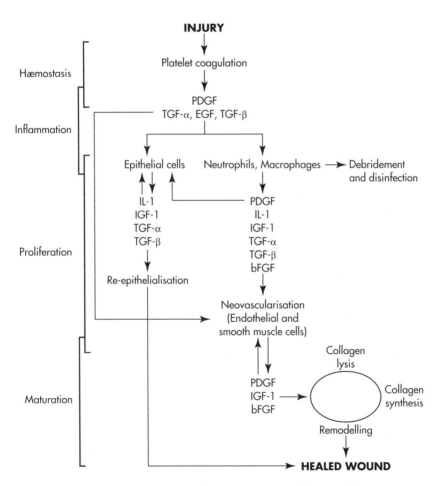

Figure 18.1   Proposed interaction of endogenous growth factors following injury to epithelium and underlying connective tissue, based on *in vitro* and *in vivo* experimental observations in human wounds. (Reproduced from Kiritsy *et al.*, 1993.)

contain smooth muscle fibrils, although the process is not universally effective. Wounds on the abdomen and on the back of the neck contract considerably, leaving only small scars. Those that are inflicted on the lower leg and on the face contract poorly, possibly due to the close interactions of the overlying skin with many underlying structures.

Epithelialisation Epithelialisation varies between wound types. Wounds that contain little or no epithelial cells will be subject to a longer and more involved process than superficial wounds, as these already contain islands of cells which rapidly proliferate. Sutured full-thickness wounds will have new epithelium within 3 days, although they will have little tensile strength. In partial-thickness wounds, the epithelial cells from hair follicles and sebaceous glands migrate towards one another, but in full-thickness wounds, where there is a lack of dermal appendages, epithelial cells must migrate from the edges of the wound.

When they meet, contact inhibition halts their lateral proliferation but they continue to proliferate vertically to produce a multicellular layer, which resurfaces the wound. The protective barrier formed is due to the migration, proliferation and differentiation of keratinocytes, which arise from the epithelium peripheral to the wound or from hair follicles. Keratinocytes (epidermal cells that secrete keratin) migrate into the area within hours of the injury. They secrete membrane components, fibronectin, collagen and laminin (Stenn and Maholtra, 1992).

The epithelialisation process is sensitive to environmental factors such as pH, moisture and temperature. Deviation from the optimum values can have a detrimental effect. Once repair has taken place the wound will still undergo a continued phase of regeneration or maturation (Schultz and Mast, 1998). In the intervening period, however, the epidermis is unable to perform its essential role as an effective barrier to the passage of water.

Initial management of veterinary wounds

The preparation of any wound before treatment is of fundamental importance. This often involves the use of restraint methods, sedatives or, in extreme cases, general anaesthesia. Regional perineural anaesthesia is recommended for wounds of the distal extremity of the horse. The hair should always be clipped from a wide area around the wound edges, as hair clippings which may enter the wound are notoriously difficult to remove. They may be regarded as a foreign body whose presence will lead to a lengthening of wound healing time. To prevent this, the wound should be protected during clipping by the insertion of either sterile moist swabs, which are easily removed, or of KY jelly (Johnson & Johnson), which will subsequently be rinsed away with sterile normal saline solution. All gross contamination should be removed if possible, but lavage should not be continued excessively as this will cause tissue maceration.

After examination of the wound, primary closure may be performed in sedated animals or under general anaesthesia. Preoperative antibiotics are important, and in the horse tetanus status must be assessed. In the horse the use of non-steroidal anti-inflammatory drugs, particularly when there is any delay in the closure of the wound, as well as bandaging with a sterile, non-adhesive dressing and plenty of support, will assist primary wound healing.

In the distal limb, particularly of the horse, large tissue deficits may lead to the production of excessive, exuberant granulation tissue (see Hypergranulation below). The precise cause of this condition is not known, but some of the factors involved are thought to be increased movement, lack of soft tissue covering, excessive contamination and a reduction in blood supply. The use of effective pressure bandaging or cast application should be encouraged.

The objective of wound care should be to prepare the wound to be surgically closed while minimising the risk of wound infection or to control wound infection, thereby promoting wound healing by second intention. If the wound cannot be closed primarily because of a large soft tissue defect or if the wound is infected, closure must be delayed and the wound bandaged. The type of bandage applied to open wounds varies depending on whether additional debridement is necessary and the degree to which movement will disrupt wound healing (see chapter 19).

The ultimate aim of any treatment is to return the animal to normal function and cosmetic appearance. The selection of the wound treatments for each particular case involves many interdependent factors:

- The duration of the injury.
- The location, depth and configuration of the wound.
- The degree of contamination.
- The amount of trauma involved in causing the wound.
- Other systemic factors.
- The intended use of the animal.
- The cost.
- The cooperation of the patient and owner.

As with human soft tissue injuries, each case should be examined carefully before a decision is made about the most apposite treatment, as many factors influence the management of wounds in the domestic species. A basic approach that uses the following procedure is normally followed in all cases:

- Carry out a complete physical examination of the animal after an initial assessment of the wound, particularly in traumatic wounds, to avoid complications such as haemorrhagic shock.
- Take the history of the wound that covers the time between occurrence of the injury and the initial examination, and record this if it is known. The so-called golden period (6–8 hours after injury) is no longer valid as it is now accepted that wounds have a better prognosis the sooner they are sutured or treated.
- The cause of the injury will influence the management of the wound and its prospect of healing as well as having an effect on the likelihood of infection. Sharp lacerations are generally less prone to infection than shearing wounds caused by barbed wire, bite wounds or extreme forms of soft tissue injury, such as degloving. Severe soft tissue injuries, such as occur when legs are trapped for considerable periods, can lead to significant alteration in the vascular pattern of the limb and increased infection susceptibility.
- Identify any previous treatment of the wound by the owner before examination by the veterinary surgeon (particularly the use of an antibiotic spray), as this may mean that the wound is no longer open to primary closure by suturing.
- Evaluate any further tissue damage that may have occurred after the initial injury.
- Consider the likelihood of infection from the surrounding environment.

Management of contaminated and infected wounds

There are many causes of tissue injury in small and large animals. The tissue insult varies from a surgeon using aseptic technique, to a dog with an open perineal wound complicated by a rectal tear and exposed pelvic bones. Both these are contaminated wounds initially, even though it is obvious that the latter injury has a significantly greater chance of becoming an infected wound.

The first important aspect of contaminated wound treatment is considered to be thorough lavage with isotonic solutions such as normal saline or Ringer's solution. It has been shown that, if the wound is less than 3 hours old, antibiotics in the lavage solution decrease the chance of wound infection. After 3 hours, antibiotics in lavage are no more effective than lavage alone.

This is followed by the removal of all debris and necrotic or obviously devitalised tissue. In most instances this entails trimming ragged skin edges and subcutaneous tissue or fragmented muscle followed by debridement, which may have to be incomplete because of the presence of vital structures or because it is not obvious whether the tissue remains viable. Multiple debridements are often necessary, and if bone has been exposed in a wound for a period of time before implementation of veterinary care, desiccation may occur, leading to subsequent death and impediment to the growth of granulation tissue over the wound area.

Wet-to-dry bandaging of veterinary wounds is still being recommended for debridement and is contraindicated. The procedure involves the use of gauze swabs which are moistened with normal saline, packed into the wound, covered by white open wove bandage or gauze and allowed to dry. When dry this packing is removed there is inevitably destruction of some regenerating healthy tissue. The modern debriding agents, such as Intrasite Gel (Smith & Nephew) and Aserbine (Forley) are designed to remove debris from a wound by the establishment of an osmotic gradient within the wound. This gentle debridement does not damage new granulation tissue and should have a place in the debridement of animal wounds.

The presence of infective bacteria in wounds is extremely common and prolongs the time required for wound healing. Decreased fibroblast activity in the presence of bacteria and the encouragement of leucocytes to release lysozymes, which destroy newly formed collagen, can delay healing. Additionally, the presence of multiplying organisms may ensure that there is competition for the available nutrients.

Infections are commonly limited to subcutaneous tissue, particularly fat. However, some may also produce systemic effects, causing a reduction in the general state of health of the patient. The most common causative organisms are *Clostridium* spp., *Streptococcus* spp., *Staphylococcus* spp., *Escherichia coli* and *Pseudomonas* spp.

The main prerequisite for the successful resolution of wound infection is adequate drainage of the wound, which in some cases will require an additional incision. The use of systemic antibiotics may assist in eliminating the infection but the use of topical antimicrobials remains controversial.

Other components of the wound and its management

Necrotic tissue and debridement

The presence of yellowish-brown or blackened tissue in the wound indicates necrosis, i.e. an area of dead material. It delays healing and promotes infection. Effective wound management requires its removal by the process of debridement. Mechanical or surgical debridement involves physical removal of the dead tissue, usually by cutting it with scissors or a scalpel and lifting it with forceps. The tissue may also be removed chemically, using keratolytic agents such as benzoyl peroxide. Dead tissue can be selectively broken down by the use of enzymatic agents (e.g. collagenase or streptokinase) but these appear to be of lower potency than chemical agents.

Slough

The accumulation of dead cells in the exudate from wounds is a natural part of the healing process. The exudate, which appears yellowish due to the presence of leucocytes, may accumulate into an unsightly mass on the surface of the wound and is termed 'slough'. The process of its removal, providing a clean area for the regrowth of new tissue, is called desloughing. Mechanical removal may be done with a swab, an absorptive wound management product, or irrigation. Great care must be taken in the process of desloughing to prevent further inflammation and damage to the traumatised skin, and the appearance of granulation tissue under the exudate must not be mistaken for unwanted slough.

Factors which influence the effectiveness of wound healing

To produce effective wound healing, the body must supply a range of materials and nutrients to the site of damage. Factors which promote healing include an adequate blood supply and a healthy diet. Both systemic and local factors may challenge the successful continuation of the wound healing stages (Levenson and Demetriou, 1992; Stotts and Wipke-Tevis, 1997). The systemic factors include, in addition to nutritional status, concurrent therapy such as corticosteroids, prostaglandin inhibition, oncolytic agents, and clinical conditions such as anaemia and diabetes. These must be monitored and the objective must be the holistic management of the animal patient and not just the wound. Optimum healing can also be encouraged by the elimination from the wound of debris which may otherwise act as an ideal environment for the multiplication of microorganisms. The presence of wound infection is to be avoided at all costs. Personal experience has shown that, once interprofessional trust has been established between a pharmacist and a veterinary surgeon, the implications for wound management of any medication being used to treat the animal can be usefully discussed in the same way as with human patients.

Blood circulation

The growing edge of new epithelium has an insatiable appetite for blood. Any reduction in the provision of an adequate blood supply considerably slows the rate of healing by reducing the levels of oxygen, cells and nutrients reaching the wound. This explains why the prevention of clinical shock is essential, both after trauma and after the loss of blood during surgery. Equally, an animal patient suffering from any disease in which the circulation is impaired may be less capable of rapid and effective wound healing.

Drugs

The importance of inflammation in the mechanism of wound healing was originally thought to contraindicate the use of anti-inflammatory drugs after trauma. However, it has been shown that therapeutic doses of most of these drugs do not retard wound healing but may in fact reduce both pain and pyrexia.

The use of corticosteroids has been equally controversial. In large doses they have been shown to suppress wound healing and reduce the effectiveness of the body's ability to respond to infection. Conversely, the stress which the body undergoes during injury results in the production of large quantities of endogenous steroids, and this is thought to have little or no effect on the efficiency of healing.

Hypergranulation

During healing the wound becomes progressively filled with granulation tissue until the base of the original cavity is almost level with the surrounding skin. At this stage the epithelium around the wound margin begins to grow over the surface of the wound, thereby restoring the integrity of the epidermis. Occasionally the production of granulation tissue continues after the wound cavity has been filled, leading to the formation of hypergranulation tissue or 'proud flesh'. This is sometimes associated with the use of occlusive wound management materials. Its management varies and includes the use of topical steroid antibiotic ointments, pressure bandaging, sharp excision or caustic agents such as a silver nitrate pencil or short-term application of a corticosteroid cream or ointment under veterinary supervision.

Many wounds of the trunk and upper limbs do heal well by secondary intention with good cosmetic results, but those of the distal extremities tend to heal slowly with production of excessive scar tissue, and here skin grafting is often useful.

Oedema

An excess of intracellular fluid reduces the effectiveness of tissue metabolism and delays wound healing. Oedema may be a consequence of any condition in which the venous return is impaired, e.g. heart failure. Appropriate measures include the administration of diuretics.

Local factors that delay healing may be avoided by providing products that will produce the optimal microenvironment for healing (Turner, 1992). This microenvironment should be moist at the wound interface but excess exudate should be removed to prevent sloughing. The tissue temperature should be maintained and the injury protected from infective organisms, foreign particles and toxic compounds. In addition, when the dressing is changed there should be no secondary trauma due to adherence.

Management of non-surgical wounds

Non-surgical wounds most frequently seen by veterinary surgeons are avulsions, bite abscesses, flaps, lacerations, puncture wounds and those caused by road traffic accidents, other trauma and pressure ulceration.

Such wounds are open, often exhibit considerable tissue damage and are frequently contaminated or infected. Injuries from road traffic accidents in which skin flaps can be repositioned often retain viable tissues when dressed with a hydrogel overlaid with a polyurethane foam (see Case study 18.1). The hydrogel rehydrates the damaged area, thereby preventing necrosis and tissue death. Hydrogel application with consequent rehydration of tissue also minimises the need for surgical debridement in many wounds. This reduces the trauma to the patient, decreases the time taken for cleansing and minimises the cost to the client. This is illustrated by the following two cases of injuries to cats.

CASE STUDY

Case study 18.1
This injury involved extensive crushing of a cat's foot and necessitated amputation of digits 1 and 5. A flap of skin had been avulsed and was attached only at the carpo–metacarpal junction. This flap was repositioned and sutured. The foot was dressed with an enclosing hydrogel sheet overlaid with a non-adherent polyurethane foam. These were retained in position by a surgical adhesive tape. On day 4 the foot was swollen, although the tissues appeared viable. It was re-dressed as before. On day 7 there was less swelling and the tissues were obviously viable. The foot was re-dressed using a polyurethane foam material as a wound contact layer, with retention materials as before. It was re-dressed in a similar manner on days 12 and 16 and by day 20 wound healing had progressed to a stage where no further re-dressing was necessary.

Case study 18.2
The flap injury was similar in size and position to that described in Case study 1 but there was less crush damage to the foot. The flap was sutured and a conventional dry, absorbent, low-adherence dressing applied postoperatively and on day 6. This dressing was overlaid with a conforming bandage. On day 10 the flap was necrotic and was surgically removed leaving a tissue deficit. The foot was dressed using a calcium/sodium alginate pad soaked in normal saline as the wound contact layer. This was overlaid with a non-adherent polyurethane foam retained in position with a cohesive bandage. On day 15 the foot had reduced in size and the wound was dressed with a vapour-permeable film overlaid with a polyurethane foam retained in position as before. On day 20 the wound was re-dressed as before and by day 25 epithelialisation was almost complete.

Comment on Case studies 18.1 and 18.2

The contrast between these two cases lies in the treatment of the wound. In the first case the sutured skin flap was dressed with a hydrogel sheet. Consequently, tissue hydration was maintained and this ensured that the tissue remained viable despite the original poor prognosis. With the second injury the wound was initially covered with a dry, absorbent, low-adherence dressing which gave no maintenance of a moist wound-healing environment. The resulting desiccation led to necrosis of the skin flap and the necessity for further surgery at day 10.

Alginates have also been used to advantage as both packing materials and sheet dressings, where they have promoted haemostasis and the formation of granulation tissue. This is shown in Case study 18.3. The

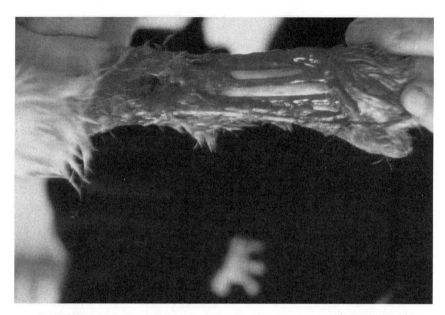

Figure 18.2   Case study 18.1, day 1.

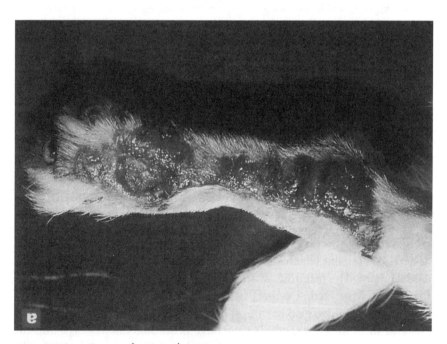

Figure 18.3   Case study 18.1, day 10.

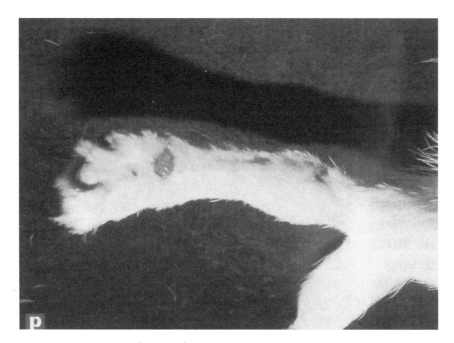

Figure 18.4 Case study 18.1, day 20.

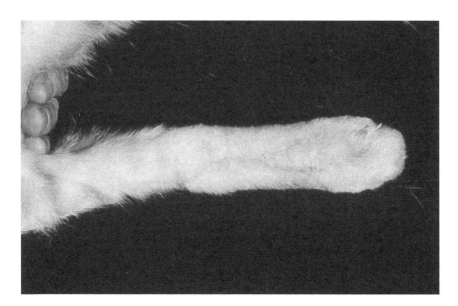

Figure 18.5 Case study 18.1, day 35.

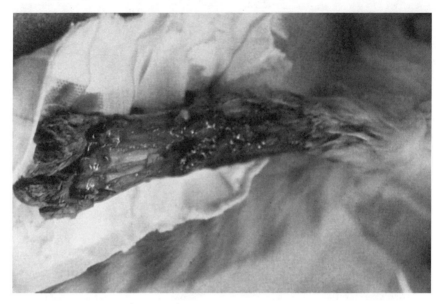

Figure 18.6 Case study 18.2, day 1.

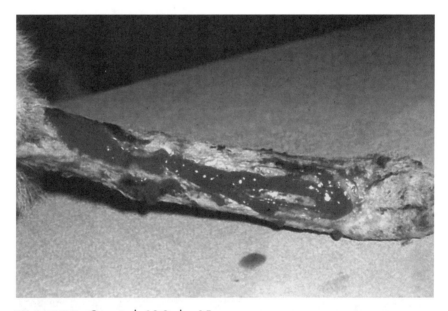

Figure 18.7 Case study 18.2, day 15.

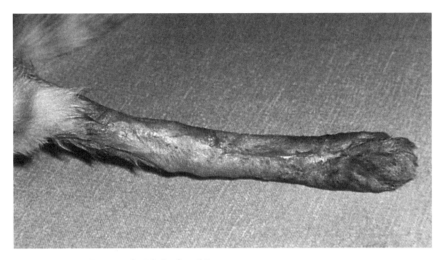

Figure 18.8 Case study 18.2, day 25.

number of dressing changes has been reduced with the appropriate use of these materials. They contribute little to wound healing if applied when the amount of exudate is declining.

Vapour-permeable films have been shown to be useful in animal wound management. However, maintenance of adhesion is often a problem because of the presence of skin secretions and hair regrowth.

 CASE STUDY

Case study 18.3
This case involved a knee injury to a horse. The initial wound had been hosed with cold water by the horse's owner and left undressed. By day 10 after injury there was significant necrosis which was treated by covering the wound with a hydrogel sheet overlaid with a polyurethane foam dressing held in position by a conforming bandage and elastic adhesive tape. Systemic antibiotic cover was given. The dressing was left in position for 48 hours after which it was removed and the necrotic tissue had rehydrated sufficiently to be removed by irrigation with normal saline. Epithelialisation was observed at the wound margins. The wound was then dressed with sodium/calcium alginate overlaid with a polyurethane foam held in position as before. The wound was re-dressed similarly three times more on alternate days after which epithelialisation had progressed and wound exudate declined sufficiently that further application of alginate was considered unnecessary. The wound was then covered with a low-adherence dressing held in position by a conforming bandage and elastic adhesive tape for a further 10 days when no further dressing was required.

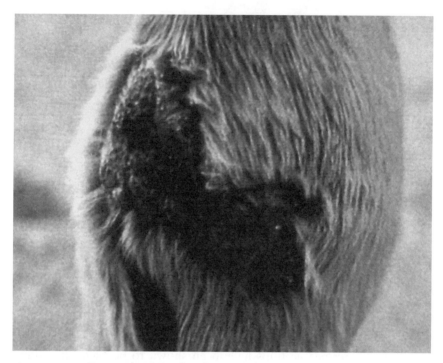

Figure 18.9 Case study 18.3, when first seen.

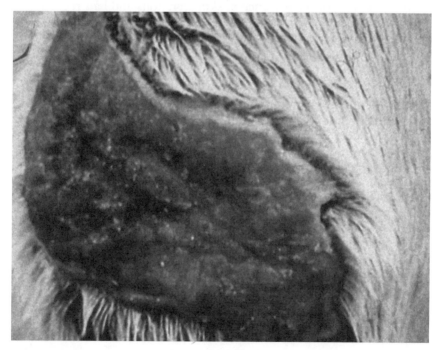

Figure 18.10 Case study 18.3, 2 days later.

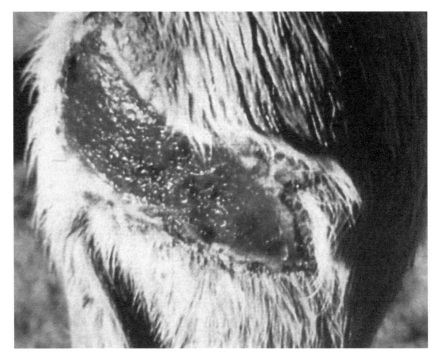

Figure 18.11   Case study 18.3, after a further 6 days.

Polymeric foams are useful retention materials as well as providing protection and thermal insulation to the wound area.

Management of surgical wounds

In surgical wound cases, the advantages of interactive contact materials are most readily observed in cases of incomplete wound closure. Alginate materials are frequently, but not always appropriately, the first choice. Vapour-permeable films and polyurethane foams have also been used to good effect in this context.

Wound management for transport

If the wound has been inflicted recently, the application of an occlusive dressing held firmly in place helps protect the wound, prevent further damage and stop all but the most severe haemorrhage. Care should be taken to ensure that all cavities are packed to aid haemostasis.

Conclusion

The paucity of literature references relating to the way animal soft tissue injuries are managed by veterinary surgeons indicates that little research has been undertaken in this area. There is an apparent lack of awareness by veterinary surgeons of the existence, appropriate use and contribution to wound healing which many of the interactive materials currently used for the management of human wounds could make to veterinary wound healing (Cockbill *et al.*, 1996; Cockbill, 1998).

These materials are individually designed to meet the different environmental stages found in the three wound-healing phases. It has been shown that their appropriate use has a positive effect on the rate of wound healing, and there is also a decrease in the number of dressing changes and a corresponding cost-effectiveness benefit for both veterinary surgeons and their clients. Whilst they are now a recognised adjunct to human medicine, they are often neglected in terms of application to veterinary injuries.

Throughout this chapter humoral substances which influence the wound-healing process have been mentioned. These include chemo-attractants, cytokines and growth factors. The relationships and interactions among these substances are complex and addressing these in detail is beyond the scope of this chapter.

As the science of wound healing progresses, the clinical application of cytokines and growth factors to wounds as topical medication will become reality. PDGF is already available commercially (Regranex, Janssen-Cilag) for application as a wound-healing stimulant. It is apparent, though, that certain characteristics of these growth factors will influence their use. Firstly, many require prolonged contact with the cells before a response is generated, and it seems as though the application of combinations of peptide growth factors may be more effective in stimulating wound healing than the use of individual growth factors. Also, a single growth factor may elicit different responses – inhibitory, stimulatory or a combination of both – depending on interactions with other factors and the cellular environment (Swaim and Henderson, 1997). It has been also shown that the concentration of growth factors also influences the rate and extent of wound healing. The type of wound and the timing of applications of these growth factors are important and this reinforces the concept that different wounds may need specific cytokines and growth factors at different times during the healing process. There is probably a delicate balance of these substances, with some overlap and phasing in or out of the cytokines as healing advances.

There could also be a variation in the balance, depending on the type of wound, and overall application at any time during healing or to all types of wound may slow the healing rate rather than benefit it.

References

Barker A T (1986). Electrical stimulation of wound healing. In: Turner T D, Schmidt R J, Harding K G, eds. *Advances in Wound Management*. New York: John Wiley, 133–135.

Bennett N T, Schultz G S (1993). Growth factors and wound healing: Part II. Role in normal and chronic wound healing. *Am J Surg* 166: 74–81.

Cockbill S M E (1998). Evaluation *in vivo* and *in vitro* of the performance of interactive dressings in the management of animal soft tissue injuries. *Vet Dermato*l 9: 87–98.

Cockbill S M E, Turner T D (1994). Management of veterinary wounds. In: Harding K G, Dealey C, Cherry G, Gottrup F, eds. *Proceedings of the 3rd European Conference on Advances in Wound Management*. London: Macmillan Magazines, 115–117.

Cockbill S M E, Turner T D (1995). Management of veterinary wounds. *Vet Rec* 136: 362–365.

Cockbill S M E, Hollinshead C M, Turner T D (1996). Veterinary wound management using contemporary surgical dressings. In: Cherry G, Gottrup F, Lawrence J C, Moffatt C J, Turner T D, eds. *Proceedings of the 5th European Conference on Advances in Wound Management*. London: Macmillan Magazines, 115–118.

Declan V (1999). The importance of growth factors in wound healing. *Ostomy Wound Manage* 45: 70–72, 74.

Desmouliere A, Geinoz A, Gabbiani A, *et al.* (1993). Transforming growth factor-beta 1 induces alpha-smooth muscle actin expression in granulation tissue myofibroblasts and in quiescent and growing cultured fibroblasts. *J Cell Biol* 122: 103–111.

Frank C, Shrive N, Huaoka H, *et al.* (1999). Optimisation of the biology of soft tissue repair. *J Sci Med Sport* 2: 190–210.

Harding C R, Scott I R (1983). Histidine rich proteins (fillagrins): structural and functional heterogenicity during epidermal differentiation. *J Mol Biol* 170: 651–673.

Haroon Z A, Raleigh J A, Greenberg C S, *et al.* (2000). Early wound healing exhibits cytokine surge without evidence of hypoxia. *Ann Surg* 231: 137–147.

Hunt T K, Hussein Z (1992). Wound microenvironment. In: Cohen I K, Diegelmann R F, Lindblad W J, eds. *Wound Healing: Biochemical and Clinical Aspects*. Philadelphia: W B Saunders, 274–281.

Kerstein M D (1997). The scientific basis of healing. *Adv Wound Care*; 10: 30–36. [Published erratum appears in *Adv Wound Care* 1997; 10: 8.]

Kiritsy C P, Lynch A B, Lynch S E (1993). Role of growth factors in cutaneous wound healing: a review. *Crit Rev Oral Biol Med* 4: 729–760.

Kunimoto B T (1999). Growth factors in wound healing: the next great innovation? *Ostomy Wound Manage* 45: 56–64; quiz 65–66.

Leaper D J (1986). The wound healing process. In: Turner T D, Schmidt R J, Harding K G, eds. *Advances in Wound Management*. New York: John Wiley and Sons, 7–16.

Levenson S M, Demetriou A A (1992). Metabolic factors. In: Cohen I K, Diegelmann R F, Lindblad W J, eds. *Wound Healing: Biochemical and Clinical Aspects*. Philadelphia: W B Saunders, 248–273.

Madlener M, Parks W C, Werner S (1998). Matrix metalloproteinases (MMPs) and their physiological inhibitors (TIMPs) are differentially expressed during excisional skin wound repair. *Exp Cell Res* 242: 201–210.

Mast B A (1992). The skin. In: Cohen I K, Diegelmann R F, Lindblad W J, eds. *Wound Healing: Biochemical and Clinical Aspects*. Philadelphia: W B Saunders, 344–355.

Moulin V, Auger F A, Garrel D, *et al.* (2000). Role of wound healing myofibroblasts on re-epithelialisation of human skin. *Burns* 26: 3–12.

Nuomeh B C, Liang H X, Cohen I K, *et al.* (1999). MMP-8 is the predominant collagenase in healing wounds and non-healing ulcers. *J Surg Res* 81: 189–195.

Peacock E E (1984). *Wound Repair*. Philadelphia: W B Saunders.

Schaffer C J, Narrey L B (1996). Cell biology of wound healing. *Int Rev Cytol*; 169: 151–181.

Schultz G S, Mast B A (1998). Molecular analysis of the environment of healing and chronic wounds: cytokines, proteases and growth factors. *Wounds*; 10 (Suppl. F): 1–9F.

Shah M, Revis D, Herrick S, *et al.* (1999). Role of elevated plasma transforming growth factor β1 levels in wound healing. *Am J Pathol* 154: 1115–1124.

Steinrech D S, Longaker M T, Mehrara B J, *et al.* (1994). Fibroblast response to hypoxia: the relationship between angiogenesis and matrix regulation. *J Surg Res* 84: 127–133.

Stenn K S, Maholtra R (1992). Epithelialisation. In: Cohen I K, Diegelmann R F, Lindblad W J, eds. *Wound Healing: Biochemical and Clinical Aspects*. Philadelphia: W B Saunders, 115–127.

Stotts N A, Wipke-Tevis D (1997). Co-factors in impaired wound healing. In: Krasner D, Kane D, eds. *Chronic Wound Care: A Clinical Source for Healthcare Professionals*. Wayne: Health Management Publications, 64–72.

Swaim S F, Henderson R A (1997). *Small Animal Wound Management*, 2nd edn. Philadelphia: Lea and Febiger, 143.

Turner T D (1992). Surgical dressings and their evolution. In: Harding K G, Leaper D L, Turner T D, eds. *Proceedings of the 1st European Conference on Advances in Wound Management*. London: Macmillan Magazines, 181–187.

Vaalamo M, Lervo T, Saarihalo K V (1999). Differential expression of tissue inhibitors of MMPs (TIMP-1, –2, –3, –4) in normal and aberrant wound healing. *Hum Pathol* 30: 795–802.

Wahl S M, Hunt D A, Wakefield L M, *et al.* (1987). Transforming growth factor type b induces monocyte chemotaxis and growth factor production. *Proc Natl Acad Sci USA* 84: 5788–5792.

Wahl L M, Wahl S M (1992). Inflammation. In: Cohen I K, Diegelmann R F, Lindblad W J, eds. *Wound Healing: Biochemical and Clinical Aspects*. Philadelphia: W B Saunders, 40–60.

Whalen G F, Zetter B R (1992). Angiogenesis. In: Cohen I K, Diegelmann R F, Lindblad W J, eds. *Wound Healing: Biochemical and Clinical Aspects*. Philadelphia: W B Saunders, 77–95.

Witte M B, Barbul, A (1997). General principles of wound healing. *Surg Clin North Am* 77: 509–528.

Yardley P A (1998). *A Brief History of Wound Healing*. Oxford: Oxford Clinical Communications.

19

Wound management materials

Sarah Cockbill

Traditional passive wound management materials used in the care of wounds were developed and used on an empirical basis, and the range of products available changed little until recently. Historically, a 'dressing' has been described as a material which covers a wound to allow healing to take place. Little thought was given to the interaction between the dressing and the processes of wound healing, as the dressing was used as a passive agent, mainly intended to protect the wound, keep it warm and hide its unpleasant appearance. Equally, a 'bandage' was an agent commonly used to keep a dressing in place at the site of the trauma, immobilise a damaged area, or provide compression of the wound and the surrounding area. Many of these traditional products are still in use today, but significant advances have been made through the development of modern *interactive* wound management products. Whilst these materials have been used successfully for the management of human wounds, there is little evidence to suggest that they have been or are currently being widely used on animals (Cockbill and Turner, 1994).

There are currently in excess of 150 product manufacturers globally who generate different brands of materials used for wound management. If brands, formats and sizes of dressings are combined, there are over 1000 products available for the management of human wounds (Ovington, 1998). These products fall into categories based on the materials from which the dressings are made and include vapour-permeable adhesive polymeric films, polymeric foams, hydrogels, xerogels, hydrocolloids and collagens. The products are made from both single components and from various combinations (Turner, 1990). There are also additional, newer categories of superabsorbents, hydrofibres and hydropolymers. All these dressings have the ability to create or maintain a moist local environment for wound healing and their performance variables include absorbent capacity, adhesive properties, conformability and their ability to rehydrate necrotic tissue. The use of two-layered systems consisting of primary and secondary materials is recommended in some instances. A primary dressing is one which is placed in direct contact with the surface of the wound, whereas a secondary dressing is a material which covers a primary dressing to hold it in place. The primary dressing should meet the requirements of permeability, non-adherence and bacterial impermeability and the secondary the need for absorption, protection and insulation.

Passive wound management products

Although considerable individual variations may exist, *passive* wound management materials can be regarded as consisting of three main components:

- A wound-facing layer. Absorbent wound-facing layers remove excess exudate, although the attraction of the dressing material for the exudate frequently causes the material to adhere to the wound. Examples of absorbent materials include absorbent gauze, muslin and lint.
- Non-absorbent materials may be produced by the impregnation of the absorbent material (e.g. gauze) with a fat-based agent (e.g. yellow soft paraffin).
- Absorbent layer. If the wound is producing large quantities of exudate, it may pass through the wound-facing layer of the dressing into a thicker layer of greater absorbency. The absorbent layer is commonly composed of a non-woven (e.g. absorbent cotton or cellulose wadding) or woven material (e.g. absorbent gauzes, rayon, or cotton).
- Outer layer. The outer layer is intended to provide support to the dressing, as an extensible material or a self-adhesive plaster.

Absorbents

Absorbent dressings remove excess quantities of exudate from the wound. They can be used in the form of swabs (e.g. to cleanse the skin and for the application of drugs), as an absorbent pad placed directly on the wound, or on top of a non-adherent material. The absorbent agent can be used individually (e.g. absorbent cotton) or in combination (e.g. gauze and cotton tissue). The material can be applied dry and may possess considerable absorptive capacity or it can be moistened before use. They are available in a number of forms:

- Fibrous (staple) absorbents.
- Fabric absorbents.
- Fibre plus fabric absorbents.
- Wound dressing pads.

Fibrous (staple) absorbents

These are made from cotton staple or from the fibres of viscose or cellulose, viscose and cotton may be admixed.

Cellulose wadding is produced from delignified wood pulp and manufactured in a multiple laminate material form. It is used in large pieces to absorb large volumes of fluid but is not used in contact with a wound.

Fabric absorbents

Absorbent lint is a close-weave cotton cloth with a raised nap on one side which offers a large surface area for evaporation when placed with the nap upwards on an exuding wound. It is generally unacceptable in modern wound management but still available for purchase.

Absorbent gauze is the most widely used absorbent and consists of a cotton cloth of plain weave bleached to a good white cotton leaf and shell that is clean and reasonably free from weaving defects. It may be slightly off-white if sterilised. It absorbs water readily but its performance may be reduced by prolonged storage or exposure to heat.

Non-woven fabrics include a wide range of products manufactured from synthetic and semisynthetic fibres. Non-woven swabs consist of a non-woven viscose fabric and are available in folded pieces of differing dimensions.

Cellulose sponge is a cavity foam cellulose-based sponge available in sheets and thin bands and may be used to absorb at small sites in surgery.

Fibrous plus fabric absorbents

Gauze and cotton tissue (Gamgee tissue) is a thick layer of absorbent cotton enclosed in a tubular form gauze. One manufacturer has produced a product recommended for veterinary use containing boric acid, which has been shown to be toxic to regenerating epithelial cells, thereby making its use contraindicated in human wound management. This toxicity must call into question the validity of boric acid incorporation into products intended for application to veterinary wounds.

Wound dressing pads

These products are widely available in a number of formulations, which include the fibrous and fabric absorbents previously described, plus other materials, combined to meet some aspects of the acceptable performance profile required. They generally consist of an absorbent pad, which may be enclosed in a sleeve of woven or non-woven fabric. This pad rapidly absorbs fluid and is therefore ideal for use on a grossly suppurating wound. It should not be used, however, if there is a risk of the wound drying out and the dressing sticking to the site of the trauma. A wound-dressing pad can be retained at the site by surgical adhesive tape or by a bandage.

The absorbent properties of wound dressing pads are due to the presence of knitted viscose, absorbent cotton and viscose, or absorbent cotton and crepe cellulose. The absorbent pad may be sleeved in a material which has been coated (e.g. with silicone, polyethylene or polypropylene) to prevent adherence to the wound. Also available are pads with wound contact faces varying from aluminium-coated fabrics to perforated polymeric films or heat-bonded polyethylene films designed specifically to be of low adherence. The wound contact film may be attached to an absorbent fibrous mat and an outer woven or non-woven fabric. They are dressings for low-exudate and drying wounds where high adherence can be expected.

Low-adherence primary dressings consist of a partially open-cell-structured nylon or viscose fabric which may be finished with a silicone coating. The open-cell structure allows fluid transmission to a superimposed absorbent dressing pad. The pad is changed when required without disturbing the primary contact layer.

The most commonly used low-adherence dressing is the perforated film absorbent dressing. The dressing consists of a dry, non-adherent, absorbent pad attached to gauze. The wound contact surface is coated with a polyethylene terephthalate film, which is perforated to allow the passage of exudate into the absorbent pad. It is a flexible dressing, available in a range of sizes, and is ideally suited for awkwardly located wounds. The pad is also available attached to an adhesive backing, and the resulting dressing is used as a primary wound contact layer for the initial management of veterinary surgical wounds. To prevent interference by the animal patient, this dressing may be overlaid by either a cohesive bandage or a conforming bandage and adhesive tape. Activated charcoal may be included in the sleeve layer. The deodorising action of the charcoal is especially useful for wounds which are infected and malodorous.

Deodorising dressings

These dressings have been formulated from the high-gaseous sorbtive material activated charcoal and are presented as a woven fabric or a fibrous mat backed by a nylon sleeve, a vapour-permeable film or a polyurethane foam. In each formulation the objective is to reduce odour and the dressings must therefore be large enough to cover the entire malodorous area. One product encourages direct contact of the carbon layer with wound exudate, and whilst this will limit gaseous absorption it is claimed that the incorporation of bound silver into the charcoal cloth inactivates bacteria that are adsorbed onto the fabric surface, thereby reducing the infective level and consequently reducing odour.

Adhesive dressings

Adhesive dressings may be permeable, semi-permeable or occlusive. Permeable adhesive dressings include elastic adhesive dressing and permeable plastic wound dressing. The permeable plastic wound dressing is designed with the self-adhesive backing perforated to allow the passage of water vapour and gases. Semi-permeable adhesive dressings are similarly constructed. However, the backing is not perforated but is semi-permeable and waterproof. It therefore allows water vapour and gases to pass from the wound surface to the external environment but prevents the movement of moisture in the opposite direction. Occlusive adhesive dressings prevent the transference of water vapour and gases from the wound surface but also minimise the inward transmission of microorganisms and dust. Their use may also prevent the spread of contamination from an infected wound to the surrounding area. They have limited use for minor human wounds, but also have limited use for protecting wounds on the paws of cats and dogs.

Adhesive dressing pads

Adhesive dressing pads consist of an absorbent pad which may be completely or partly surrounded by an adhesive plaster.

Elastic adhesive dressing consists of an absorbent pad attached to an extension plaster coated with zinc oxide adhesive. It may be supplied as a wound dressing or as a strip dressing and can be used as a protective covering for many types of wound.

Perforated plastic wound dressing is similar to the elastic adhesive dressing (see above). However, the adhesive dressing is a perforated plastic self-adhesive plaster which is permeable to water vapour and oxygen. A waterproof version is also available which is occlusive and prevents the outward transmission of infection and the inward transmission of bacteria or dirt. A further variation is the waterproof microporous plastic wound dressing. This can promote wound healing by allowing the passage of water vapour from the wound while still providing a waterproof environment.

Bandages

Bandages can be classified for use as dressing retention materials, for support and for compression according to their structure and predicted performance.

Retention bandages

Retention bandages can be used to keep absorbent dressings in place, or on their own to provide support. This is particularly important with animal wounds, as adequate and efficient adhesion of materials to animals' skin is one of the major problems to be overcome by dressing manufacturers. Consequently, retention bandages are commonly used in veterinary practice.

Non-extensible retention bandages include open-weave bandage, which is made of cotton or cotton and viscose. Retention bandages may also be made of stretch fabrics. Cotton conforming bandage is a two-way extensible bandage whose shape can be easily adapted to cover difficult sites of application. The elasticity may also provide some support and this assists the bandage to keep an underlying wound management product in place. The warp threads in polyamide and cellulose contour bandage are composed of crimped polyamide, which gives the bandage a longer life than a crepe bandage. Tubular bandages may be made of gauze, stockinette (in which a cotton/viscose yarn is interspersed with a rubber thread) or cotton. Most are available in a range of sizes.

Support and compression bandages

Support and compression bandages commonly consist of fibres which stretch only along the length of the bandage. One-way stretch imparts support and pressure to the bandaged area, and the degree of support varies according to the material of composition. Support and compression bandages can also be classified as non-adhesive and adhesive:

- Non-adhesive support and compression bandages. Crepe bandage, cotton crepe bandage, and cotton stretch bandage are appropriate in situations where light support is required. A crepe bandage contains wool and can provide warmth and insulation on exposed surfaces.

- Adhesive support and compression bandages. These may be self-adhesive bandages or diachylon bandages. Elastic adhesive bandage consists of an elastic cloth which may be completely spread with an adhesive (e.g. zinc oxide elastic self-adhesive bandage) or partially spread (e.g. half-spread zinc oxide elastic self-adhesive bandage). These bandages are used to provide support and compression. They are also commonly used to secure other appliances and wound management products but are notoriously difficult to remove from hirsute surfaces.

One further product which may be considered to be self-adhesive but which does not have an adhesive coating is the cohesive extensible bandage. This bandage clings to itself, preventing slippage during use. It is commonly seen when applied over absorbent cotton to act as a support for the tendons of cross-country competition horses.

Medicated bandages

Medicated bandages combine the benefits of a cotton dressing with the use of an agent such as zinc oxide, coal tar, ichthammol, calamine and clioquinol to reduce inflammation or promote healing, or both. These bandages can be kept in place for 3–7 days but particular care must be taken to ensure that the animal/patient does not react adversely to the incorporated agent. These bandages have limited use in veterinary practice.

Surgical adhesive tapes

The classification of surgical adhesive tapes depends on the properties of the materials of construction. The backing material may be woven, non-woven or plastic. The adhesive may produce a tape which is permeable, allowing the passage of oxygen, water, and bacteria; semi-permeable, allowing the passage of oxygen and water vapour only; or occlusive. The choice of tape depends on the requirements for use and the type of skin surface to which it is to be applied.

Permeable surgical adhesive tapes may comprise a woven backing fabric and are available with a range of adhesives. Adhesives containing zinc oxide are available on non-extensible (zinc oxide surgical adhesive) or extensible (elastic surgical adhesive) tapes.

Non-woven synthetic materials are also used as the tape backing material. They are often preferable to woven fibres as their application permits the transmission of water vapour and oxygen while minimising the damage to healthy skin. Permeable non-woven surgical synthetic adhesive tape possesses less inherent strength than woven tapes but has the advantages of easy removal and handling. It has little practical use in veterinary practice.

Plastic film tapes may be perforated (producing a permeable tape) or non-perforated (producing an occlusive tape). They may be used to cover sites of infection while allowing the continued passage of oxygen and water vapour (e.g. permeable plastic surgical adhesive tape), or to cover sites where total exclusion of water and water vapour is required (e.g. impermeable plastic surgical synthetic adhesive tape and impermeable plastic surgical adhesive tape).

Tulle dressings

Tulle dressings (*tulle gras* = greased net) are non-adherent wound-contact dressings consisting of an open-weave fabric impregnated with white or yellow soft paraffin, but not with enough to produce a totally occlusive dressing. The dressing may be non-medicated (e.g. paraffin gauze dressing) or medicated (e.g. with chlorhexidine, framycetin, sodium fusidate, or povidone–iodine).

Close-weave gauze and open-weave tulles are used as carriers of medicated and non-medicated 'ointments' to the wound surface. These materials coat the area of the wound with hydrophobic paraffin spread on an open-mesh gauze, thereby providing both insulation and partial occlusion but allowing excess exudate to be absorbed by a super-imposed absorbent pad. The product has the advantage of low adherence and allows gaseous diffusion but the disadvantages include the incorporation of the soft paraffin or loose cotton fibres into the healing wound, thereby producing a 'foreign body' response within the wound, leading to an extended inflammatory phase with consequent delayed wound healing. These products also, when used excessively, retain wound exudate, causing maceration to the surrounding, otherwise healthy, tissue.

Non-medicated tulle dressings

Paraffin gauze is bleached cotton or combined cotton and rayon cloth impregnated with yellow or white soft paraffin. It is available as sterile single pieces or multipacks. The paraffin is present to prevent the dressing adhering to a wound. The gauze is coated so that all the threads of the fabric are impregnated but the spaces between the threads are free of paraffin. The material is used primarily in the treatment of wounds such as burns and scalds, where the protective function of the stratum corneum is lost and water vapour can escape. Paraffin gauze dressing functions by reducing the fluid loss while the water barrier layer is reforming. In addition to burns and scalds, the dressing is used as a wound contact layer in lacerations and abrasions. The two properties of the paraffin gauze that are most useful are those of non-adherence and semi-occlusiveness.

Medicated tulle dressings

Povidone–iodine 10% w/w, chlorhexidine 0.5% w/w, sodium fusidate 2% w/w and 1% w/w framycetin sulfate are some examples of available impregnations which are recommended for the reduction of infection. Diffusion of the antibacterial agent into or onto an infected and exuding wound has been shown to be minimal. The possibility of development of resistant strains of infective organisms has reduced the use of these products.

Chlorhexidine is a relatively non-toxic antiseptic with activity against many Gram-positive organisms, some Gram-negative bacteria, and fungi.

Framycetin sulfate is a broad-spectrum aminoglycoside antibiotic almost identical to neomycin. It may be used in a wide range of infected wounds. Although there is normally minimal systemic absorption of the antibiotic, the application of the dressing to large tracts of skin (>30% of body area) in which the epidermal barrier layers have been lost may lead to the characteristic ototoxicity of aminoglycosides. This is a factor which should be taken into consideration when managing animal wounds.

Sodium fusidate gauze dressing contains sodium fusidate ointment. It can be used in the treatment of wounds infected with Gram-positive organisms, particularly staphylococci. Unlike other tulle dressings, it may not require the outer application of an absorbent dressing and it should not be applied around or near the eye because of the risk of conjunctival irritation.

A non-adherent dressing containing povidone–iodine may be used to prevent the development of infection, particularly in burns. However, its activity is less than that of chlorhexidine because the antiseptic is inactivated by exudate from the wound. This material has a place in the management of veterinary wounds as its wide spectrum of activity helps to overcome the bacterial hazards encountered in animal living environments, particularly stables, fields and byres.

Contemporary wound management products

Advances in the design and efficacy of wound management products was spasmodic and limited to the adaptation of available materials until 1959. Up to 1959, wound management products were primarily of the 'plug-and-conceal' variety, exemplified by lint, gauze, cotton wool and tow, which were considered to be passive products that took no part in the healing process. Little or no attention was paid to the functional performance of a product and minimal consideration was given to the different healing environments required for different wound types. It was in 1959 that perforated film absorbent dressing (Melolin, Smith & Nephew Healthcare) was developed and marketed as the first 'non-adherent' dressing, and since that date there have been both technological and clinical advances in the design and use of dressing materials. Melolin was closely followed by products which were derived from the advances in the development of synthetic polymers. A statement of required performance could now be considered as a possible specification for a polymeric product.

Polymeric wound management product developments have resulted in more successful management of soft tissue injuries of different aetiologies and has led to the present range of *interactive* and *bioactive* dressings available. The former are designed to maintain the optimum microenvironment for wound healing at the surface of the wound, and the latter are used to potentiate the healing cascade in different wounds. This microenvironment should be moist at the wound interface, but should be such as to remove excess exudate in order to avoid irritation and excoriation of the surrounding skin. This philosophy applies to the healing of both animal and human wounds.

The new generation of products was a rejection of the traditional passive 'cover all' dressing philosophy and was potentiated by the advances in knowledge of the humoral and cellular factors associated with the healing process and the realisation that a controlled microenvironment is necessary if wound healing is to progress at the optimum level. Such environmental-control dressings could be classified as *interactive*. Vapour-permeable adhesive polymeric films, polymeric foams, hydrogels, xerogels, hydrocolloids, collagens, superabsorbents, hydrofibres and hydropolymers fall within this classification and mark the progression towards the production of an ideal wound dressing, as does the emergence of *bioactive* materials, such as those derived from fibroblasts by tissue cell culture, artificial skin derived from keratinocytes and an extracellular matrix dressing derived from the submucosal layers of the porcine small intestine.

Interactive dressings are individually designed to meet the different environmental stages found in the three phases of wound healing. It should, however, be emphasised that no single dressing will produce the optimum microenvironment for all wounds or for all of the healing stages of one wound. The spectrum of performance requires that the wound is diagnosed and the treatment progressed by prescribing the most suitable dressing at each stage of the healing process. Careful selection based upon knowledge and experience is necessary if rapid healing of the injury is to be achieved with minimum discomfort to the patient. Whilst interactive materials are now a recognised adjunct to human medicine, they have been neglected in terms of application to veterinary injuries.

It is recognised that both the acellular and the cellular activities involved in the healing cascade are optimised by a wound microenvironment which will allow the free movement of cells and effective response to bioactive compounds, such as growth factors which have cellular activity and are used to potentiate one or more steps in the healing cascade. These products will be further developed for use in both human and animal wound management. Their optimal response can be expected where environmental factors such as temperature and humidity are at subdermal levels.

In contrast with the management of human soft tissue injuries, the commercial value of the animal plays more than a significant part in the perceived cost-effectiveness of any new treatment. It follows that the principal areas where there will be veterinary interest in the use of modern wound management materials will be the small-animal and equine, as most farmers will consider sending casualty cattle and sheep straight to the abattoir before extra expenditure on veterinary fees and materials (Cockbill and Turner, 1995).

Performance criteria and properties of an ideal wound management product

The concept of moist wound healing is generally attributed to George Winter, after his much cited publication in *Nature* in 1962, although Bull and his co-workers in 1948 (Bull *et al.*, 1948) published results showing enhancement of healing under a 'film' dressing but no explanation was given. In 1975, Winter (Winter, 1975) expressed his initial concern with the secondary trauma produced at the wound surface by removing the strongly adhesed fibrous and fabric dressings of the 1960s, and described his attempts to produce a moist wound environment and thereby reduce dressing adherence by using polythene sheets as wound covers. This gave an unacceptable 'wet' environment that resulted in tissue maceration, but an alternative microporous polyvinyl chloride material, which he reported as having a permeability to water vapour of 'about 2500 g/m^2 24 hours' proved more successful. He showed that the mitotic rate of regenerating epidermal cells in a wound covered by a gas-permeable membrane could be increased by a factor of 5–10 by exposing them to an oxygen-enriched atmosphere. Similar effects were reported by Silver (1972), who demonstrated that low-exudate wounds healed more rapidly in the presence of the oxygen found beneath the so-called permeable dressings than under hypoxic conditions. In heavily exuding or grossly contaminated wounds, the partial pressure of oxygen (pO$_2$) beneath these dressings was found to be extremely low and disappeared within an hour of applying the dressing. It was suggested that the reason for this was the metabolism of this oxygen, together with the oxygen that may have diffused through the dressing material, by macrophages or bacteria in the exudate before it could reach the tissues beneath (Thomas, 1990). The assumption could be made, therefore, that the use of a dressing with high oxygen permeability would contribute positively to the wound healing process. However, angiogenesis is also fundamental to healing and Knighton *et al.* in 1983 demonstrated, by the use of a rabbit-ear-chamber technique, that a hypoxic tissue gradient was essential for angiogenesis, and they postulated that capillary formation in hypoxic conditions is stimulated by a secondary angiogenic factor produced by hypoxic macrophages. This theory is supported by further work which has shown that a reduced oxygen (pO$_2$) promotes the growth of fibroblasts and the production of angiogenic factors from tissue macrophages *in vitro* (Hunt *et al.*, 1984).

The process of wound healing is an active process and therefore optimum conditions must be created within and around a wound to obtain effective and efficient wound healing. Although these optimum conditions may vary according to the site, type and depth of the wound and associated physiological and pathological factors, an ideal wound management product may be recommended to meet the requirements of the majority of animal and human wounds.

Local factors which delay healing may be avoided by providing products which will produce the optimal microenvironment for healing. The tissue temperature should be maintained and the injury protected from infective organisms, foreign particles and toxic compounds. In addition, when the dressing is changed there should be no secondary trauma due to adherence.

Turner in 1979 (Turner 1979 a, b) identified the performance criteria for a wound dressing product that would successfully contribute to an acceptable microenvironment. These were:

- To maintain a high humidity at wound/dressing interface.
- To remove excess exudate and toxic components.
- To allow gaseous exchange.
- To provide thermal insulation.
- To afford protection from secondary infection.
- To be free from particulate or toxic contaminants.
- To allow removal without trauma at dressing change.

These criteria are still valid and have not been greatly modified. An additional requirement with the advance in our knowledge of the growth factors involved in the healing process is that the product should be compatible with the humoral and cellular factors involved in healing.

Humidity levels and removal of exudate

Human or veterinary partial- or full-thickness wounds exposed to the air will have a lower temperature than ambient because of the loss of latent heat through tissue fluid evaporation. The clotting process and fibril development produce an occlusive dry eschar or scab which effectively seals and insulates the wound, thereby limiting the transmission of moisture and gases and restricting the migration of epithelial cells to the moist sub-scab tissue (see Figure 19.1).

The maintenance of a high level of humidity between the wound and the dressing is therefore a requirement for rapid epidermal healing. A drying wound will result in a gas-impermeable eschar and will require epithelial cell penetration to a moist lower level, resulting in prolonged healing time.

The absorption of excess exudate not only prevents tissue maceration but also removes exotoxins or cell debris, which may retard growth or extend the inflammatory phase of the healing process. The balance between humidity and absorption is critical and excessive wicking must be avoided to prevent drying and necrosis.

Gaseous exchange

Gaseous permeability will allow water vapour transmission, which may be particularly important in a high-exudate wound such as a burn. Of equal significance will be the effect of gaseous exchange on oxygen (pO_2) and hydrogen ion (pH) levels. Movement across the dressing of

Wound covered   **Wound exposed**

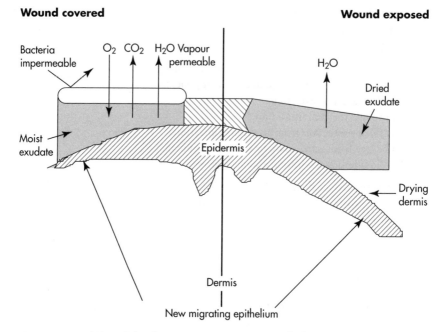

Figure 19.1 Wound healing response to a controlled microenvironment versus exposure. The result of exposure is slow healing with a high risk of contamination and infection, together with possible excessive scarring in an excised wound from closure without full cavity granulation. This is important when show animals are involved.

oxygen and carbon dioxide will relate directly to cellular and humoral factor activity. Epithelialisation of the wound is greatly accelerated by the availability of atmospheric oxygen, which dissolves in the serous exudate to supplement the oxygen that is transported to the wound area by haemoglobin and which is subsequently directly utilised by the migrating epidermal cells. This applies to both human and animal burns.

Thermal insulation

Thermal insulation will assist in maintaining the wound temperature at a level as close to body core temperature as possible. Phagocytic and mitotic activity are particularly susceptible to temperatures below 28 °C. Thermal insulation and 'warm' dressing-change conditions are very important if the optimum healing rate is to be maintained. Long exposure of wet wounds may reduce the surface temperature to the point where mitotic activity ceases and the recovery of that tissue may take up to 3 hours. Temperatures of 30 °C and above may be found beneath a good insulating dressing, and this will result in high mitotic activity with rapid epithelialisation and improved granulation.

Impermeability to microorganisms

Bacterial impermeability has a dual role. The wound will not heal if it is heavily infected. The inflammatory phase will be extended and, unless topical or systemic antibacterial agents are used, a more general infection could result. However, a limited number of microorganisms are tolerated by most wounds and the destructive or cleansing phase produced by phagocytic activity should result in a self-sterilised environment. The wound should now be protected from secondary infection or, if still contaminated, be prevented from transmitting the infective organisms.

A dressing should, therefore, be impermeable to airborne microorganisms which may fall on its surface and penetrate to and infect the wound. It should also act as a barrier to any wound organisms which may be transmitted to the dressing surface and become airborne and may thus cause cross-infection. Organism transmission occurs most frequently in dressings which exhibit 'strike-through' of the exudate to the wound surface, providing a wet pathway to or from the wound surface. The passage of organisms can take as little as 6 hours from the time of strike-through.

Freedom from particulate and toxic wound contaminants

Both the particles and the toxic compounds that may contaminate a wound will be responsible for disrupting the healing pattern. The incorporation of fibrous particles into a wound may result in a granuloma which could subsequently reduce the wound strength and induce keloid scarring. It is well documented that particulate contamination can also reduce the infection resistance levels by a factor of 1.0×10^{-6}; thus, organism levels which would previously have been self-sterilisable are infective and colonise the wound to produce a gross infection.

Trauma during dressing change

The wound environment may be optimally maintained with a product which has the preferred performance parameters but, nevertheless, is disrupted during the dressing change. The hazards of temperature change and secondary infection may be accompanied by a secondary trauma caused by the dressing adhering to the wound and, on removal, stripping newly formed tissue.

This adhesion is normally caused by the adhesiveness of the drying exudate, and the trauma can be exaggerated on removal by the destruction of capillary loops which have penetrated the dressing material. This produces a bleeding surface which, at most, may revert the wound to the primary inflammatory phase and, at least, delay epithelialisation.

Although not associated with the production of an acceptable microenvironment, there are certain physical characteristics which are required to assist in the overall dressing procedure. The dressing should have:

- A size range of and shape to match the wounds for different animal species.
- An absorption range for dry and heavy exudate wounds.
- Good conformability and good handling when both dry and wet.
- Sterility and be stable in storage.
- Easy disposal.

The use of antiseptics is still common in the cleansing process associated with wound healing (see chapter 3). This is a practice not to be recommended as it has been demonstrated that agents such as hypochlorites (contained, for example, in Eusol) interfere with the synthesis of new collagen and the budding of new capillaries.

There are significant deficiencies in the presentation, packaging and available size ranges of the products when considering their potential use for the management of veterinary wounds, all of which could be remedied. There are also problems of dressing retention, hirsutism, protection of the dressing against patient and environmental abuse, and ease of application and removal (Cockbill *et al.*, 1996). It is to be hoped that manufacturers will meet the challenges presented, to thereby ensure a wider veterinary use of these important materials.

A new range of debriding agents is now available which remove bacteria and dead cells and promote the formation of new granulation tissue. The presence of a defined structure in these new wound management products allows the cleansing process to be regulated, permitting effective removal of exudate but preventing drying out of the wound.

Polymeric dressings

The following descriptions will include examples of some, but inevitably not all, of the products available within each group. Many are found in veterinary practices and are used commonly for the management of wounds in animals.

Vapour-permeable adhesive films

Vapour-permeable films are of use in those wounds in which granulation tissue has been formed and wound exudate is reducing (Ovington, 1998; Thomas, 1990, 1994). These products were developed as materials which would in part mimic the performance of skin. Film dressings are transparent, thin but very resilient semi-permeable membranes, generically described as vapour-permeable adhesive films formed from elastomeric copolymer, whose wound contact surface is evenly coated with a synthetic adhesive. The adhesive is cohesive and inactivated by contact with moisture and will not, therefore, stick to moist skin or the wound bed. The films are also permeable to water vapour, oxygen and carbon dioxide but occlusive to the inward passage of bacteria and water. They have highly elastomeric and extensible properties which contribute to both their conformability and their resistance to shear and tear. The products are sterile and particle-free.

In the treatment of burns, less water vapour passes through the film than is lost from the traumatised skin surface, and a moist environment at the wound surface is therefore maintained. A significant advantage is the transparency of the film, which allows healing to be monitored without disturbing the wound site.

The moist interface at the wound surface allows the rapid migration of new epithelium across the wound surface, precludes trauma due to adherence when the dressing is changed and contributes to gaseous diffusion in the damaged tissue. Oxygen and carbon dioxide transfer are accomplished by intramolecular diffusion through the membrane and by solution in the moisture at the wound surface. The oxygen permeability of the films is variously described as 4000 to 10 000 $cm^3/m^2/24$ hours at ambient atmospheric pressure. The pO_2 and pH levels of the wound surface are directly related to the gaseous permeability and contribute to cellular activity. The wound is protected against secondary infection by the bacterial impermeability of the film.

The physical performance is applicable to the management of superficial tangential wounds, such as dermabrasions, split-skin-graft donor sites and burns. In a dermabrasion, haemostasis must first be obtained and the margin of the wound dried before the film is applied. Provided the film is correctly positioned, it may be left *in situ* until epithelialisation is complete. In its application for the treatment of burns, careful disinfection must precede the positioning of the film. It is only recommended for superficial and clinically clean burns and contraindicated for deep burns, where it retards the separation of necrotic tissue.

Preparation of the skin before the film dressing is applied is important. If the skin is wet or greasy the film will not stay in place. The skin can be degreased with an alcohol swab. The presence of hair may also reduce adhesion and therefore wet shaving of the skin surrounding the wound is recommended before application of the dressing.

Film dressings are used in the treatment of a wide range of conditions, including pressure ulcers, burns, abrasions and donor sites. Recently, film dressings have been introduced that are impregnated with an antibacterial (silver) for the management of infected wounds or a deodoriser (charcoal) for malodorous wounds.

The method of applying film dressings varies according to the manufacturer.

Recommended use

It has been shown, as with human wounds, that re-epithelialisation of a partial-thickness wound occurs more quickly when it is covered by a vapour-permeable film which maintains a moist environment at the surface of the wound. The rate of animal hair growth, which is acknowledged to be up to three times as high as that of human hair, can prove to be a problem both in the maintenance of adhesion and, ironically, in the removal of the dressing (Cockbill, 1998). Therefore, careful monitoring of the film whilst it is in use is essential. Adhesion of the vapour-permeable film to the wound area can be enhanced by the initial use of a vapour-permeable film spray such as Opsite (Smith & Nephew) around the perimeter of the wound before application (manufacturer's recommendation).

Examples

- Bioclusive (Johnson & Johnson Medical).
- Cutifilm (Beiersdorf, UK).
- Opsite Flexigrid (Smith & Nephew Medical).
- Tegaderm (3M Healthcare).

Polymeric foams

Polymeric foam dressings are a diverse group of products with a wide range of properties. At their simplest they are foamed polymers which have been made into sheets. The first foam dressing developed was a partially expanded, modified polyurethane foam. It comprised a lower layer of open cells and an upper hydrophilic surface with closed impermeable layers which reduced the loss of water vapour and prevented strike-through of absorbed fluid (Lock, 1979).

These materials are useful for filling cavities as they assume the shape of the wound, exert pressure and absorb exudate within the wound to stimulate the granulation process of wound healing. The most common polymer used is polyurethane, the absorbency and water vapour permeability of which are varied either by a physical modification to the foam or by combining the foam with an additional sheet component. The wound contact layer is often heat-treated to give a smooth surface which absorbs fluids by capillarity (Ovington, 1998; Thomas, 1990, 1994). Foaming the polymer creates small, open cells which are able to hold fluids, and the cell size may be controlled during the foaming process. Their structure and softness also provide a cushion which protects and contributes to the thermal insulation of the wound. They may also be tailored for particular applications without particle loss to the wound and with the retention of their conformable characteristics. They are available with or without an integral charcoal cloth to assist in the deodorisation of malodorous wounds, and in a wide range of sizes. The non-adhesive foams will require a secondary dressing and the formulations may require a retention dressing when they are applied to animal wounds, both to keep it in position and to discourage interference with the material by the animal patient.

The dressings are available as sheet dressings and as *in situ* formed foams. The sheet dressings have a non-adherent wound contact surface and are also available as adhesive island dressings and cavity fillers (Ovington, 1998).

Absorption of exudate is limited to the wound/dressing interface. This primary dressing expands when it becomes wet and conforms to the contours of the wound, producing an environmental chamber with entrapped solutes and cell debris. It is claimed that this function enhances the inflammatory response of the wound and subsequently stimulates the production of granulation tissue and revascularisation. In use, the absorptive capacity of the hydrophobic portion will be exceeded in a high-exudate wound, and although moisture vapour transmission occurs through the dressing frequent changes may be required until the exudate level diminishes. The superpositioning of a secondary absorbent pad will solve the problem of excess exudate whilst retaining the non-adherence, bacterial impermeability, gaseous and water vapour permeability functions and the additional cushioning and thermal insulation properties of the foam. The dressing combines the function of absorbency with that of producing an acceptable micro-environment which will allow healing to take place at the fastest rate with the total clinical condition of the patient.

Primary foam dressings with low absorptive capacity have been produced from a carboxylated styrene butadiene rubber latex foam. The foam is bonded to a non-woven fabric coated with a polyethylene film which has been vacuum-ruptured. The basic foam is naturally hydrophobic and a surface-active agent is incorporated to facilitate the uptake of wound exudate. The polyethylene foam layer is particularly effective in preventing adherence and the dressing is recommended for minor wounds and abrasions where exudate levels are low and adherence is a hazard.

Recommended use

Absorbent dressings are recommended for moderate to heavy exudation. They are also recommended for the management of dry sutured wounds and minor lacerations.

Examples

- Allevyn (Smith & Nephew Medical Ltd).
- Cutinova Foam (Biersdorf UK).
- Lyofoam (SSL International).

In situ foam

One of the major problems in wound management is the treatment of large cavity wounds. It is necessary to occlude the cavity by packing to absorb excess exudate and to stimulate the production of granulation tissue, neovascularisation and collagen deposition. The traditional procedure is to pack the cavity with ribbon gauze (see Fabric absorbents) variously impregnated. The subsequent removal of such a dressing is difficult and the pain and stress associated with the dressing change may require low-level anaesthesia for both human and animal patients.

An *in situ* formed foam it is now available as Cavi-Care (Smith & Nephew). Cavi-Care Foam Dressing is a two-part foam composed of a filled polydimethylsiloxane base and a catalyst. The two components are mixed together immediately before use. The reaction is slightly exothermic and over a period of 2–3 minutes the dressing expands to approximately four times its original volume and sets to a soft spongy foam stent accurately conforming to the contours of the wound cavity. When used to manage human cavity wounds, this stent is normally removed twice daily, soaked in a mild antiseptic (0.5% aqueous chlorhexidine) rinsed in cold running water, squeezed dry and replaced. A new dressing is formed after a week or more to match the reduction in size of the cavity. The product does not adhere to granulation tissue. It maintains free drainage around the wound and has a low but significant absorptive capacity at the dressing surface.

Hydropolymer

This material appears visually as a foam and is made from polyurethane but is described as a foamed gel. The material expands into the contours of the wound as it absorbs fluid. The material is used in an island configuration with an adhesive portion which is unique in that it has the ability to re-adhere once lifted, thereby enabling manipulation of the product for fit or assessment of the wound without dressing change. The hydropolymer wicks fluid into the upper layers of the dressing, where it escapes through the backing (Ovington, 1998).

Recommended use

Hydropolymer is recommended for the dynamic fluid management of heavily exuding wounds or when extended periods between dressing changes are desirable.

Example

- Tielle (Johnson & Johnson Medical).

Fibrous polymers

This group of dressings includes synthetic, semi-synthetic and naturally occurring products embracing a range of polysaccharide materials.

Xerogels

The xerogel dressings may be regarded as a subgroup of products within the larger group of polysaccharide dressings. The latter contains the well-known cellulosic dressing products, such as gauze and absorbent cotton (see Absorbents), but the products, which consist of dextranomer beads, dehydrated hydrogels of the agar/acrylamide group, calcium alginate fibres and dehydrated granulated Graft T starch polymers, are identified specifically as xerogels (Schmidt, 1986); the material remaining after the removal of most or all of the water from a hydrogel (or the disperse phase from any type of simple gel). These materials therefore have no water in their formulation but swell to form a gel when in contact with aqueous solutions.

Alginate dressings

The alginates are produced in fibre form and presented as a fleece or layered needled fabric. When applied to a bleeding surface, both the availability of the calcium ions and the fibrous matrix contribute to coagulation, and serum absorption produces a gel-like mass. Calcium alginate dressings are flat, non-woven pads or either calcium sodium alginate fibre or pure calcium alginate fibre. The alginate wound-contact layer may be bonded to a secondary absorbent viscose pad. Alginate hanks are also available, as are packing and ribbon for deeper cavity wounds and sinuses.

Alginates have been shown to be effective in the management of injuries where there has been substantial tissue loss, as in degloving injuries (those where limb tissue has been completely removed and bone exposed). They have reduced the number of surgical procedures which could normally have been expected, and have accelerating healing. The non-adhesive formulations will require a secondary dressing.

Alginic acid is a polyuronic acid composed of residues of D-mannuronic acid and L-guluronic acid and is obtained chiefly from algae belonging to the Phaeophyceae, mainly species of *Laminaria*. The isomeric acids are present in varying proportions according to the seaweed source. The guluronic acid forms an association with calcium, providing the stimulus to produce the continuous disperse phase of a hydrogel. A biodegradable gel is formed when the calcium alginate fibre is in contact with exudate and the released calcium ions and a phospholipid surface promote the activation of prothrombin in the clotting cascade. The gel may be firm or soft depending upon the proportions of calcium and sodium in the alginate fibre, and may be removed from the wound with saline. Calcium alginate products are used as the source of calcium ions to arrest bleeding, both in superficial injuries and as an absorbable haemostat in surgery. The rate of biodegradation is related to the sodium/calcium balance in the preparation. The dressings may be removed with a sterile 3% sodium citrate solution followed by washing with sterile water, or with sterile normal saline.

The 'wet' integrity of the dressing, which facilitates removal from the wound, may be improved by incorporating fibres of greater strength, such as viscose (rayon) staple fibre, or fibres which interact with the alginate fibres when wet, such as chitosan staple fibres (Gilchrist *et al.*, 1986).

The primary haemostatic use of calcium alginate is in the packing of sinuses and fistulae. The alginate dressings have recently become widely used as a soluble wound packing for a number of additional wound types. They have been used as a useful non-adherent for lacerations and abrasions and are effective in the management of hypergranulation tissue (proud flesh), interdigital maceration and heloma molle.

Alginates have proved to be useful debriding agents. When used for this purpose, the alginate must be covered by a secondary dressing of foam or film. Some proprietary products bond calcium alginate to a secondary backing, such as an absorbent viscose pad or semi-permeable adhesive foam, to produce an island dressing.

Recommended use As a haemostat in lacerations, post-operative wounds, donor sites and in the management of non-bleeding wounds, such as second-degree burns and heavily exuding wounds, where long periods are required between dressing changes. These materials are becoming widely used in veterinary practice to treat small- and large-animal soft tissue injuries.

Examples

- Algosteril (Biersdorf UK), Comfeel Seasorb (Coloplast).
- Kaltostat (Convatec).
- Sorbsan (Steriseal).
- Tegagen (3M Healthcare).

Collagen dressings

The collagen used in these dressings is usually derived from cowhide and this bovine material is non-antigenic due to enzymatic purification. It is available as sheets, particles, pastes or gels. It is believed that addition of collagen to a wound bed accelerates wound repair by the provision of a matrix for cellular migration. The dry materials absorb exudate to form a gel and the example quoted on page 570 contains 10% alginate. These materials all require a secondary dressing.

Recommended use

Any recalcitrant wound, moist sloughy wounds whether clean or infected and small-area burns.

Example

- Fibracol (Johnson & Johnson Medical).

Hydrogels

Hydrogels, or water polymer gels, are modified cross-linked polymeric formulations which form three-dimensional networks of hydrophilic polymers prepared from materials such as gelatin, polysaccharides, cross-linked polyacrylamide polymers, polyelectrolyte complexes and polymers or copolymers derived from methacrylate esters. These interact with aqueous solutions by swelling to an equilibrium value, and retain a significant proportion of water within their structure. They are insoluble in water. Hydrogels are available in dry or hydrated sheets or as a hydrated gel in sachets. When hydrated they contain up to 96% water and have additional, high, absorption properties.

Their high moisture content maintains a desirable moist interface which facilitates cell migration and prevents dressing adherence. Water can be transmitted through the saturated gel whilst the unsaturated gel will have a water vapour permeability comparable with that of vapour-permeable membranes.

The absorption, transmission and permeability performance result in the maintenance of a moist wound with a continuous moisture flux across the dressing and a sorption gradient which assists in the removal of toxic components from the wound area. The high moisture content allows dissolved oxygen permeability, which varies between products but will allow the continuation of aerobic function at the wound/dressing interface and have an effect upon both epithelialisation and bacterial growth. It has been observed that the positioning of a hydrogel frequently results in a marked reduction in pain response. It is suggested that the high humidity protects the exposed neurons from dehydration and also produces acceptable changes in pH. A secondary effect which may contribute to this response is the ability of the gels to immediately cool the wound surface and maintain a lower temperature for up to 6 hours (Turner, 1985). This lowering of temperature could result in a reduction of the inflammatory response.

Sheet hydrogels

These dressings are sheets of three-dimensional networks of cross-linked hydrophilic polymers, generally polyethylene oxide, polyacrylamides, polyvinylpyrrolidone, carboxymethylcellulose or modified corn starch. Their formulation may incorporate up to 96% bound water but they are insoluble in water and interact by three-dimensional swelling with aqueous solutions. The polymer physically entraps water to form a solid sheet, which may make them feel moist, but compression of the sheet will not release any water. They have a thermal capacity which provides initial cooling to the wound surface. A secondary dressing is required (Thomas, 1990, 1994; Ovington, 1998).

Recommended use The recommendation for use of these products includes the management of donor sites and superficial operation sites, and also the treatment of fresh chronic damaged epithelium, such as degloving, thermal and other painful wounds and dermatitic skin, for which the avoidance of topical agents is indicated.

Examples

- Geliperm (Geistlich Sons).
- Intrasite Conformable (Smith & Nephew Medical).

Amorphous hydrogels

Many of these hydrogels are similar in composition to sheet hydrogels but the polymer has not been cross-linked. They may have additional ingredients, such as alginate, collagen or complex carbohydrates, besides water and a polymer. These amorphous preparations do not have the cooling properties of the sheet dressings. Again, a secondary dressing is required. They have been used in animal wound management to treat cavity wounds and, admixed with antibacterial agents, to treat abscesses, particularly those commonly found in rabbits.

Recommended use Amorphous hydrogels are recommended for the hydration of dry, sloughy or necrotic wounds and autolytic debridement.

Examples

- Intrasite Gel (Smith & Nephew Medical).
- Nugel (Johnson & Johnson Medical).

- Purilon Gel (Coloplast).
- Sterigel (SSL International).

Hydrocolloids

Hydrocolloid dressings consist of composite products based on naturally occurring hydrophilic polymers. Generally these dressings are flexible, highly absorbent, occlusive or semi-occlusive adhesive pads formulated from biocompatible hydrophilic polymers, such as sodium carboxymethylcellulose, hydroxyethylcellulose pectins and gelatin incorporated into a hydrophobic adhesive. Hydrocolloid dressings with formulations consisting of sodium carboxymethylcellulose combined with karaya gum or sodium carboxymethylcellulose on its own have been manufactured, and the products are also available as pastes, powders gels or granules of similar formulation, allowing a continuous fill for cavity wounds. The dressings may be backed by a polymeric film and may be contoured to fit difficult areas without shedding particles into the wound. The pads do not require a secondary dressing.

The adhesive formulation of hydrocolloids gives initial adhesion greater than that obtained with some surgical adhesive tapes. After application, the absorption of transepidermal water vapour modifies the adhesive flow to maintain a high tack performance throughout the period of use. *In situ*, the dressings provide a gaseous and moisture-proof environmental chamber strongly adhesed to the area surrounding the wound and offering protection against fecal or urinary contamination plus that from other sources, such as the environment in which the animal is kept.

In the wound contact area the exudate is absorbed to form a gel that swells in a linear fashion, with a higher moisture retention at the contact surface. This results in expansion of the gel into the wound cavity with the continued support and increasing pressure from the remainder of the elastomeric dressing. The larger the volume of exudate, the greater the expansion into the cavity up to the limitation imposed by the availability of the gel. The advantage of this system is that it applies firm pressure to the floor of a deep wound, thereby helping to stimulate the production of healthy granulating tissue.

The formed 'colloidal' gel also produces a sorption gradient for soluble components within the serous exudate and allows the removal of toxic compounds arising from bacterial or cellular destruction. The moist gel is soft and conforms to the wound contours. When the dressing is removed, the gel remains in the wound and can be washed away with normal saline. During use, the dressing in contact with the wound liquefies to produce a pus-like liquid with a somewhat strong odour. The hydrocolloids are suitable for desloughing and for light- to medium-exuding wounds, but are contraindicated if an anaerobic infection is present.

When used to treat veterinary wounds, hydrocolloid dressings applied to relatively immobile muscular areas, such as the rump of a horse, have evinced an improvement of up to 30% in healing time from injury to hair regrowth (personal observation) and will remain *in situ*. The dressings are removed by soaking with normal saline. When positioned on muscular areas of greater flexion, such as the neck and shoulders, the conformability and adhesiveness of hydrocolloids are inadequate in their present form for veterinary use and fail to adhere for any significant period.

Examples

- Comfeel (Coloplast).
- Granuflex (ConvaTec).
- Granugel (ConvaTec).
- Tegasorb (3M Healthcare).

Superabsorbents

These are hydrocolloidal compounds which have a high absorbent capacity and entrap exudate so that it cannot be squeezed out once absorbed. One product incorporates this material into an island pad which is covered by a non-woven absorbent and surrounded by an extra-thin hydrocolloid as the adhesive portion. The covering acts as a transfer layer while its surface stays dry.

Example

- Combiderm (ConvaTec).

Hydrofibres

Hydrofibres are fibres of carboxymethylcellulose formed into flat, non-woven pads with the facility to form a gel on contact with fluid. The absorbent rate and capacity is approximately three times that of calcium alginate. The resulting gel is similar to a sheet hydrogel which does not dry out or wick laterally. Therefore there is no maceration of the skin surrounding the wound but moisture is maintained in contact with the wound bed. The high absorbent capacity reduces the frequency of dressing changes.

Example

- Aquacel (ConvaTec).

Biodressings

Biodressings are composed of materials which originate almost exclusively from living tissue and are said to 'participate actively and beneficially in the biochemistry and cellular activity of wound healing' (Lofts, 1986). They can be identified as biological dressings and biosynthetic dressings, and the biological dressings can be further subdivided into natural or cultured according to their origin.

These materials are being developed extensively for wound management, but there is little indication that they will ever have a meaningful role to play in the management of veterinary wounds as their use is limited, their application specialised and their cost prohibitive. Most owners would not be prepared to accept these costs when, to date, there is little evidence of cost-effectiveness.

Conclusion

This chapter has described some of the *passive* materials which are still used extensively for the management of animal soft tissue injuries in many veterinary practices, and has outlined the performance parameters of the *interactive* dressings which are now routinely used for human wound management. There are vast areas of ignorance about the mechanisms of wound healing in different animal species. Assumptions have been made that some of these *interactive* products will be equally successful, after appropriate modification for veterinary use, in the management of animal injuries. Preliminary evaluations (Cockbill and Turner, 1995; Cockbill *et al.*, 1996) have indicated that these assumptions are not wholly erroneous. Current developments have confirmed that the next generation of products will participate actively in the wound healing process by contributing growth hormones, chemotactic agents, angiogenic agents and other growth factors, either in a depot-release mode or as sequentially released compounds (Turner, 1989) or by controlling the microenvironment surrounding the wound.

Each wound management product will eventually be designed to meet the environmental, nutritional and growth requirements of particular wound types and will probably be based on biodressings. They will be designated 'bioactive' wound management products. These biodressings must be the precursors of the many more exciting products being developed, which will improve the morbidity of wound healing and must eventually have a place in veterinary wound management. This will be to the advantage of patient, owner and veterinary surgeon.

References

Bull J P, Squire J R, Tophey E (1948). Experiments with occlusive dressings of a new plastic. *Lancet* 2: 213–214.

Cockbill S M E (1998). Evaluation *in vivo* and *in vitro* of the performance of interactive dressings in the management of animal soft tissue injuries. *Vet Dermatol* 9: 87–98.

Cockbill S M E, Turner T D (1994). Management of veterinary wounds. In: Harding K G, Dealey C, Cherry G, Gottrup F, eds. *Proceedings of the 3rd European Conference on Advances in Wound Management*. London: Macmillan Magazines, 115–117.

Cockbill S M E, Turner T D (1995). Management of veterinary wounds. *Vet Rec* 136: 362–365.

Cockbill S M E, Hollinshead C M, Turner T D (1996). Veterinary wound management using contemporary surgical dressings. In: Cherry G, Gottrup F, Lawrence J C, Moffatt CJ, Turner T D, eds. *Proceedings of the 5th European Conference on Advances in Wound Management*. London: Macmillan Magazines, 115–118.

Gilchrist T, Mitchell D C, Burrows T R, *et al.* (1986). Sorbsan™ – The Natural Dressing. In: Turner T D, Schmidt R J, Harding KG, eds. *Advances in Wound Management*. New York: John Wiley, 73–82.

Hunt T K, Knighton D R, Thakral K K, *et al.* (1984). Studies on inflammation and wound healing: angiogenesis and collagen synthesis stimulated *in vivo* by resident and activated wound macrophages. *Surgery* 96: 48–54.

Knighton D R, Hunt T K, Scheuenstuhl H, *et al.* (1983). Oxygen tension regulates the expression of angiogenesis factor by macrophages. *Science* 221: 1283–1285.

Lock D M (1979). The effect of temperature on mitotic activity at the edge of experimental wounds. In: Lundgren A, Soner AB, eds. *Symposia on Wound Healing: Plastic, Surgical and Dermatological Aspects, Molndal, Sweden*. Mölindal: A. Lindgren and Söner A B, 103–109.

Lofts P M (1986). Biodressings. In: Turner T D, Schmidt R J, Harding K G, eds. *Advances in Wound Management*. New York: John Wiley, 127–131.

Ovington L G (1998). The well-dressed wound: an overview of dressing types. *Wounds* 10 (Suppl. A): 1A–11A.

Schmidt R (1986). Xerogel dressings. In: Turner T D, Schmidt R J, Harding K G, eds. *Advances in Wound Management*. New York: John Wiley, 65–72.

Silver I A (1972). Oxygen tension and epithelialisation. In: Maibach H I, Rovee DT, eds. *Epidermal Wound Healing*. Chicago: Year Book Medical Publishers, 291–305.

Thomas, S (1990). *Wound Management and Dressings*. London: Pharmaceutical Press.

Thomas S (1994). *Handbook of Wound Dressings*. London: Macmillan Magazines.

Turner T D (1979a). Hospital usage of absorbent dressings. *Pharm J* 22: 421–426.

Turner T D (1979b). Products and their development in wound management. In: Sundell B, ed. *International Symposium on Wound Healing, Espoo*. Mölindal: A. Lindgren and Söner AB, 75–84.

Turner T D (1985). Current and future trends in wound management. *Pharm Int* 6: 131–134.

Turner T D (1989). The development of wound management products. *Wounds* 1: 155–179.

Turner T D (1990). The development of wound management products. In: Krasner D, ed. *Chronic Wound Care*. Health Management Publications Inc, 31.

Turner TD (1992). Surgical dressings and their evolution. In: Harding K G, Leaper D L, Turner T D (eds). *Proceedings of the 1st European Conference on Advances in Wound Management*. London: Macmillan Magazines, 181–187.

Winter GD (1962). Formation of the scab and the rate of epithelialisation of superficial wounds in the skin of the young domestic pig. *Nature* 193: 293–294.

Winter GD (1975). Epidermal wound healing. In: Turner T D, Brain K R, eds. *Proceedings, Conference on Surgical Dressings in the Hospital Environment*. Cardiff: Surgical Dressings Research Unit, University of Wales Institute of Science and Technology, 47–83.

Further reading

Goldsmith L A, ed. (1983). *Biochemistry and Physiology of the Skin*, vols 1 and 11. Oxford: Oxford University Press.

Najano G (1975). *The Healing Hand*. Cambridge (MA): Harvard University Press.

Bucknell T E, Ellis H, eds. (1984). *Wound Healing for Surgeons*. London: Baillière Tindall.

Leaper D J, Harding K G, eds. (1998). *Wounds: Biology and management*. Oxford: Oxford University Press.

Peacock E E (1984). *Wound Repair*. London: W B Saunders.

Royal Society of Medicine (1984). *An Environment for Healing*. International Congress Series, No. 88. London: Royal Society of Medicine.

Turner T D, Schmidt R J, Harding K G, eds. (1986). *Advances in Wound Management*. New York: John Wiley.

Westaby E S, ed. (1985) *Wound Care*. London: William Heinemann Medical Books.

Index